THE
PRIMAL
PRESCRIPTION

DOUG McGUFF, MD
AND
ROBERT P. MURPHY, PhD

Mention of specific companies, organizations, or authorities in this book does not imply endorsement by the author or publisher. Information in this book was accurate at the time researched. The author received no incentives or compensation to promote the item recommendations in the book.

Library of Congress Control Number: 2015945803
Library of Congress Cataloging-in-Publication Data is on file with the publisher
McGuff, Doug 1962 - ; and Murphy, Robert 1976 -
The Primal Prescription/Doug McGuff, MD and Robert Murphy, PhD

ISBN: 978-1-939563-09-5
1. Health Care Reform—United States 2. Medicine & Health Sciences Policy
3. Health Services Economics 4. Patient Education 5. Health Care Advice

Editor: Denise Minger
Design and Layout: Caroline De Vita
Illustrations & Cartoons on pages 8, 18, 129, 147, 225, 246, 270, 287, 326:
© Caroline De Vita
Cartoons on pages 6, 36, 38, 44, 82, 104, 124, 216, 238, 292, 332:
© cartoonresource - Shutterstock.com
Cartoons on pages 68, 150, 252, 270: © andrewgenn - iStock.com
Cover Design: Janée Meadows
Index: Tim Tate

Publisher: Primal Blueprint Publishing.
23805 Stuart Ranch Rd. Suite 145 Malibu, CA 90265
For information on quantity discounts, please call 888-774-6259,
email: info@primalblueprint.com, or visit PrimalBlueprintPublishing.com.

DISCLAIMER
The ideas, concepts, and opinions expressed in this book are intended to be used for educational purposes only. This book is sold with the understanding that the authors and publisher are not rendering medical advice of any kind, nor is this book intended to replace medical advice, nor to diagnose, prescribe, or treat any disease, condition, illness, or injury. It is imperative that before beginning any diet program, including any aspect of the diet methodologies mentioned in *The Primal Prescription*, you receive full medical clearance from a licensed physician. The authors and publisher claim no responsibility to any person or entity for any liability, loss, or damage caused or alleged to be caused directly or indirectly as a result of the use, application, or interpretation of the material in this book. If you object to this disclaimer, you may return the book to publisher for a full refund.

This book is dedicated to William Allen, MD, my mentor and friend since my days as a resident. Dr. Allen taught me how to think in principles and opened the world up for me, and without him, this book could not have been written. I also dedicate this book to J. Lance Reese, MD, my best friend since residency, who has also benefitted from Dr. Allen's teaching and has contributed more to my life than he will ever know. Also, and especially, to my beautiful wife Wendy, who has stood by me every step of the way and fought *for* me as an entire system fought *against* me. There is no greater love than that which you have shown. Finally, to my son Eric and daughter Madeline: thanks for being such amazing human beings and making me realize why I want to continue to fight for my profession.
—*M. Doug McGuff, MD*

I dedicate this book to those Americans struggling to maintain liberty in their lives—in all of its dimensions.
—*Robert Murphy, PhD*

Table of Contents

Acknowledgments..vi
Foreword by Mark Sisson...ix
Introduction..1

PART I: UNDERSTANDING U.S. HEALTH CARE, UP THROUGH OBAMACARE

1. How We Got Here: A Brief History of
   US Health Care Through 2009...............................7
2. The Deadly FDA...45
3. The Medicare Ponzi Scheme...............................69
4. The Perverse Economics of US Medicine........................83

PART II: OBAMACARE, THE FUTILITY OF HEALTH REDISTRIBUTION

5. The Inner "Logic" of the Affordable Care Act...............105
6. Fatal Flaws of the ACA.......................................125
7. Paving the Way for "Single Payer".....................151

PART III: SAVE YOURSELF

8. Ken Korg Battles the Beast................................187
9. Lead By Your (Primal) Example...........................217
10. Choosing Your Doctor..239
11. Getting Off Your Meds.......................................253
12. Surviving the Hospital..271
13. Medical Screening & Elective Procedures:
    Worth the Risk?...293

PART IV: FREEDOM IS THE ANSWER

14. Rolling Back Big Government and Big Pharma............327
15. Living Healthy and Free......................................333

Acknowledgments

Special thanks go out to Mark Sisson. I am honored that you thought of me when you contemplated taking on an exposé of the American "sick care" system. To my co-author Robert Murphy, PhD, thank you for your tireless work in bringing rational principles to the field of economics and for integrating your vast knowledge into this book. To my partners at Blue Ridge Emergency Physicians (made extinct by the Affordable Care Act), I would like to acknowledge your twenty years of friendship and professionalism and assure you that our beloved founder, Dr. Jack Warren, is looking down upon you with a cup of black coffee in hand . . . smiling. To Ed Garbe, Sherry Edwards, and Joe Byers (my team at Ultimate Exercise, Inc.), thank you for your boundless energy and enthusiasm in teaching our clients that prevention really is the best medicine. Finally, to Denise Minger, thank you for your excellent work in editing the manuscript for this book and turning my submissions into something worthy of Mark's high standards.

—*M. Doug McGuff, MD*

I would like to thank Mark Sisson for introducing me to my co-author for this important project. (Economic theory is great, but I felt much more confident when Doug's ER experience confirmed my analysis.) I am also very grateful for the tremendous work Denise Minger did on our manuscript, to help us make it more accessible for the lay reader.

—*Robert Murphy, PhD*

Foreword

BY MARK SISSON

When I wrote *The Primal Blueprint,* my mission was simple: I wanted to explain the trap into which Americans had fallen, where even those trying to do the right thing for their health (as dictated by the "experts" in government and big business) were only falling deeper into the throes of disease. In addition to diagnosing the problem—a modern world at odds with our ancient genes—I gave people practical steps they could implement to achieve *immediate results.* They didn't have to reform the system, they just had to understand what was happening and alter their behavior accordingly.

In *The Primal Prescription,* the subject is broader—the entire health care industry—but the approach is the same. It diagnoses the problem so we can understand how and why things have gone so terribly awry, but it also provides practical solutions that we can implement *immediately* to gain independence, as much as possible, from the broken system. We're led through an uncomfortable tour of American health care's unseemly innards, but we're just as swiftly escorted out and given a set of tools to navigate the labyrinth on our own. Instead of being asked to wait for a legislative miracle to fall from the heavens and fix the sorry state of affairs (don't hold your breath), we're empowered to make our own changes *now,* regardless of how long it takes for the rest of the world to catch up. And best of all, those changes are already well within our reach.

Few people are better suited to guide us through this book's shocking and enlightening material than the two authors, Doug and Bob. An emergency room physician and economist, respectively, Doug and Bob have a collective breadth of knowledge that encompasses all angles of America's health care industry—the bloody and medicated, the politically wayward, the financially futile. Their combined experience exposes the intersection of Conventional Wisdom from both the health and economic sectors, and it's a sad sight indeed.

By joining forces, Doug and Bob allow their unique insights to benefit you, the reader, as you flee America's sinking health care ship and swim safely ashore.

Mark Sisson
July, 2015

Introduction

BY THE AUTHORS

L
ike virtually all Americans, you have probably sensed that something is terribly wrong with the US health care system. Feeling helpless, you may have reluctantly agreed with the academics, public policy wonks, and politicians who promised that a massive round of legislation from Washington would set the country back on track.

Yet the Patient Protection and Affordable Care Act—also known as the ACA or simply "ObamaCare"—is only the most recent of a string of government initiatives, going back at least to the Great Depression, aimed at improving the delivery of health care to Americans. This history forces us to ask: is the ACA actually *working*? Or is it, instead, exacerbating the very problems it was supposed to solve, setting us up for another crisis down the road? In the meantime, while the politicians and pundits bicker, what can Americans do to keep their families healthy?

The book you are holding answers just these questions. It contains the *real* history of what went wrong with US health care and insurance, and explains why so many people thought massive new legislation was necessary. Once you realize exactly how and why American health care had fallen into such a hole on the eve of the Affordable Care Act, you will understand that the new legislation is only making things worse. Indeed, we will use the government's own estimates to show how *all* workers—not just "the rich"—are going to pay hundreds of billions more in taxes to make the legislation "pay for itself." Furthermore, you the reader will be shocked to see how many millions of people the *government itself* predicts will be paying fines rather than obtaining the "universal" and "affordable" health insurance that is now supposedly a federal guarantee. With relentless arguments, data, and real-world examples from an ER doctor, we will convince you that the delivery of US health care will only become more inefficient, frustrating, and bureaucratic over the coming years.

In this book, we argue that each round of increased government intervention within the health care and health insurance sectors has further hobbled the ability of the market economy to provide quality service at affordable prices. Yes, health care is a crucial component of a person's lifestyle, and that might make Americans hesitant to rely on "the free market" to deliver it. But food, clothing, and shelter are even *more* fundamental staples of life, and most Americans would agree that having the government act as a "single payer" for all of their purchases at the grocery store and The Gap would be an absolute disaster. And if a giant new government agency—perhaps called "Housicare"—were given the power to tax all paychecks in order to pay for all home purchases and apartment rentals (according to an official schedule of prices corresponding to family size and job location), the disruption in the market would be mind-boggling. By severing the direct connection between buyer and seller, consumers' satisfaction with their homes and apartments would suffer while prices would soar. After a few years of such a nutty system, the housing market would be just as screwed up as . . . well, as the health care and health insurance markets currently are.

Make no mistake: though we have strong views on the political drama in Washington and its disastrous fallout for average Americans, this book is not partisan. Indeed, our historical journey will show you that the problems with US health care are a *bipartisan affair*, the fault of legislation signed into law by both Democrats and Republicans, including the conservative icon Ronald Reagan. Seen in the proper historical perspective, "ObamaCare" is simply an extension of the trends that have been in motion for decades.

Fortunately, there is a way out for you and your family. The primary purpose of this book is *to educate you, the reader, so that you're better equipped to take control of your own health.* We are strong advocates of the "primal" lifestyle of diet and exercise (as popularized most notably by Mark Sisson) as a baseline for promoting the default status of wellness in your life. The best way to avoid the problems of a faulty health care system is *to stay healthy*.

Yet sickness and sometimes even hospitalization are unavoidable parts of life, and this book offers a complete introductory guide for these topics as well. We provide a framework for choosing your doctor, picking an insurance plan, surviving a hospital stay, reducing (or eliminating) your medications, evaluating the merits of medical screening procedures such as mammograms, and getting accurate information on elective procedures. Our goal here is not to tell you "the answers," but instead to give you a *framework*—or a blueprint—for making the right decisions for you and your family.

An added virtue of our recommendations is that they can be implemented immediately, without the need to convince politicians (or other voters) to change their own views or actions. We do offer some policy solutions for the broader US health care system, but these are given mostly for the sake of logical completeness, and to avoid charges that we are mere complainers. The overall delivery of US health care and health insurance could be improved very quickly with those solutions, but the great news is that *you have the power to take charge of your own health* regardless of what others do.

We have certainly promised you a lot in this book, so let's take a moment to explain why we are qualified to deliver on those promises. The problems with US health care are obviously medical in nature, but they *also* involve economics—especially because one of the biggest problems is how *expensive* care (and insurance) has become. That is why the two authors of the book you are currently holding decided to join forces: one of us (McGuff) is an MD with years of experience in the trenches of the emergency room, while the other (Murphy) holds a PhD in economics and has experience in academia, the financial sector, and DC-based policy analysis.

To put it simply, in this book the doctor co-author will give his firsthand account of what has been happening on the ground, while the economist co-author will explain how the policies adopted by government and insurance providers are causing these absurd—and heartbreaking—outcomes. Although we will be taking (well-deserved) swipes at some of the "experts" in our respective fields, our criticism will be of their *hubris*—of failing to appreciate the complexity and self-regulating properties of both the human body and the market economy. We are not here to criticize intellectualism, per se, but instead puncture the myths that the cutting-edge research has toppled.

There is so much we want to tell you from our respective fields of medicine and economics. As bad and shocking as the rumors about "ObamaCare" or hospital practices may be, we promise you: the reality is worse. Yet we understand that your time is valuable, which is why we have boiled down our report to include only what you most imperatively need to know. *The Primal Prescription* will first walk you through exactly what went wrong with US health care, and in so doing will turn the conventional wisdom upside down. Then, armed with the truth, you will learn what practical steps you can take to navigate the health care debacle that will—for those who aren't prepared—only get worse before getting better.

Doug McGuff, MD
Robert P. Murphy, PhD

PART I

UNDERSTANDING U.S. HEALTH CARE, UP THROUGH OBAMACARE

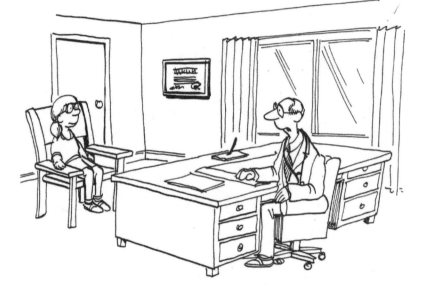

"Don't worry, the healthcare mess
will be solved by the time you retire."

Chapter 1

HOW WE GOT HERE:
A Brief History of
US Health Care Through 2009

In the debate over government health care policies, partisanship and the desire to win the argument often leads both sides to talk past each other. Conservative Republicans proudly proclaim that Americans had enjoyed "the best health care system in the world," but now President Obama's radical legislation is interfering with the free market's ability to deliver medical services. Liberal Democrats reject this naïve vision, arguing that the very real problems of skyrocketing costs and sporadic coverage that existed in 2009 were precisely why President Obama pushed for his sweeping overhaul of the whole system.

Both sides are partially right—but mostly wrong—in this typical battle along partisan lines. The conservative Republicans are correct when they warn that the Affordable Care Act is making medical care worse, but the liberal Democrats are correct when they say the pre-ACA system was broken. Yet when we study the history of US health care and insurance, we can understand exactly *why* the system was broken as of 2009. We will see that far from being a revolutionary "paradigm shift," the Affordable Care Act (ObamaCare) is instead merely a ramping up of trends that have been in place for decades.

There was no "free market" in US health care or health insurance circa 2009. That is precisely why so many Americans were legitimately scandalized with the system and hence demanded drastic reforms. Yet it also demonstrates that the Affordable Care Act is only making the problem worse.

To fully understand these claims, we need to review the actual history of US health care and insurance up through 2009.

EARLY HEALTH CARE: NO "SYSTEM"

Before the twentieth century, there was no health care system in the United States or anywhere else. Of course physicians and medical care existed, but there was not really a *system* the way we conceive of it nowadays. Part of our current problem, as we'll see, comes from the organization of our modern "system," which is why it's important to realize that things weren't always this way. In these opening sections, we draw from the history of medicine as laid out by John F. Fulton in the *British Medical Journal*.[1]

The existence of physicians has been recorded as far back as 500 BC Early Sanskrit literature documents the story of a physician and teacher named Charaka who, like Hippocrates, endorsed an apprenticeship system of medical education. The apprenticeships could be a simple one-on-one relationship between teacher and student, but as early as the fifth century BC, a medical school had been established to organize the process for larger groups of students. This ancient model persisted into medieval times, with a medical school established in Salerno sometime around the ninth century AD Throughout the Middle Ages, the apprentice model of training within organized schools of medicine remained the predominant form of medical education.

During the Renaissance, medical education began to aggregate around the great Italian schools in Padua, Bologna, Ferrara, and Pisa. Most practicing physicians in England had trained at one of these institutions. Cambridge and Oxford offered theoretical studies in medicine, but these courses mostly consisted of memorizing the works of ancient writers like Galen or Hippocrates.

Medical education in colonial America was strongly influenced by the European apprentice system. Not surprisingly, the most ambitious American medical students went to the established schools in Edinburgh, London, Paris, or Leyden to complete their training. Two such students, William Shippen and John Morgan, returned to Philadelphia where they established the first American medical school at the College of Philadelphia. In a graduation address in 1765, Morgan laid out what would become the model for university-based medical education. The lecture was titled, *A discourse upon the institution of medical schools in America; delivered at a public anniversary commencement held in the College of Philadelphia May 30 and 31, 1765*. Based on the content of this lecture, university-based medical schools sprung up at Yale, Columbia, Harvard, and Dartmouth.

The system that emerged from Morgan's elevated vision proved very popular and quite lucrative for the official universities and the professors who instructed in them. Seeing this trend, private schools without formal "university" affiliation began to materialize seemingly everywhere. Some of these institutions functioned on a high plane and churned out competent practitioners, while others were substandard and produced less competent, or even incompetent, practitioners.

Throughout the eighteenth century in the United States, there was no system of formal government licensure of doctors. Some schools granted an MD or MB degree, but many were simply apprentice programs. It was even possible to announce oneself as a physician without any formal training. To be sure, a degree from one of the better schools would confer a competitive advantage in the market, other things being equal; but such practitioners still faced numerous rivals, many of whom achieved great competence through the apprentice system and word-of-mouth advertising.

"THERE OUGHTA BE A LAW": THE ORIGINS OF THE AMA AND U.S. MEDICAL LICENSURE

Alarmed by the proliferation of unregulated rivals, the university-trained physicians organized into county and state medical societies and lobbied to enact licensure legislation, which would ultimately eliminate much of their "amateur" competition. By 1821, the state of Connecticut was granting licenses to all of the "properly" trained physicians and forcing all unlicensed practitioners to pass state-administered examinations. This movement spread to other states, and ultimately the American Medical Association (AMA), founded in 1847, picked up the ball and ran with it.

Of course, the *official* goal of the AMA was to ensure minimum levels of quality of medical education and practice. They set standards for admission to medical schools and established examinations for licensure. Yet we cannot ignore the obvious fact that when the AMA met its goal of raising standards, this success rather conveniently served to protect the entrenched medical practitioners from competition. Anyone trying to gain entrance into the profession from one of the private institutions was blocked, while even those coming up through the approved pathway had to do so with much more stringent entrance requirements, as well as a longer and more rigorous period of training.

To reiterate, the stated purpose of these regulations was to protect potential patients and to ensure high standards for the medical profession. While the measures certainly achieved these noble goals, they also served the personal interests of the established doctors, shielding them from the competition of those who obtained their education through less prestigious means, as well as those who offered alternatives to traditional medicine. To point out these facts is not to impugn the motives of every individual agitating for the requirements, but we must not be naïve when studying the history of medical regulation.

Regardless of intentions, it is a simple matter of economics that the government restrictions had—at best—a mixed effect on the customers, i.e., the patients. On the one hand, patients receiving medical treatment obviously benefited from the more rigorous hurdles that their doctors had to surpass. On the other hand, the stricter standards just as surely *harmed* patients of modest means who would have preferred to hire the services of a cheaper provider, an option that was now illegal.

To adopt the analogy of Milton Friedman: government licensing of doctors is a double-edged sword, equivalent to mandating that all cars sold in the United States are as good as Cadillacs or better.[2] Yes, such an absurd regulation would naturally raise the quality of vehicles on the road, and in that sense would "help" American motorists. Yet clearly there is also a very real sense in which such a regulation would be harmful to the poor, many of whom would now be priced out of the car market altogether, having to walk or take the bus instead.

What is crystal clear in Friedman's fictitious Cadillac analogy holds true in the real world for medical regulations: even "sensible" government licensing of doctors that improves the quality of care will nonetheless restrict the *amount* of care offered to the public, thereby raising prices and making care less affordable for the poorest patients. (Of course, things are even worse if the government standards are somewhat arbitrary, and/or forbid legitimate medical techniques and products.)

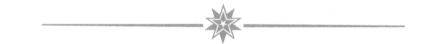

THERE ARE ALWAYS TRADE-OFFS, EVEN IN MEDICINE

"Under the interpretation of the statutes forbidding unauthorized practice of medicine, many things are restricted to licensed physicians that could perfectly well be done by technicians, and other skilled people who do not have a Cadillac medical training... Trained physicians devote a considerable part of their time to things that might well be done by others. The result is to reduce drastically the amount of medical care."

—Milton Friedman[3]

A GREAT LEAP FORWARD IN REGULATION: THE FLEXNER REPORT

In the United States, the regulatory movement in medicine gained major momentum as a result of the Flexner Report. In 1910, Abraham Flexner of the Carnegie Foundation published his comprehensive report of the state of medical education in the US and Canada. He concluded that many of the 155 schools he surveyed were substandard, and that the freestanding institutions in particular were underfunded and inferior to the university-based institutions. He recommended that minimum admission standards should include at least two years of university education, that medical school should last four years (two years of basic science and two years of clinical training), and that the proprietary schools should be closed or incorporated into university-based programs. The osteopathic schools (which rely on the body's self-healing capacity through focus on bones, muscle, ligaments, and connective tissue) were hit particularly hard. To this day, many feel the exclusion of osteopathy was a deliberate effort by Flexner and the AMA to bring harm to a competing discipline of "alternative" medicine.

DOCTOR SHORTAGE?! GOVERNMENT CREATES THE VERY PROBLEMS IT THEN "SOLVES"[4]

The heightened standards recommended by the Flexner Report (1910) and the American Medical Association (AMA) were implemented by law through various government licensing requirements. Although touted as a way to protect the public from medical quacks, the other obvious effect was to reduce the number of practicing doctors, from about 175 physicians per 100,000 of the population in 1900 down to about 125 by 1930. (During this same period, more than 30 medical schools closed.) This dearth of physicians was not rectified until the 1960s, when the federal government used Medicare funds to subsidize graduate medical education. Try to get used to this pattern, for we will see it throughout the book: a government intervention into medicine leads to a problem, but rather than repeal the initial measure, the government simply slaps on further interventions.

THE DISMANTLING OF THE DOCTOR-PATIENT RELATIONSHIP: THE RISE OF THIRD-PARTY PAYMENT FOR MEDICAL CARE

Thus far, our historical sketch has focused on the transformation of medical *education*, which began as spontaneous master-apprentice relationships with open entry into the field, and only gradually morphed into standardized schools with compulsory government licensing requirements to practice medicine. Yet despite this change on the educational front, the actual doctor-patient relationship had remained intact, as it was originally intended in the Hippocratic oath. This relationship was a fiduciary one, where the patient compensated the doctor for his services directly, and the doctor proceeded with the patient's best interest in mind. All negotiations about the extent and expense of treatment were between the patient and his doctor. From the time of Charaka and Hippocrates, this ancient tradition had remained sacred. But in the early part of the twentieth century, it too would begin to wither.

As we will soon see, this relationship deteriorated into a third-party arrangement where payment is carried out by a distinct entity (an insurance company, the government, or both), which inserts its interest between the provider and the consumer. In this third-party system, the provider eventually becomes coerced into placing the needs of the collective over the needs of the individual patient.

HEY DOCTORS:
GOVERNMENT MAKES A DANGEROUS
SERVANT AND A FEARFUL MASTER

As we sketch the history of US health care, it will be very easy to paint doctors as the victims. While ultimately both doctors and their patients suffer under our current system, we must emphasize that even though some of their motives may have been pure, to some extent *doctors brought the present mess upon themselves.* Even though it is the political officials who are directly responsible for harmful government interventions into medicine, we must not be naïve by minimizing the role that the medical establishment plays in our narrative. The politicians didn't slap the industry with each round of new regulations amidst howls of protest; many influential doctors welcomed the restrictions because they gave them a relative advantage over their competitors. Tragically, the willingness of some doctors to embrace government encroachment into their industry for short-term gain facilitated the unintended consequences that would eventually imprison all doctors.

A CRUCIAL DISTINCTION: HEALTH CARE VERSUS HEALTH INSURANCE

Before summarizing the rise of third-party payment in the United States, we must make a clear distinction between health *care* and health *insurance*, terms that Americans nowadays have been trained to think are interchangeable. In fact, health care is distinct from health insurance, and we must recognize the difference in order to have any chance of understanding what went wrong with US medicine. *Health care* describes the services and products provided by doctors, hospitals, and other medical professionals. *Health insurance* is simply a means to pay for these services and products.

NOTHING NEW UNDER THE SUN

In 1932, the Committee on the Costs of Medical Care, funded by private organizations such as the Rockefeller Foundation and the Carnegie Corporation, issued its final recommendations (five years in the making) on how to reorganize the medical sector to contain rapidly rising costs (sic!). The majority report proposed the consolidation of medical care through hospitals and other group practices, as well as dispersed payment through insurance, taxation, or both. Newspapers announced that the report urged "socialized medicine." According to a 2002 retrospective: *"[E]ight private practitioners and one representative of the Catholic hospitals . . . composed Minority Report No.1. They denounced the majority's promotion of group practice as the technique of big business and mass production, and further projected that such a plan would establish a medical hierarchy that would dictate who might practice in any community. . . .They argued throughout Minority Report No.1 that government should be removed from medical care in all instances except in the care of the medically indigent and that the general practitioner should be restored to the central place in medical practice."*[5]

One of the central messages of this book is that *there is nothing magical about health insurance* that would make us treat it differently from other types of insurance. In our uncertain lives, we are beset by all sorts of risks, many of them catastrophic: a person can suddenly drop dead of a heart attack, total his car in a collision, witness his house burn to the ground, become disabled and unable to work, and on and on. The institution of insurance evolved to pool similar risks so that unlucky individuals (or their survivors) were not devastated when one of these outcomes struck. In reference to the previous examples, people can buy life insurance, car insurance, fire insurance, and disability insurance.

The common element here is that people pay premiums to be financially compensated in an *unlikely but catastrophic* event. The point of car insurance, for example, is to provide indemnification in the rare and expensive event of a car crash; you don't use your car insurance to pay for a routine oil change.

Health insurance originally evolved in this vein. The insurance was to cover major, unexpected health care events, such as a hospitalization for a severe illness or injury. Even when health insurance was limited in this way, Americans didn't really enjoy a full-blown free market in health care, because government tax policy and regulations could allow politicians to play favorites with one insurance company over another. Still, health insurance in its original form served merely to augment the underlying financial relationship between patient and doctor, so that medical care responded to market prices. This approach began its breakdown during the Great Depression of the 1930s, as the United States moved toward a system of default third-party payments for medical expenses.

KEY DATES IN U.S. MEDICINE AND HEALTH INSURANCE[6]

1765: John Morgan's address at College of Philadelphia lays out vision of formal medical training.

1847: Founding of the American Medical Association (AMA).

1847: The Massachusetts Health Insurance Company becomes first to issue sickness insurance.

1853: A "mutual aid society" offers prepaid hospital care plan in San Francisco.

1863: The Travelers Insurance Company offers accident insurance for railway injuries.

1877: The Granite Cutters Union provides its members with first national sick benefit program.

1910: Flexner Report calls for stricter standards for doctors.

1910: Montgomery Ward & Co. offers one of the first group insurance policies.

1927: The Committee on the Costs of Medical Care (funded by private foundations) begins its five-year task of studying the industry and suggesting reforms to ensure affordability, especially hospital care.

1937: The Blue Cross Commission is established.

1943: The War Labor Board rules that wartime wage freeze doesn't include fringe benefits (such as premiums for employee health insurance).

1954: Revenue Act of 1954 (Sec. 106) clarifies that employer contributions to employee health insurance plans are, and had always been, tax-deductible business expenses.

1965: Passage of Medicare and Medicaid legislation.

1974: Employee Retirement Income Security Act of 1974 (ERISA) establishes uniform standards for employers to maintain tax-favored status of employee benefit plans.

1986: Consolidated Omnibus Budget Reconciliation Act (COBRA) requires large employers to maintain coverage for terminated employees and dependents for specified period. Includes EMTALA mandates on hospitals.

1996: The Health Insurance Portability and Accountability Act (HIPAA) strengthens mandates on insurance portability between jobs as well as privacy safeguards.

2003: The new Medicare Part D provides prescription drug benefits to seniors (regardless of income), costing half a trillion dollars in its first decade alone.

2010: The Patient Protection and Affordable Care Act—aka ObamaCare—provides options for health insurance to all applicants and imposes increasingly heavy fines on (most of) those who choose not to purchase it.

AMERICANS GET THE BLUES: THE GREAT DEPRESSION AND THE GREAT HEALTH INSURERS

Everyone has heard the romantic stories of Depression-era doctors working long hours and receiving payment in the form of chickens, eggs, or baked goods. These stories, though likely embellished, are to a great extent true. It was likely a very personally rewarding way to practice medicine, but not very financially rewarding for such demanding and grueling work. It was during this time that doctors, and the hospitals with which they were affiliated, came up with the idea of organizing their own insurance companies. The idea was that the premium pool would provide funds that would pay them for their services. Patients could be protected from the expense of a catastrophic health event and doctors could be paid for their services, just as an auto body shop gets a check from the car insurance company for repairs made after a collision. So far, so good.

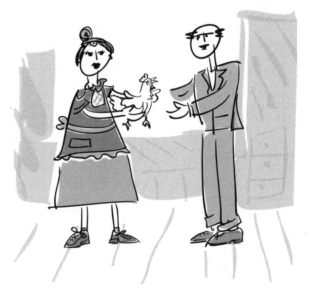

But times were hard, and even *routine* (not just catastrophic) medical care was still significantly underpaid (unless you really liked chicken and eggs). The doctors and hospitals that began this venture saw an opportunity for expansion: they devised a system where premiums would not just pay for major hospitalization, but would also cover all routine medical care such as office visits and preventive care such as check-ups and screening. In order to provide this much coverage and still keep premiums affordable, the doctors and hospitals sought the help of the government. This was the beginning of the largest health insurers of that time period, organized under the auspices of Blue Cross/Blue Shield (also known as the Blues).

What the Blues sought from the government was a tax-exempt status on all of their premiums, which would make those premiums affordable to the public.[7] The Blues could then provide what was advertised as a public good: health care for Americans. In this new approach, once people paid an affordable premium, they wouldn't have to worry about their health care needs, regardless of whether they were routine or catastrophic. During the uncertainty of the Great Depression, this new approach seemed very appealing. As a further benefit, it would also ensure that doctors would be compensated promptly in dollars (rather than in kind), which encouraged the development of a solid pool of physicians and hospitals to provide the care. It seemed like a win-win innovation for the industry.

A FAUSTIAN BARGAIN: THE BLUES AGREE TO "COMMUNITY RATING"

Of course, the government never gives out a favor without strings attached. By agreeing to exempt their health insurance premiums from taxation, the government was clearly providing a major benefit to the Blues, and in exchange the government insisted on *community rating*. In the beginning, this meant that plans administered under Blue Cross/ Blue Shield had to charge the same premium to all applicants within a given geographical region, regardless of the applicant's age, sex, or medical history.[8]

We will return to the issue of "community rating" in Part II of this book, in our discussion of the Affordable Care Act (ACA), because it plays such a large role in the problems with ObamaCare. For now, we should stress that under traditional insurance models, an individual's premium is determined by his or her own particular level of risk. Or, if you have a long list of speeding tickets and a few fender-benders on your record, then you should expect your automobile insurance premiums to be higher. If you skydive and hang glide for fun, your life insurance premiums should be a little higher. Likewise, if you are 75 pounds overweight and smoke a pack of cigarettes per day, then your *health* insurance premiums should be higher. What "community rating" means is that everyone within a given community or geographical region will be given the same risk rating and pay the same premium, based on the aggregate risk of the community. Effectively, the community rating established early on for Blue Cross/Blue Shield meant that the lower-risk customers were subsidizing the higher-risk ones. Nonetheless, the whole thing seemed to work for a while, as the doctors and hospitals got paid for their services while the politicians took credit for making affordable premiums available to everyone.

Although having low-risk customers subsidize high-risk ones might strike some Americans as only fair—it is this mentality that drove passage of the ACA, after all—it actually sets in motion a destructive process that ends up hurting everybody because of what economists call *moral hazard*. Moral hazard refers to the fact that people take on greater risks when they are personally shielded from the negative consequences. It is the difference between how you behave when you walk on a slack line or tightrope when it is two feet off the ground, versus how you behave on the same wire when it is ten *stories* off the ground. The consequences influence behavior.

Your health behaviors are also subject to moral hazard. You are much less likely to avoid risky health behaviors if you know that it won't affect your personal premiums, and when you know all of your health care costs will be covered regardless of what illness or injury befalls you. Less dramatically, if all medical expenses—even routine office visits—are fully covered by insurance, then the consumer has no reason to shop around, and will be much more likely to, say, visit the emergency room for even routine problems. Our point isn't that *everyone* will suddenly change his or her behavior dramatically when facing a new set of incentives, but merely that many people *will* do so. In a country the size of the United States, these effects add up.

The health insurance model adopted early on by the Blues—which covered *all* medical expenses, not just catastrophic ones, and where premiums were based on a community rating—set in motion the problems in US health care that would fester over subsequent decades. The problem of moral hazard led to a vicious cycle, in which (community-rated) premiums had to rise because the participants in the system lacked the incentive to hold down costs. But the rise in premiums then drove out the healthiest individuals, and encouraged those who remained in the system to seek out more medical care in order to "get their money's worth" from their insurance coverage. This is why we claimed earlier that "community rating" can actually end up hurting even the people who would pay relatively high premiums under traditional insurance.

If this principle is hard to grasp when it comes to health insurance, consider it in the context of auto insurance: it would obviously degrade the system if auto insurers had to charge the same premiums to all drivers, regardless of their vehicle, age, sex, and driving record. When the dust settled, even the people who drove expensive cars and frequently got speeding tickets might end up paying a higher auto insurance premium under community rating.

THE WHOLE INDUSTRY FALLS IN LINE

As Blue Cross/Blue Shield was given a competitive advantage by the government, its model of third-party payment for all health care expenses became the gold standard for the industry, as doctors and hospitals could refuse to work with insurers who didn't follow suit. After World War II, this standardization cut off consumer choice. Since all medical fees were set ahead of time by the third-party payer (the insurance company), it meant that the consumer (the patient) had no way of negotiating prices with his or her doctor. This cut off any real possibility of comparison shopping, which is one of the major elements of the price system that keeps costs down. Economist Milton Friedman illustrated the general phenomenon (not specifically relating it to health care) using four quadrants, showing the combinations of the *source* of money and the *beneficiary* of the spending:

Table 1-1. Milton Friedman's Categories of Spending[9]

You Spend Your Money **ON YOURSELF** **Economize and Seek Highest Value**	You Spend Your Money **ON SOMEONE ELSE** **Economize But Don't/Can't Seek Highest Value**
You Spend Someone Else's Money **ON YOURSELF** **Don't Economize But Seek Highest Value**	You Spend Someone Else's Money **ON SOMEONE ELSE** **Don't Economize and Don't/Can't Seek Highest Value**

In the upper left quadrant, you are spending your money on yourself. Here you care very much about quality *and* price. In this quadrant you will make the best economic decisions. If we're considering food, for example, you will only occasionally go out to dinner, and when you do, you will be sure to patronize restaurants that provide a good meal in light of its cost.

In the left lower quadrant, in contrast, you have access to someone else's money, but you still get to spend it on yourself. For example, suppose you are on a business trip and know that you can spend up to $150 on dinner. In this case, you won't worry about holding down expenses—you'll blow the whole $150. Yet at the same time, you'll still be picky about the quality of the meal. You'll end up spending the $150 getting a great steak and bottle of wine; you won't agree to buy a pretzel from a street vendor for $150.

In the upper right quadrant, you are spending your money on behalf of someone else. In this case, you will watch prices like a hawk—it's your money—but you won't be as attentive to quality. For example, if you're making a donation to a local food pantry at Thanksgiving, you're still going to respond to sale items and you will definitely limit the total amount you spend. Yet you probably won't put as much thought into the particular items you grab as you would have if you were preparing your own meal.

Finally, in the lower right quadrant, you are spending someone else's money on behalf of someone else. For example, your boss may have given you a $1,000 budget to take care of the catering for a reception you won't even be in town to attend. In this scenario, you have little personal incentive to watch costs or quality (except for the ramifications coming from your boss if you do a really bad job). You might pick the caterer that is closer to the office (to minimize your drive) even though she's more expensive than the one across town, and furthermore, you might not do a lot of research on which menu items are the best from that caterer. So long as you spend the $1,000 on a selection that nobody can yell at you for, you can call it a day and get back to your other work responsibilities.

Of course we are slightly exaggerating for rhetorical effect, and we can come up with many examples where people behave in a fiscally responsible and altruistic manner regardless of the external incentives. Yet hopefully it is clear that Friedman's fourfold classification contains a great deal of wisdom, especially when it comes to designing systems governing large expenditures and involving millions of people.

With this generic discussion as backdrop, let's return now to the context of US health care. Before the rise of the Blues, virtually all medical service had been in the left upper quadrant—the one that promotes an efficient use of resources. Yet with the new third-party payment system, the *patient* now operated in the left lower quadrant, while the *insurance company* was operating from the right upper quadrant. This placed the patient and insurance company in opposition to each other. The patient is very attentive to the *quality* of medical care he or she receives, but is relatively unconcerned about its official *price*. In total contrast, the insurance company will establish procedures to hold down total spending, with little regard to the impact these rules have on the quality of care that the patient receives.

Thus the rise of the Blues and third-party payment set up an adversarial relationship between the consumer and the provider. Over thousands of years, the doctor-patient bond had been a fiduciary relationship that was mutually beneficial. Within a few short years doctors and patients had taken the first steps of breaking down that bond. It would take a few more decades, as government assumed more and more of the medical payments, before the system moved into the right lower quadrant that represents the worst of both worlds—escalating costs with little to show for it in terms of quality.

WHOEVER PAYS THE BILLS
CALLS THE SHOTS

"[H]ealth insurance is not fundamentally about a relationship between the insurer and the insured. It's about a relationship between the insurer and the healthcare providers.

Home insurers are not in the roofing business. Automobile insurers are not in the car repair business. But modern health insurance is very much in the business of healthcare. In fact, it originally began not as a way to compensate patients for their losses, but as a way to make sure providers got paid for the services they rendered. In such a world, the providers came to view the third-party payers, rather than patients, as their clients."

—Health economist John Goodman[10]

As the Blue model developed, there was a reinforcing trend due to the war effort, which we explain in the next section.

WAGE AND PRICE CONTROLS DURING WORLD WAR II

Labor—like anything else in limited supply—has a price, and that price is termed "wages." Wages are like any other price, in that they are determined by supply and demand. If demand for labor is high and supply is low, wages will have to be high to attract workers. During World War II, a very large segment of the labor supply was off to war. Simultaneously, there was an incredible demand for labor not only for the jobs vacated by soldiers, but also for new jobs of production to supply the war machine. Wishing to suppress the most obvious signs of the strain on the economy, the government passed the 1942 Stabilization Act, which (among other things) froze wages.

Unable to outbid each other with promises of higher pay, employers competed for scarce labor resources by offering more attractive fringe benefits, including employer-provided health insurance. (The government did not include such benefits as being subject to the wage freeze.) The seeds of the medical-industrial-government complex had been planted, and as usual, a major intervention by government was a chief culprit.

As an addendum to the 1942 Act, the government decreed that insurance premiums were a legitimate cost of doing business and could be deducted from the employer's taxable income. However, insurance purchased by an individual outside of an employment benefit program was *not* a tax-deductible expense. This gave industry even more bargaining power to entice employees, and provided an enormous incentive for employees to have their health insurance premiums paid by employers (with pre-tax dollars) rather than buying it themselves out of their wages (with after-tax dollars). In addition, this development was a major step in the collectivization of medicine. These tax advantages were available only to those who purchased health care collectively. This created a situation where very few insurers were responsible for huge numbers of "covered lives," amplifying their bargaining power with doctors and other health care providers.

THE NEXT STEP: MEDICARE

The government, knowingly or not, had sent a Trojan horse into the medical and insurance industries when it required the Blues to offer a community rating in exchange for their tax-exempt status. As we have discussed, the third-party payment system created incentives for medical costs to rise unchecked. At the same time, demographic trends meant that the United States population was skewing more toward the elderly as the decades passed. Naturally, as people age, they tend to require more health care interventions, and these interventions are more complex and costly. This is where the community rating issue came back to haunt the Blues. While the community rating prevented the Blues from charging a higher premium on the elderly, the other insurers (who were not able to trade tax-exempt status for a community rating) could charge higher premiums and thus began developing a competitive advantage.

However, as the private insurers started to compete on equal ground with the Blues, health care costs continued to soar, and thus premiums for the elderly went up concordantly. The problem was that this segment of the population was very likely to be living on a fixed or declining income; more and more elderly began to fall through the cracks. Formerly, the elderly indigent were cared for largely on a charity basis, but because of price expansion in the medical industry, this became very costly for doctors and hospitals. The entire situation created significant public pressure that "something had to be done." Previously, most hospitals and the smaller insurers had opposed government intrusion into health care, but the business model they were using by the 1960s—which was most certainly *not* a "free market in medicine"—was untenable, making a political solution seem necessary.

Thus, two major players in the health care industry now had a vested interest in the government taking over health care. The Blues and the American Hospital Association would eventually lend support for the establishment of Medicare. All the while, the elderly were getting more complex and chronic illnesses that were driving costs ever higher. The ultimate result was that President Lyndon Johnson signed Medicare into law on July 30, 1965. At the time, dubious physicians were reassured that the government did not wish to dictate how medicine was practiced; it just wanted to pay the bill.

In the stroke of a pen, anyone over the age of 65 was removed from the private sector's insurance pool. This improved the profit potential for private insurance by transferring the highest cost and highest risk segment of their business to the taxpayers.

As soon as this became the law of the land, demographics were already conspiring to cause problems. We will explain the situation, with numerical precision, in Chapter 3.

DRGS = PRICE CONTROLS

During the period between 1965 and 1980, the costs of Medicare saw a dramatic rise. Payments were made retrospectively: the doctor or hospital would submit a bill and Medicare would send the reimbursement. Under this model, consumption of medical services expanded rapidly. Since the providers knew they would be reimbursed, the supply of services expanded to meet this demand. The new incentives under Medicare had caused both consumers and producers to drastically change their behavior, something that had not been fully appreciated by the proponents of the "reform" measure at its inception.

Politicians sought to control costs *not* by limiting treatment, as that would offend the electorate, but instead by limiting payment to the providers. To accomplish this, payment would have to be curtailed on a prospective basis, before the service was actually provided. The government found a model for doing this through the work of two Yale University professors. John D. Thompson, MPH of the Yale School of Public Health, and Robert B. Fetter, PhD of the Yale school of management had been working on a model that determined the effectiveness of hospitals by measuring the types and severities of illnesses that they treated. These researchers eventually developed *diagnosis-related groups* (DRGs), which prospectively modeled what a hospital should be paid based on the mixture and severity of cases within each institution. Diseases were given specific codes and registered in a compendium called ICD-9, with ICD standing for the "international compendium of diseases."

Doctors and hospitals had to prospectively accept the payment calculated by the DRG system for the patients' primary discharge diagnosis. The amount calculated by the DRG was a best-case scenario based on the hospital's severity of illness index. The system was designed to incentivize efficiency and cost containment. The problem was, the patients seldom cooperated. Many had co-morbidities (more than one medical problem) for which the DRGs did not effectively account. Caring for such patients meant that complications could arise, or that other acute illnesses could manifest during the treatment of the primary diagnosis. In general, the mathematical model of the severity index was based on ideal conditions, whereas the delivery of actual medical care occurred under the conditions of Murphy's Law. Doctors and hospitals quickly came to recognize the DRG system for what it really was: a system of price controls.

PRICE CEILINGS CAUSE SHORTAGES, EVEN IN MEDICINE

One of the standard lessons in an introductory economics course is that price ceilings lead to shortages. By definition, the market-clearing price balances supply and demand. Therefore, if the government makes sellers charge less than this amount, then the customers will try to buy more of the product or service than producers want to provide at the (artificially) low price. History is replete with examples of well-intentioned price controls leading to shortages and rationing, hurting the very people who were supposedly the beneficiaries of the policy.

In medicine, the government instituted a form of price ceilings through Medicare's DRG reimbursement formulas, which were soon adopted by commercial insurance companies as well. The response was a contraction in the amount of inpatient services offered and an expansion of services in the outpatient arena: doctors and hospitals naturally adjusted their output to cater to those areas where they had more flexibility in charging adequately for their own costs and time.

To this day, we can see the results of these pseudo-price controls. Drive by most any community hospital and you will see dilapidated inpatient buildings surrounded by beautiful, modern outpatient facilities, such as outpatient surgery centers, heart centers, cancer treatment centers, medical imaging centers, and blood donation centers. The cumulative square footage of the outpatient centers greatly exceeds that of their parent hospital.

SLEEPING ON THE JOB
(NOT WHAT YOU THINK)

Prior to 1965, medical school graduates would typically undergo a year of training where they would rotate through various specialty areas in a hospital. Such doctors-in-training were called "interns" or "residents" because they literally lived in the hospital. In essence, these doctors were given room and board plus invaluable real-world experience in exchange for working grueling hours at the hospital. After a year of a rotating internship, most doctors would then go into general practice. A small number would go on for more specialized training under a similar structure.

DOMINOES KEEP FALLING: MEDICARE FUNDING OF GME LEADS TO EMTALA

We have already explained how the tightened government rules on medical schools and licensing, combined with the expanding number of elderly patients, led to a relative shortage of doctors that was supposedly "solved" in 1965 when the new Medicare legislation included provisions for funding of graduate medical education (GME). These funds were split into direct and indirect funding. Direct funding was for the salaries of the residents and faculty, as well as the hospital expenses directly related to GME. Indirect funding was to subsidize the higher operating costs of teaching hospitals, including increased test ordering and length of stays.

From 1965 to the 1980s, hospitals used this as a means for funding their indigent care. Teaching hospitals and residents became the sole source of care for poor and underprivileged populations, and were compensated accordingly. Private hospitals were well aware of the funding discrepancies and would divert indigent patients toward the teaching institutions. It was an unspoken understanding that the county teaching hospital was where such people would go for care.

By the mid-1980s, the workload related to indigent care was reaching a critical level at teaching institutions, even though residents typically worked over 100 hours per week. Especially taxing was the practice of "dumping," in which a private hospital would occasionally transfer an unstable indigent patient to a teaching hospital without first providing any stabilizing treatment.

As the public outcry over "wallet biopsies" and patient "dumping" grew, Congress was also facing concerns that the DRGs they had recently passed would lead hospitals to provide fewer services. Further, the late Senator Edward Kennedy pointed out that many teaching hospitals' obligations to provide indigent care under the Hill-Burton Act of 1946 were going to expire in 1986.

Consequently, in 1986, President Reagan signed into law EMTALA, the Emergency Medical Treatment and Active Labor Act. EMTALA was a mere section of the much larger Congressional Omnibus Reconciliation Act (COBRA), which you may recognize because of its employer requirements to provide health insurance for a period after termination. Even so, EMTALA is a crucial piece of our story, necessary for understanding what went wrong with US health care.

EMTALA imposes three distinct duties on hospitals. First, ERs must provide a medical screening exam (MSE) on anyone who presents requesting care and determine whether an emergency medical condition (EMC) exists. This must be done regardless of the patient's ability or intention of paying for care. Second, if an EMC exists, the hospital staff must either stabilize that condition or arrange transfer to another hospital that can. Third, if a hospital possesses specialized capabilities or facilities, they are required to accept transfer of patients in need of their specialized services (again, regardless of capability or intent of paying for these services). This third component of the statute is referred to as the "reverse-dumping" statute.

If a given hospital cannot stabilize an emergency medical condition, the hospital cannot transfer the patient unless the individual requests a transfer after being informed of the risks of transfer and the hospital's obligation to stabilize. If this cannot be achieved (if the patient is unconscious, for example), then the physician has to sign a certification that the medical benefits of transfer outweigh the risks to the patient and, in the case of labor, the unborn child. Finally, the transfer must meet the statute's definition of "appropriate."

Immediately after passage, critics warned that the law would be crippling for physicians and hospitals because of its vague definitions of an emergency condition, medical screening exams, and what constitutes "stabilization," which the Act defined as "no medical deterioration should occur from or during the transfer." As the law took effect and cases started to accumulate, it became evident that the courts interpreted these terms so strictly that nearly *any* patient could be considered unstable. This is because almost any complaint from an ER patient could conceivably be attached to a dangerous diagnosis that the originating hospital, per the statute, had to rule out before transferring the patient. For example, a complaint of a sore throat *could* be a retropharyngeal abscess or epiglottitis, and the complaint of a crick in the neck *could* be a vertebral artery dissection.

As ridiculous as it may sound, *under EMTALA no actual illness or injury needs to be proven for a violation to have occurred.* Thus all transfers are fraught with danger, as the courts might interpret that deterioration *could* have occurred, or that the benefits *might* not have outweighed the risks. There was no burden of proof that harm actually occurred in order for a physician or hospital to be shown guilty. Further, the definition of "transfer" does not just mean moving the patient from one hospital to another. Under the law, "transfer" can mean discharge home, or admission to the hospital with subsequent discharge. Further, it can mean admission of a patient for an extended period of time, followed by a transfer to a long-term care facility (nursing home). Even sending the patient to another facility from any part of the hospital for testing, even when the patient will return afterwards, is considered a transfer. Thus if the hospital's CT scanner goes down, and a patient is going to be sent to an outpatient imaging center across the street, a full EMTALA procedure must take place.

THE SEVERE PENALTIES UNDER EMTALA

The penalties associated with the 1986 law were the most severe in the history of medicine, and they applied to all patients (not just those covered under Medicare). Here were some of the potential consequences for violating EMTALA:

• Medicare/Medicaid program termination for up to two years. This is a financial death sentence to a hospital or physician, especially an emergency physician who is hospital-based.

• Monetary penalties of $50,000 for each *violation* (not merely each patient—multiple violations can be levied with each patient). These fines are not covered by malpractice insurance.

• Hospital pays hospital. The hospital that is "dumped" on can have all costs of the patient's care covered by the transferring hospital.

• Hill-Burton Act funds. The government may take action to recover loans and grants made to the violating facility.

• Civil rights action. If the violation is interpreted as discrimination, the violating doctor and facility can face criminal prosecution under the Civil Rights Act.

EMTALA IN THE LONG RUN

Despite the sentiment to the contrary, EMTALA did not just apply to emergency physicians and hospital ERs. The law also applied to on-call specialists for the hospital. Such specialists were obligated under EMTALA to see anyone within their specialty at the hospitals they were on call for. It didn't take specialists long to realize that when the ER paged them, there was a very significant chance it would be for a complicated case with no chance of being paid for their services. Furthermore, despite providing uncompensated care, they were still exposed to considerable liability. Many specialists felt that the non-paying patient was also the most litigious. It is no wonder that specialists began to develop a negative attitude about their call responsibilities.

The DRG payment system had already caused a contraction of inpatient beds, which contributed significantly to ER crowding. EMTALA exacerbated the problem by opening the floodgates at the front door. The government had essentially made ERs across the nation the free clinic and safety net for the American health care system. If you liken the ER overcrowding problem to an overflowing bathtub, then DRGs could be visualized as the drain plug that prevents patients (water) from exiting the tub. What EMTALA did was turn the faucet on full blast while the drain plug remained in place.

"IN CASE OF AN EMERGENCY . . ."

Edwin Leap, MD coined the term "moral diversion," referring to EMTALA's removal of any impediment or inconvenience related to referring someone to the ER. If any situation is too complicated to be bothered with, you can simultaneously get out of the situation and yet be reassured that the problem will be addressed in a way that releases you of any risk. Examples abound. If a nursing home resident is acting unruly he can be sent over to the ER. If someone checks his blood pressure at the pharmacy and asks the pharmacist what to do about a pressure of 190/100, the pharmacist can say, "Go to the ER." Get in a fender-bender? The cop (or your attorney) may tell you to go to the ER "just to get checked out." Feeling depressed and call a local suicide helpline? Be prepared for law enforcement to show up at your door to take you to an ER for a mental evaluation. When you get the answering machine at your doctor's office, listen for the ever present . . . "If you think you may be having a medical emergency, dial 911 or go to your nearest emergency department."

Any attempts to deflect this onslaught of patients has been tamped down by expansions of EMTALA's power. One of the most famous cases revolved around the tragic fate of Christopher Sercye, a 15-year-old boy who was shot in 1998 by gang members while playing basketball near Chicago's Ravenswood Hospital Medical Center. Sercye's friends dragged him to within 50 feet (reports differ about the exact distance) of the hospital. Despite being informed of Sercye's location and condition, hospital staff did not leave the building to retrieve him, choosing to wait for police. By the time Sercye was finally brought in for treatment, it was too late; he was pronounced dead (about an hour and a half after he had been shot) from bullet wounds that punctured his abdominal aorta and other large blood vessels.

The Sercye case received national attention, with even President Bill Clinton threatening to yank the facility's Medicare funding. The hospital responded that its staff had simply been following policy (keep in mind that there had just been a shooting nearby), and that it would amend the policy to prevent such a tragic repeat. It's worth noting that part of the delay was due the on-scene police officers *also* initially refusing to move the injured teenager from outside into the facility, citing their *own* policy that they had to wait for paramedics to arrive. A spokesman for Ravenswood also claimed that police had told their staff that an ambulance would take Sercye to a trauma center that was better equipped than the Ravenswood ER for dealing with gunshot wounds. Despite these mitigating circumstances to what everyone agreed was a tragic event, the hospital ultimately settled a lawsuit in 2003 for $12.5 million with the victim's family, and additionally was fined $40,000 by the federal government for an EMTALA violation.[11]

The result of this case and EMTALA conviction was an expansion of the law. H.R. 3937, the Christopher Sercye Emergency Hospital Care Zone Act of 1998, prohibited any "hospital limitations on emergency room workers treating emergency cases in immediate vicinity of emergency room entrance." The Act defined the immediate vicinity as "within 150 feet or such other reasonable distance as the Secretary may specify."[12] (Apparently the secretary must have specified 250 yards, because that now seems to be the national standard.) As a result of this 1998 expansion to EMTALA, now emergency physicians and nurses must not only provide uncompensated care to anyone who shows up *in* the ER, but they must go *outside* the hospital (into potentially life-threatening situations) to *retrieve* patients.

Although one can understand each incremental tweak to the federal government's interventions in medicine, the cumulative result has been disastrous: as a result of the massive financial burden imposed by EMTALA, emergency departments and hospitals across the country have shut down. The remaining ERs and hospitals have developed a severe shortage of subspecialty on-call backup. Due to DRGs, there was already a shift toward outpatient centers. Most surgical specialists relied on hospital operating rooms to perform the elective cases that made up the bulk of their income. In exchange, the hospital required these specialists to provide on-call coverage for emergency cases that occurred in the hospital or that presented to the ER. With the influence of EMTALA, the cases that came through the ER were much more likely to be uncompensated. It did not take long for specialists to figure out that there would be a significant return on investment if they built their own outpatient elective surgery centers as means of avoiding EMTALA exposure. It is a testament to the size of the financial burden of EMTALA that specialists would spend or borrow millions of dollars in order to build a place to perform their elective cases.

The consequences for emergency physicians and ER patients have been dire. Across the country, ERs are required by law to take all comers, but have no specialty backup to help care for these patients. It is not uncommon for even tertiary care centers to lack coverage in surgical subspecialties such as opthalmology, ENT, neurosurgery, and others.

An additional consequence is cost-shifting. With so many people using the ER as a free source of care but with no intent of paying, hospitals and physicians try to partially recoup these losses by charging higher fees to those who do pay. This partly explains the horror stories about $150 hospital charges for a Tylenol. Under EMTALA even illegal immigrants are covered. In fact, ERs are now required to have professional translators for those patients who do not speak English.

Even if a doctor is fluent in the patient's language, he or she is none-theless required to use a "professional" translator.

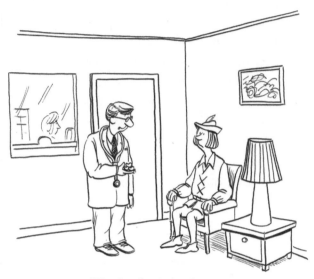

"Typically, I don't accept magic beans for payment."

ELECTRONIC MEDICAL RECORDS (EMRS)

Let's keep in mind that EMTALA was signed into law by an icon of conservatives, Ronald Reagan. Likewise, the next government inter-vention to get between you and your doctor was driven very much by former Speaker of the House and Presidential hopeful, Newt Gingrich.

Before we discuss Mr. Gingrich's contributions, we must first pro-vide a little background. DRGs are not the government's only attempt at price control. In order to prop up a system that promises so much to so many, they must always be thinking of ways to avoid paying for services rendered by providers. On the *inpatient* side of medicine, this was done through DRGs using a compendium of approved diagnoses. Clinicians had to document how they had satisfied complex require-ments in order to get full payment for their services.

Starting in the 1990s, a similar requirement for *outpatient* care—called E&M (Evaluation and Management) coding—began to emerge.

This based reimbursement on each medical case's level of complexity. That level was not drawn from the doctor's estimate (as it had been in the past), but instead was determined by how many elements from a Chinese menu of documentation requirements were included in the medical record. For instance, under the "history of present illness" section of a medical record, there are elements such as duration, location, character, intensity, associated symptoms, relieving factors, and aggravating factors, among others. Under "review of systems," the patient is asked about potential problems in areas not related to the chief complaint. This is divided into body systems such as head, eyes, ears/nose/throat, neck, respiratory, cardiac, gastrointestinal, genitourinary, and so on. Likewise, a certain number of body areas on the physical exam were required for a given level of complexity. The E&M coding system allows for levels of billing from the most simple (Level I) to the most complex (Level V). In order to bill at higher levels, you have to rack up more elements in each segment of the medical record.

In the past, if you had a complex trauma case, you could just circle a Level V on the chart or indicate it in your record to determine the level of billing. This was done somewhat on an honor system (with severe penalties for fraud), but it was fairly easy to tell if the case on the chart jived with the level billed. Coding an ankle sprain a Level IV would not fly. Suddenly, the new rules forced doctors to record five elements in the patient's history, complete almost all elements of the review of systems, and record almost all elements of a physical exam in order to code a Level V charge.

While the system might seem fair at first glance, it really had little clinical relevance and was often very counterproductive to the ultimate goal of providing medical care. Imagine you are an ER doctor and receive an unconscious patient wheeled in with a knife sticking out of his chest in the area over his heart. As the patient loses his vital signs, you have to quickly open his chest with a scalpel and rib spreader while one of your partners inserts a breathing tube. You then clamp his aorta, open the heart sac, empty out the blood clot, and place a purse string suture in the laceration in the left ventricle. The cardiothoracic surgeon arrives and the patient is wheeled off to the operating room.

In the past, this event could have been recorded on a handwritten chart quickly, and anyone in his right mind would have agreed that this was a Level V case. But the new protocols make things much more difficult. How is it possible to get five elements of history from a patient who cannot talk? How are you supposed to include seven or nine body areas in the physical exam when all you are trying to do is reach the heart? How do you conduct a review of systems in such a case? In this type of scenario, is it even important if this patient has had ringing in his ears, burning with urination, or recent weight loss? If an element is omitted, the health care provider must explain the reason for each omission (e.g. "patient unconscious, patient in cardiac arrest, patient intubated"), even though common sense would indicate that a single note could have conveyed the situation to anyone reviewing the event.

All of these documentation hoops are time consuming and greatly increase the workload. This slows down clinical care in the outpatient environment and adds an administrative burden to deal with the extra paperwork.

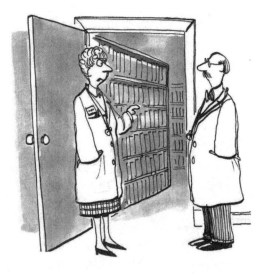

"Doctor, we have some new forms for you to fill out."

A cynical (though we believe accurate) way to interpret these ever-shifting reimbursement requirements is that the government wanted to make things too complex for health care providers to receive full compensation for their services. However, the doctors and hospitals proved to be incredibly intelligent, adaptable, and industrious, relying on professional transcription services and other techniques to handle the enormous increase in administrative overhead. Yet this very adaptability proved to be a giant bull's eye for cronyism, as we will now explain.

As computer technology advanced, it became a new requirement to file electronically with government payers and many other third-party payers. The dot-com boom was in full swing, and everyone thought computers would improve efficiency in all realms, including medicine.

One of the strongest proponents of this notion was Newt Gingrich, former Speaker of the House and founder of The Center for Health Transformation (a health policy think tank). The Center generated policy papers and provided experts to appear at congressional hearings and other forums in favor of numerous pieces of legislation. Coincidentally enough, the measures that Gingrich's Center supported would financially benefit its clients, who paid up to $200,000 a year for its services. In 2006, Gingrich testified before a House subcommittee about the benefits of using health information technology, citing his Center's member companies favorably 48 times. He even specified certain companies (including Siemens, GE Health Care, and Allscripts) that he felt should take the lead in implementing this technology. The Center's project director, David Merritt, testified before the Department of Labor urging the Secretary of Labor to require doctors and hospitals to upgrade to electronic recordkeeping systems.

Ultimately, President Obama's Affordable Care Act would include billions in funding to "encourage" adaptation of electronic medical records.[13] This episode is one more in a long line suggesting the stereotypes of "conservatives" and "liberals" in US politics are an illusion: in practice, *both* camps support government interference with business practices, and *both* camps funnel taxpayer money to large corporations.

Regardless of the dubious motivations, what can we say about the results? One would assume that the use of computerized medical record documentation would be a boon to doctors and hospitals. This would be true if EMRs had evolved in a bottom-up and *voluntary* fashion, with medical providers adopting the new technology wherever it offered a genuine improvement over the old way of doing things. Yet instead, the electronic "revolution" in medical records was foisted upon the industry through a top-down and involuntary series of proclamations. As a result, medical records can now balloon into hundreds of pages. Further, simple mousing errors can introduce mistakes into the record that range from the ridiculous (such as a six-month-old baby who smokes two packs of cigarettes per day) to the dangerous (incorrect drug allergy). As these records get shared between treating physicians, the errors are "populated" into other charts and duplicated over and over.

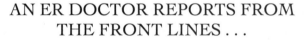

AN ER DOCTOR REPORTS FROM THE FRONT LINES . . .

"In my own case in emergency medicine, our experience with EMR [electronic medical records] has been pretty abysmal. Seeing the writing on the wall, we implemented an EMR four years before 'meaningful use' criteria were instituted. We did this so that we could select the best emergency medicine-specific EMR. While its prescription-writing and discharge instruction functions were an improvement, the actual process of charting has been appalling. Prior to the EMR, we used voice dictation to generate a chart, and we used a grease-board system to track the status of patients within the emergency department. Using the old approach, I could see patients at almost double the pace that I can muster under the EMR. More importantly, if there is any computer malfunction, the entire department can cease to function. In the dynamic environment of a busy emergency room, this is one of the greatest dangers of EMR."

—Co-author Doug McGuff

Finally, we should stress the most obvious drawback of the new rules: doctors and other health care providers are chained to a computer screen, tapping away and dutifully filling required documentation, rather than focusing on the patient and using common sense in each encounter. The next time you are frustrated by the apparent lack of attention from your doctor or nurse, keep in mind that this system has been foisted upon them. It aggravates *them* more than *you*, because your temporary annoyance during a procedure is what they now must endure for the rest of their careers (assuming they stay in mainstream medicine).

HIPAA

HIPAA (The Health Insurance Portability and Accountability Act) evolved along with the development of electronic medical records, and in the most basic sense, the bulk of the law deals with enforcing privacy issues that arise with the use of electronic health information. It was originally signed into law in 1996 by President Clinton to protect health insurance coverage for workers and their families if they changed or lost jobs. This was to address a problem again created by government intervention: the fact that the vast majority of people obtained their health insurance as a benefit through their employer. That part of the law, title I, was relatively simple.

Title II addressed health care fraud and abuse, and it tried to make uniform all diagnosis coding for billing purposes. Section 2.5 is the enforcement rule that sets civil and monetary penalties for violating HIPAA. These penalties can be quite severe. An example is a hospice organization fined $50,000 because an unencrypted laptop with patient information was stolen from a van. A similar theft occurred at a Massachusetts eye infirmary and resulted in a $1.5 million fine.[14] In May 2014, the largest HIPAA settlement to date occurred, when New York Presbyterian Hospital and Columbia University agreed to pay $4.8 million. Here is how the government's Health and Human Services website describes the case:

The investigation revealed that the breach was caused when a physician employed by [Columbia University] who developed applications for both NYP [New York Presbyterian] and [Columbia] attempted to deactivate a personally owned computer server on the network containing NYP patient ePHI [electronic personal health information]. Because of a lack of technical safeguards, deactivation of the server resulted in ePHI being accessible on internet search engines. The entities learned of the breach after receiving a complaint by an individual who found the ePHI of the individual's deceased partner, a former patient of NYP, on the internet.[15]

DON'T TAKE OUR WORD FOR IT—SEE FOR YOURSELF

To appreciate the day-to-day threat that health care providers face from the federal government, go to the HHS.gov website, click on the "News" tab at the top, and then select the "HIPAA" filter (from a pull-down "Category" menu). You will likely see several stories involving major fines (some exceeding $1 million) for HIPAA violations within just the past year. (You may have to click on the headline to read the story and see the size of the payment.) In some cases, the news stories discuss medical entities paying major fines to settle what are described as "potential" HIPAA violations!

Among doctors' fears about these government mandates, one of the greatest was the potential for inadvertent violations of the duty of confidentiality as spelled out in the Hippocratic oath. After enacting expensive mandates requiring unnatural and counterproductive use of EMRs, the government then finished its one-two punch under HIPAA by severely punishing health care providers for data vulnerabilities that the government's own rules created in the first place.

CONCLUSION

In this opening chapter we have provided a crash history course in US health care and insurance. You are now well on your way to understanding what went wrong in these fields. However, you still only have the big picture. In the following chapters we will walk through some specific issues in much greater depth, offering you an exact diagnosis of how health care gradually spun out of control.

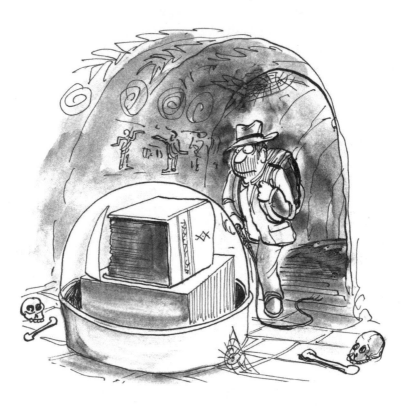

At last he had found the Regulatory Guidelines.

Chapter 2

THE DEADLY FDA

"This country has a new public health problem—Congress and the FDA."
— Dr. Joel J. Nobel, 1993

"We will surely live to regret the day we gave the FDA the kind of arbitrary power it is now exercising."
— James O. Page, editor of *Journal of Emergency Medical Services*, 1992[1]

I f you asked the average American to name the single biggest problem with US health care, he would probably answer, "It costs too much." Indeed, from 1960 to 2009, the "medical care" component of the Consumer Price Index grew an average of 1.8 percentage points more per year than the overall CPI. Measured in 2009 dollars, US per capita expenditures on health care rose from $1,066 in 1960 to a staggering $8,170 in 2009. Finally, expressed as a share of the economy, total American health care spending ballooned during this same period from 5 percent of GDP to 17.4 percent.[2] This seemingly unstoppable growth in both the unit price and total expense of US health care was undoubtedly one of the main reasons for the passage of the Affordable Care Act in 2010. As President Obama and his supporters framed the issue, it seemed that "the private sector" couldn't provide affordable medical care to Americans.

After our historical survey in the first chapter, we know that such claims are completely erroneous. Even before the New Deal, time and again the government has ratcheted up its interventions in the markets for health care and insurance, driving up cost far above what it would be in a freer environment.

Broadly speaking, the government's interventions in the market for health care can be grouped into two categories: (1) those that *increase demand* and (2) those that *restrict supply*. Putting these two together obviously pushes prices up; the laws of economics work the same in health care as in any other sector. (If the government started buying up apples at the same time it burned down half of the apple trees, what would happen to the price of apples at the grocery store?)

The first category of intervention, in which the government boosts demand for medical services and products, includes direct government payments (through Medicare and Medicaid). However, it also includes the tax code's encouragement of third-party payment arrangements, which—as we have seen—weaken the incentives for end consumers to "shop around" and do their part to control medical costs.

The second category of intervention, in which the government restricts supply, is also important when considering what went wrong with US health care. One obvious culprit here is government-enforced medical licensing, which makes it literally illegal for people to provide various types of medical care without first jumping through numerous and expensive hoops. Another obvious culprit is the Food and Drug Administration (FDA), which erects enormous hurdles in the way of companies trying to bring new drugs to market.

This chapter focuses on the FDA because it is a perfect example of how top-down government planning fails when it comes to medicine. As we will see, the FDA hits Americans with a double whammy. On the one hand, it prolongs the development of potentially useful drugs, leading to delayed treatment and artificially inflated prices. On the other hand, the FDA also fails to protect Americans from unacceptably *dangerous* drugs, even when experts in the private sector have raised alarm bells.

The FDA thus gives Americans the worst of both worlds: it makes it harder and more expensive to obtain quality treatment, while at the same time promoting the use of unacceptably dangerous products. By analyzing the operations of the FDA and its impact on drug development, this chapter will help explain why US health care costs have been rising so dramatically, and why more government intervention is *not* the answer.

THE FOOD AND DRUG ADMINISTRATION: RHETORIC VERSUS REALITY

The Food and Drug Administration was not organized under that name until 1930, but its regulatory functions were laid out in the 1906 Pure Food and Drugs Act.[3] According to its website, the FDA's current mission includes:

> . . . protecting the public health by assuring the safety, effectiveness, quality, and security of human and veterinary drugs, vaccines and other biological products, and medical devices. The FDA is also responsible for the safety and security of most of our nation's food supply, all cosmetics, dietary supplements and products that give off radiation.[4]

Most Americans have been taught to believe that the creation of the FDA was an obviously necessary event in US history. In the bad old days before the FDA, so the story goes, Americans had little protection from snake oil salesmen pushing poisonous products on an ignorant public. The normal market forces of competition could not be trusted to weed out greedy hucksters, because when it comes to medicine (and food), a dangerous product can mean death. This is why, so the usual narrative concludes, we need an agency like the FDA to set minimum standards of safety and efficacy, above which private companies can then compete for sales. The problem with this typical understanding of the FDA's role is that in reality, there's no such thing as a "safe" drug. Even *water* can kill you if you drink too much of it, too quickly. To take a less flippant example, imagine a new drug that promises an 80 percent chance of curing a certain type of cancer, but will cause a stroke in 1 percent of the patients who use it. Should the FDA approve such a drug? With these hypothetical numbers, it definitely seems "effective," but is it "safe"? What if we kept reducing the percentage of cancer victims it would cure, while increasing the percentage of patients who would suffer a stroke? It's not obvious where the dividing line should be drawn, and indeed readers would no doubt offer different opinions. Just as the FAA (Federal Aviation

Administration) can't really guarantee "safe" air travel—the only way to ensure zero plane crashes would be to ban all flights—the FDA can't truly guarantee a "safe" supply of drugs. To completely eliminate the possibility of an impure drug causing a harmful side effect, the FDA would need to ban *all* drugs, which is clearly a cure worse than the disease.

A BEDROCK CONCEPT: THE NUMBER NEEDED TO TREAT (NNT)

At this point we need to briefly suspend our analysis of the FDA in order to provide you with a bedrock concept: the *number needed to treat,* or NNT. We urge you not to skip this section, even though at first you might not think the material is necessary to follow the historical discussion. We will return to the concept of NNT time and again throughout this book; it is critical that you give us a chance to explain the basics. Along with shedding light on the skullduggery of the FDA, awareness of this concept will allow you to far more knowledgeably evaluate the pros and cons of medications in your own life.

When it comes to pharmaceuticals, we have a natural tendency to give them a lot more credit than they deserve. We tend to think that a given drug is designed to produce a certain therapeutic effect—in other words, an effect that addresses a specific disease condition or symptoms—and that the therapeutic effect will be expressed in anyone who takes it. We also tend to think that the drug's most dominant feature is its therapeutic effect and that side effects are minor nuisances that occur rarely or intermittently. We have even reached the point where we believe a well-crafted drug can produce a therapeutic effect devoid of unwanted side effects.

The actual truth is quite different. Therapeutic effects are intrinsically linked to side effects, and the degree of therapeutic effect has a lot more to do with the individual taking the medicine than with the intrinsic properties of the drug itself. As Hippocrates said, *"It is more important to know what sort of person has a disease than to know the sort of disease a person has."*

For this crash course in NNT, we will first summarize Keaton's Laws of Pharmacology, named in honor of one of our (McGuff's) Pharmacology professor from Medical School, T. Kent Keaton, PhD.

Keaton's Laws:
1. Not all drugs have a therapeutic effect, and those that do depend on the presence and severity of a disease.
2. All drugs have side effects.
3. No drug has a single effect.
4. Side effects are proportionate to therapeutic effect.
5. Drugs can kill you.

Now let us elaborate on each of these laws. First, for a drug to have a therapeutic effect, there has to be an objective disease condition. Furthermore, the more serious the disease condition, the greater the likelihood that a therapeutic effect will be realized. When a disease condition is not present, what would have been a therapeutic effect has now become a side effect. For example, a person with very high blood pressure has a high likelihood of experiencing a therapeutic benefit from the administration of a blood pressure medicine, but a person with normal blood pressure will only experience the side effect of hypotension. A person with mild disease—such as borderline hypertension with only transient elevations of blood pressure—has a much lower likelihood of experiencing the drug's benefit when his pressure intermittently spikes, and a much greater chance of hypotension during the majority of the day when his blood pressure is normal.

If we look at all people being treated with a particular medication for a particular disease, and view the disease as being expressed across a spectrum of severity, we can derive a number called the number needed to treat. This figure represents the number of patients with a condition that you would need to treat in order to confer benefit to one patient. This is called NNT-B (number needed to treat to benefit). Typically, a NNT-B of five is considered a pretty good therapeutic ratio, meaning you have to treat five patients in order to benefit one patient.

Now Keaton's second law states that all drugs have side effects. This is not dependent on the presence of disease (at least not directly). With regard to a person with a disease state, there is a single desired "side effect" that addresses the disease state in question. When the disease state is present, the desired side effect *becomes* our therapeutic effect. The more severe the disease state, the more likely you are to have a therapeutic effect. When the disease state is less severe, there is a greater chance that the therapeutic effect will just revert to one of the drug's side effects. In other words, we can simply state that a drug has a constellation of effects. If one of those effects improves upon a disease state we call it *therapeutic*, while all the other effects we call *side effects*.

Keaton's third law is related to the second law. It is not possible to create a drug that has a single effect (the therapeutic effect). Human physiology is not that simple. It is impossible to isolate a single effect of a medication and eliminate all the others. When someone tells you a drug or supplement has a therapeutic effect, but no side effects, you are being lied to. In fact, this leads us to our fourth law.

The fourth law states that side effects are proportionate to therapeutic effects. This is true because a drug simply has a collection of effects bundled together. When one of these effects is directed at a disease state (or a marker of disease), it becomes a therapeutic effect and all the others become side effects. A popular TV ad for an over-the-counter antihistamine once claimed "side effects similar to placebo." Well, guess what? If side effects were similar to placebo then the therapeutic effect also had to be similar to placebo.

The fifth law states, quite simply, that drugs can kill you. This law is related to the inverse benefit law we've described and requires an understanding of NNT. The number needed to treat is simply an expression of the power of the medication: it is the number of people that you need to give the drug to in order to see the effect in one patient. The NNT-B is the number needed to show benefit, as we mentioned previously. NNT-H is the number needed to show harm. NNT-B is dependent on the presence and severity of the disease state that the drug is supposed to treat. If a disease state is severe, the NNT-B will be small (it may take only five patients being treated in order to show benefit to one). If the disease state is mild, the NNT-B may be much larger (25 patients treated in order to show benefit to one).

Here is the problem: NNT-H does *not* depend on the presence of disease, because it is an effect that occurs independent of the disease state. Also, the other effects that contribute to NNT-H are additive, meaning that they can reinforce each other, lowering the threshold needed to cause harm to a patient. When a patient is taking two or more drugs, this additive effect can be greater than the sum of its parts because many drugs are metabolized by common pathways. When multiple drugs are metabolized in the same organ, they are eliminated more slowly and the circulating drug level rises, which disproportionately affects the NNT-H.

NNT-B and NNT-H are interrelated. Because there will always be a greater number of side effects than therapeutic effects, we must be careful to use a drug only in a situation where the NNT-B is a smaller number than the NNT-H. Since NNT-B is at a numerical disadvantage right out of the gate, the only way it can gain this ground back is to be given *only* to patients with the most severe disease. If someone has a severe disease, the NNT-B of a drug may be three and the NNT-H may be 10, but in someone with mild disease, the NNT-B may be 15 and the NNT-H remains 10. The simple presence of a disease is *not* an indication to use a drug; only if the disease is of sufficient severity should the patient consider doing so.

Now that we've given you a basic framework with which to think about the possible benefits and harms of pharmaceuticals, we can return to our analysis of the FDA.

SINS OF OMISSION: HOW THE FDA DELAYS DRUG DEVELOPMENT AND INFLATES PRICES

When assessing the ways in which the FDA might be harming Americans, economists typically focus on the onerous restrictions it places on the development of new drugs. Economists are wont to focus on incentives, and when they consider those facing the FDA, they see reasons to expect the agency to err on the side of restriction rather than approval. As a recent study explained:

[T]he FDA faces asymmetrical incentives. Damage can occur when bad drugs are approved quickly or when good drugs are approved slowly. However, the cost to the FDA of these two outcomes is not the same. When bad drugs are approved quickly, the FDA is scrutinized and criticized, victims are identified, and their graves are marked. In contrast, when good drugs are approved slowly, the victims are unknown. . . . We know that some people who died would have lived had new drugs been available sooner, but we don't know which people. As a result, premature deaths from drug lag and drug loss create less opposition than deaths from early approval, and the FDA's natural stance is one of deadly caution.[5]

From our discussion of NNT, we know that the language in this quotation is a bit imprecise; in reality it's too simplistic to classify drugs as either "good" or "bad." Nonetheless, the authors of the study *are* pointing to an important phenomenon regarding incentives, which we can illustrate by studying the FDA's response to two tragedies: thalidomide in the 1960s and Vioxx in the 2000s.

Let's begin with thalidomide. Even though the FDA never approved commercial distribution—indeed President Kennedy would later honor the FDA reviewer who had denied the drug company's application—American physicians nonetheless had received millions of tablets of thalidomide for clinical testing, and had distributed them to some 20,000 patients (though fewer than 1,000 of them were pregnant women). Though the impact in the US was fortunately contained, in the late 1950s and early 1960s more than 10,000 children in 46 countries were born with birth defects due to their mothers' use of thalidomide during pregnancy.[6] Ultimately the thalidomide tragedy increased the scope of the FDA's powers, which the FDA itself explains in the following historical treatment taken from the *FDA Consumer* magazine:

All they wanted was a good night's sleep, and a drug called thalidomide gave it to them. It brought a quick, natural sleep for millions of people who had trouble drifting off, and it also gave pregnant women relief from morning sickness. The drug's German manufacturer claimed it was . . . safe for pregnant women. . . .

By 1957, thalidomide was sold over-the-counter in Germany. By 1960, it was sold throughout Europe and South America, in Canada, and in many other parts of the world. To introduce it into the United States, the Richardson-Merrell pharmaceutical company of Cincinnati submitted an application to FDA in September 1960 to sell thalidomide under the brand name Kevadon.

The application was assigned to medical officer [Frances Oldham] Kelsey, who had joined FDA just one month earlier. It was her first drug review assignment...

Kelsey had concerns about the drug from the beginning. . . After Kelsey detailed these deficiencies in a letter to Richardson-Merrell, the company sent in additional information—but not enough to satisfy Kelsey.

. . . Kelsey did not cave under the pressure.
"I think I always accepted the fact that one was going to get bullied and pressured by industry," says Kelsey. "It was understandable that the companies were very anxious to get their drugs approved."...

The headline read "'Heroine' of FDA Keeps Bad Drug Off of Market." The story appeared on the front page of *The Washington Post* on July 15, 1962. Reporter Morton Mintz told the tale of "how **the skepticism and stubbornness of a Government physician prevented what could have been an appalling American tragedy,** the birth of hundreds or indeed thousands of armless and legless children."...

In the wake of the furor these articles created, **the American public soon came to realize how narrowly they had averted**

a major tragedy. And politicians who had been fighting for years for tighter drug controls were finally taken seriously. A controversial bill introduced by Sen. Estes Kefauver of Tennessee several years earlier was resurrected from its congressional committee graveyard and rewritten. **President Kennedy signed the bill generally known as the Kefauver-Harris Amendments into law on Oct. 10, 1962. This landmark drug law, which modified the earlier Federal Food, Drug, and Cosmetic Act of 1938, strengthened FDA's control of drug experimentation on humans and changed the way new drugs were regulated.**

Under the 1938 law, drug manufacturers had only to show that their drugs were safe. Under the 1962 law, for the first time, they also had to show that all new drugs were effective. . . .

FDA grew along with its increased regulatory responsibilities. In 1960, Kelsey was one of only seven full-time and four young part-time physicians reviewing drugs at the agency. Today [in 2001—eds.] there are nearly 400 medical officers at FDA, but they are not as accessible to the drug companies as they were in the 1960s when Kelsey was pressured by the thalidomide manufacturer.[7]

We have included the lengthy quotation from the *FDA Consumer* magazine because it so perfectly epitomizes the image of itself that the FDA wants to inculcate in the minds of the American public. The FDA is portrayed as a band of heroic, selfless scientists and supporting staff doing their best to keep the American public safe from the unscrupulous sales efforts of big pharmaceutical companies.

Yet even on its own terms, this tale is somewhat odd. After all, the FDA *hadn't* approved thalidomide, so it's not clear why the 1938 scope of its powers was deemed inadequate. It would make sense for the *other* governments (such as Germany's) that *had* approved thalidomide to review their procedures, but the US government was drastically changing the organization and mandate of the FDA at the same time President Kennedy was giving an award to Kelsey for doing such a great job under the old framework.

Adding to the irony, the obvious problem with thalidomide was that *it clearly wasn't safe for use during pregnancy*. Why then, in response to the thalidomide tragedy, would the FDA's powers be beefed up in 1962 to include the criterion of proof of efficacy, in addition to the long-standing proof of safety? To repeat, the problem with thalidomide was that it was *dangerous* for certain populations; Kelsey hadn't been asking the manufacturer for evidence that thalidomide was *effective*.

Whether or not it was a rational response to the thalidomide experience, the 1962 expansion of the FDA's powers came with a significant downside. Once again we turn to Milton Friedman, who explained the trade-offs in his bestselling book, *Free to Choose*. Writing in 1979, Friedman explained:

> [T]he number of "new chemical entities" introduced each year has fallen by more than 50 percent since 1962. Equally important, it now [in 1979—eds.] takes much longer for a new drug to be approved and, partly as a result, the cost of developing a new drug has been multiplied manyfold. According to one estimate for the 1950s and early 1960s, it then cost about half a million dollars and took about twenty-five months to develop a new drug and bring it to market. . . . By 1978, "it [was] costing $54 million and about eight years of effort to bring a drug to market"—a hundredfold increase in cost and quadrupling of time, compared with a doubling of prices in general. As a result, drug companies can no longer afford to develop new drugs in the United States for patients with rare diseases. Increasingly, they must rely on drugs with high volume sales.[8]

As Friedman makes clear, the post-thalidomide expansion and transformation of the FDA's powers in 1962 drastically curtailed the introduction of new drugs on the market. The enormous increase in development costs also changed the strategy of drug makers, who now had to focus on drugs with mass-market appeal in order to have any hope of turning a profit. The whole episode drives home the standard point that economists make when criticizing the FDA: because the public will be outraged if the FDA allows a drug with unacceptably dangerous side effects on the market, the agency has the incentive to proceed too cautiously, holding up potentially beneficial drugs for too long and artificially driving up the cost of drug development. In contrast to the quite visible victims of thalidomide, it's not as obvious to identify the Americans over the years who have suffered or even died because the FDA stifled the development of a new drug that would have provided relief.

In addition to the thalidomide episode, we can see another illustration of this pattern with the 2004 voluntary recall of Vioxx by its manufacturer, Merck. But first we need to explain the historical context.

Largely because of the 1962 transformation of the FDA's procedures in reaction to the thalidomide tragedy, the time it took the agency to review a New Drug Application (NDA) had grown excessively long: a typical NDA review took two and a half years, while some applications took eight years. The problem was *not* that any particular review involved such long consideration, but rather that the FDA was understaffed; applications might sit in a queue for years.

To address this problem, Congress passed the 1992 Prescription Drug User Fee Act (PDUFA) "establishing renewable five-year periods of mandatory fees submitted by pharmaceutical companies along with their applications (as well as product and establishment fees)."[9] Those fees allowed the FDA to hire hundreds of new employees. Because of the vast new manpower at its disposal, in the post-1992 PDUFA era the FDA tackled the backlog of drug applications, leading to a surge of approvals in 1996.

However, disaster once again struck in 2004—this time concerning Vioxx, a popular anti-inflammatory drug. The manufacturer, Merck, voluntarily pulled Vioxx from the market after a long-term study on patients at risk of developing recurrent colon polyps had to be halted "because of an increased risk of serious cardiovascular events, including heart attacks and strokes, among study patients taking Vioxx compared to patients receiving placebo."[10]

DON'T LEAVE YOUR HEALTH IN THE HANDS OF GOVERNMENT "EXPERTS"

The sordid Vioxx episode led an FDA whistleblower, David Graham, to declare that the agency was complicit in *"what may be the single greatest drug safety catastrophe in the history of this country or the history of the world."*[11]

As with thalidomide, following the Vioxx bombshell the FDA reduced the approval rate of new drugs. Specifically, from 1993 through 2004—a period *after* the PDUFA reforms but *before* the Vioxx scandal—the FDA approved an average of 33.4 new molecular entities (NMEs) and new therapeutically significant biologics each year.[12] Yet from 2005 through 2013, in the wake of the Vioxx public relations disaster, the FDA only approved an annual average of 25.3, a decline of 24 percent.[13]

"WHEREVER THERE IS MISLEADINGLY LABELED ORANGE JUICE, I'LL BE THERE.."

David A. Kessler, M.D. was Commissioner of the FDA from 1990 to 1997. According to the FDA's bio page, *"Dr. Kessler was sworn in on the same day that the Nutrition Labeling and Education Act (NLEA) was signed. Early in his tenure, he took action to protect consumers from misleading uses of the term 'fresh' in conjunction with processed or partially processed orange juice and tomato products, gaining himself the name 'Elliot Knessler.'"*[14]

What this cutesy description fails to convey is the absurd destruction unleashed under Kessler's tenure. To take an example, on one occasion US marshals seized and destroyed 12,000 gallons of

Procter & Gamble's orange juice because it was labeled "Citrus Hill Fresh Choice." (For what it's worth, the juice had the disclaimer "Made from Concentrate" on the packaging, but FDA officials said the print was too small.) Kessler timed this raid to take place during a speech he was giving at a convention of food and drug attorneys, ensuring they realized there was a new sheriff in town.

Just to make sure the entire industry got the message, associate FDA Commissioner Jeff Nesbitt later announced, *"The agency expects any and every company to make sure that its labeling is consistent with FDA policy, which has been in place for several decades. And if they don't, and if the FDA finds out about it, then those companies can expect similar action."* [15]

In summary, we see that in response to public scandals, the FDA clamped down on its approvals, raising the barriers to the delivery of new drugs (and biologics) to patients. These episodes illustrate an incentive problem facing the FDA: because it receives far more negative feedback for approving drugs with dangerous side effects than for withholding drugs with useful therapeutic effects, the FDA will end up delaying or even totally preventing many suffering patients from receiving relief. If someone dies because the FDA does *not* approve a drug that would have saved his life, that death will be attributed to the illness, not to the FDA.

ADVERTISING ITS ABSURDITY: THE FDA TREATMENT OF ASPIRIN AND ROGAINE

One mechanism of the harm (and silliness) of the FDA's arbitrary power flows through its regulation of advertising. (Our account in this section draws on the analysis of Paul H. Rubin, in his contribution to a volume on the deadliness of FDA regulations.[16]) By the late 1980s, there was substantial evidence that a daily dose of aspirin could significantly reduce the risk of heart attack in middle-aged men. At the time, a package of BAYER would instruct the consumer, "Ask your doctor about new uses for BAYER ENTERIC Aspirin." But the package itself did not specify exactly what these "new uses" might be!

The reason was that on March 2, 1988, the FDA Commissioner Frank Young told the relevant companies that if they advertised the use of aspirin to prevent first heart attacks, they would face legal action. Rubin describes the Catch-22 nature of the aspirin manufacturers in this situation, and explains why they didn't go through the formal process to win FDA approval for the use of aspirin in first heart attack prevention:

> The FDA's approval process is costly, and it would cost some tens or hundreds of millions of dollars to obtain approval for aspirin as a heart attack preventative. Indeed, because the benefits of aspirin are so well documented, it might be impossible for ethical reasons to undertake such a study at all; researchers would probably be unwilling to deny any patients the benefits of aspirin, as is required in such a study. The one study cited previously . . . was terminated early because of the overwhelming evidence of the benefits of aspirin.[17]

Let us reiterate the Kafka-esque absurdity (and tragedy) of the situation: the FDA would not allow aspirin manufacturers to tell their customers about the medical benefits of their product in preventing first heart attacks, because these benefits had not been empirically validated in accordance with FDA protocol. Yet the *reason* the manufacturers couldn't provide such evidence was that the benefits were so obvious, it would have been professionally unethical for researchers to conduct the relevant studies!

Later in his paper, Rubin also touches on the humorous aspects when discussing the FDA's requirement of a "brief summary" in almost all advertisements of a drug. (The brief summary must include the "uses, side effects, and contraindications" of a drug.) However, the FDA allows that if an ad merely mentions the name of the drug but not its purpose, then the "brief summary" may be omitted. This rule led to some funny situations, such as a TV actor who "was forbidden from scratching his head during a Rogaine® commercial because the FDA believed that this indicated that the product was related to hair."[18]

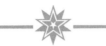

WARNING! SIDE EFFECTS MAY INCLUDE TUNING OUT...

Nowadays, it is commonplace for TV ads for a new drug to hire a professional speed-reader to zip through all of the horrible things that could happen to you if you use the product. When this practice first began, it struck many people as hilarious and also foolish: why in the world would a drug company pay good money to let people know its pill could give you diarrhea?

Yet in retrospect, it's clear what has happened: precisely because the public is overwhelmed with every *possible* danger associated with *every* drug on the market, the information is drowned out. Nobody bothers trying to parse the actual warning. The assumption is: "If the FDA is letting them advertise this on TV, it must be safe."

SINS OF COMMISSION: HOW THE FDA DOES A HORRIBLE JOB OF KEEPING UNACCEPTABLY DANGEROUS DRUGS OFF THE MARKET

Although the standard economist discussion of the FDA is correct in pointing out its "deadly caution," this is only half the story. At the same time that the FDA systematically keeps beneficial drugs off the market—or at least delays their introduction and makes them needlessly expensive—the FDA *also* approves unacceptably dangerous drugs, and is very reluctant to admit its mistakes even when the evidence is obvious. At first it might seem as if we are contradicting ourselves, but the two patterns are simultaneously true: the FDA gives Americans the worst of both worlds; it commits sins both of omission and commission.

Perhaps the best example we can give of the FDA ignoring clear evidence that it had approved an unacceptably dangerous drug is the tragic case of Vioxx, to which we've already alluded but will now give a fuller account. In the late 1990s, COX-2 inhibitors were the new darling of the drug market. They inhibited cyclooxegenase, an enzyme integral to the inflammation present in osteoarthritis. There was obviously a massive market for such drugs. Vioxx was approved for sale by the FDA in 1999. One year later, Merck, the maker of Vioxx, sent the results of a study (titled "**V**ioxx **G**astrointestinal **O**utcomes **R**esearch" or "VIGOR") to the FDA. Although there was much controversy over this study (and how Merck allegedly tried to spin its results in a positive light), the VIGOR results certainly raised red flags suggesting that Vioxx carried significant risks for heart attack, stroke, and sudden cardiac death. Yet it was not until April 2002 that these risks were even mentioned on the drug label, a shocking delay of two years that critics say indicates the cozy relationship between Merck and the FDA.

Then in 2004, reviewing the preliminary results of another trial (the APPROVe study), Merck shut down the study early and pulled Vioxx from the market—an action they took voluntarily without FDA direction. This was an extraordinary decision, making rofecoxib (the generic drug which Merck sold under the brand name of Vioxx) one of the most widely used drugs to be withdrawn from the market.

Even more alarming was a study performed by veteran FDA employee David Graham, MD, which was slated for publication in the November 17, 2004 issue of the British medical journal *The Lancet*. Graham's study showed that Vioxx had caused 140,000 cases of coronary artery disease, with 60,000 of those cases being fatal. Yet for some reason, the article never appeared. Dr. Graham alleges he was threatened by the FDA. In an interview Dr. Graham gave with *Newsweek*, he stated:

> *I believe there were multiple levels of FDA management who wanted to keep the information of the magnitude of harm caused by Vioxx from the public and wanted to damage my credibility as*

a scientist. There's no question in my mind that, had Merck not withdrawn Vioxx, it would still be on the shelves today and Americans would still be dying of heart attacks because of it. And this would be with the FDA's full knowledge and complicity.[19]

The tragic case of Vioxx is extreme, but it is not isolated. Indeed, there are institutional biases in the current regulatory framework that prevent the FDA from achieving its ostensible function of protecting the public from dangerous drugs. We'll explain the main forces at work in the remainder of this chapter. In doing so we rely heavily on the NNT framework explained earlier, which you may need to review to understand the discussion that follows.

NOT EVEN GOOD PEOPLE CAN FIX
A BROKEN SYSTEM

"Since November [2004], when I appeared before the Senate Finance Committee and announced to the world that the FDA was incapable of protecting America from unsafe drugs or from another Vioxx®, very little has changed on the surface and substantively nothing has changed. The structural problems that exist within the FDA, where the people who approve the drugs are also the ones who oversee the post-marketing regulation of the drug, remain unchanged. The people who approve a drug when they see that there is a safety problem with it are very reluctant to do anything about it because it will reflect badly on them. They continue to let the damage occur. America is just as at risk now, as it was in November, as it was two years ago, and as it was five years ago."
—2005 interview with David Graham, MD, 20-year FDA employee and senior drug safety researcher[20]

To understand why the FDA ends up giving a false signal of safety regarding some drugs, we need to review the rules governing the introduction and marketing of pharmaceuticals. During the FDA approval process, a new drug's efficacy is assessed in patients with more severe disease, and furthermore, the drug is likely to be investigated in isolation and therefore not exposed to the effects of other medications that drive down the NNT-H.

Once a drug receives FDA approval, the manufacturer now has permission to advertise it as an "approved treatment" for a certain disease state. Once a drug gets marketed to physicians and patients, its use becomes more widespread; now people with milder disease are taking the drug, compared to those with more severe cases who were involved in the initial testing. Because of this change in the population taking the drug, there is an increase in the NNT-B (the number of people who need to take the drug in order to experience one case of benefit) and a simultaneous decrease in the NNT-H (the number of people who need to take the drug in order to experience one case of harm). Amplifying this problem is the fact that in the real world, most patients are on multiple medications for which their side effects are additive, which drives the NNT-H even lower. The end result is that the medication's side effects become evident as the NNT-B and NNT-H become increasingly out of balance. This process explains why we so often find out a couple of years later about the dangerous effects of medications that started out as the "next great thing."

FDA approval is based on a stepwise process that involves animal or basic science data (IND or investigational new drug), followed by clinical trials in humans, followed by provisional approval (NDA or new drug application).[21] These studies are usually carried out by the manufacturer and are submitted to the FDA. This process naturally has the potential for conflicts of interest, a situation that was greatly exacerbated with the 1992 Prescription Drug User Fee Act (PDUFA) in which the drug manufacturers began to literally provide the funding for the FDA to hire the staff who would then review their drug applications.

To be clear, we are *not* alleging that there is systematic manipulation of data involved, or that the researchers employed in the pharmaceutical industry on the whole are more dishonest than those in other fields. Rather, we are pointing out that the current system—with the FDA sitting atop a pyramid of control by the power of law—suffers from institutional biases that would be weeded out in a more competitive arena with multiple "authorities" providing expert product review. Under the current framework, the data about therapeutic effects and side effects for a new drug are collected under controlled and ideal circumstances. To repeat, what typically happens in a study (conducted by and reviewed by people who are all ultimately on the payroll of the manufacturer) is that a new drug will be tested on a population with severe disease who are not using other medications. This unrealistically places the NNT-B and the NNT-H in the best possible light, relative to the population of consumers to whom the drug eventually will be marketed.

It is not mere speculation on our part to suggest that a voluntary system of private review would produce better results than the current approach. For example, since 1993 the "Worst Pills, Best Pills" newsletter successfully predicted all 20 of the FDA's withdrawals, in some cases *years* before the FDA actually reversed its initial decision. "Worst Pills, Best Pills" warned consumers about Meridia 12.5 years before its withdrawal, Zelnorm 2.8 years, Tequin 3.8 years, Bextra 2.4 years, Vioxx 3.5 years, Baycol 3.4 years, Propulsid 1.7 years, Rezulin 2.2 years, Raxar 1.4 years, Duract 0.6 years, and Redux 1.2 years before FDA withdrawal.[22]

No system is going to be perfect, but we can definitely improve upon the current framework in which the FDA simultaneously saddles pharmaceutical companies with arbitrary hurdles while giving the seal of approval to some drugs that have blazing red flags. Consumers would make more informed medical decisions in an open environment with competing medical "authorities" providing information on the potential benefits and dangers of new drugs, where reputation and track record determined the "power" of an opinion. It is commonplace for government agencies to waste money and underperform private-sector counterparts. Why would we expect anything different from the FDA?

A DRUG IN SEARCH OF A DISEASE

The misunderstanding of NNT is behind a lot of polypharmacy (the use of four or more medications by a patient) and the harm that can come from it. Not understanding NNT also explains why so many physicians and laypeople tolerate the concept of inventing diseases to fit a medication. What if you are a drug company that develops a medication whose therapeutic effect is supposed to be a lowering of blood pressure, but you notice that one of the side effects is that it grows hair in balding patients? Well, you simply change it into a baldness medication that now has a side effect of lowering blood pressure (Minoxidil). What if you are working on a medication to treat a certain type of disease state and notice that a major side effect is an erection lasting a couple of hours, or that it makes eyelashes grow longer? Then you invent diseases that are really just normal parts of life ("male pattern baldness" or "erectile dysfunction" or "PMDD"), in the process creating a much larger cohort of people taking the medication. When greater numbers take a medication, the NNT-H shrinks. Inventing diseases creates a much broader market for a drug than exists with most legitimate diseases, which is why this has become such a common practice. The problem is, when there is *no* legitimate disease, the NNT-H will always exceed NNT-B.

BIG GOVERNMENT AND BIG BUSINESS: A PERFECT MATCH

What you should now be starting to see is a particular pattern that develops when the government is given the power to regulate. There is an immediate alliance that develops between the government and the dominant players in the industry to be regulated. A naïve observer might expect all private companies to adamantly resist government interference with their business. However, the biggest companies in an industry often recognize the advantages of costly new regulations. For one thing, they can more easily absorb the fixed compliance costs of filing reports and other mundane requirements. Yet more ominously, the dominant players can often gain credibility in the eyes of the public by obtaining the government's "seal of approval"—a seal that is all too easy to acquire, because the government needs the expertise of industry leaders in order to develop those very regulations.

Having been placed in the prestigious consultant role, the industry leaders can then help frame regulations that hamstring the competition. The advantage that ensues gives the industry leaders even more dominance, which makes these companies incredibly rich. The money generated by government-favored companies gets funneled back to the government in the form of lobbying and regulatory fees. This entire process matures in a feed-forward fashion until ultimately there develops a "revolving door," whereby CEOs of the dominant corporations end up serving a stint as the czar of a given regulatory agency that oversees their industry. It is hardly a "conspiracy theory" to suggest that this process invites corruption and fails to protect the public.

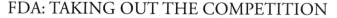

FDA: TAKING OUT THE COMPETITION

Another pattern of the FDA's activities is that their most severe actions seem to be directed at non-pharmaceutical companies. Supplements in particular are a prime target for the FDA's punitive powers. This seems odd given that the safety record for even the sketchiest supplements (such as those containing ephedra) is far superior to the safety records of pharmaceuticals. Certainly no supplement has ever caused 140,000 cases of heart attack or stroke with 60,000 fatalities, as did Vioxx!

Indeed, there is growing evidence that supplements may in some cases prove superior to pharmaceuticals.[23] (For example, research suggests that SAM-e works as well as selective serotonin reuptake inhibitors (SSRIs) and that omega-3 supplementation works better than statins.) Many critics plausibly argue that the FDA attacks the supplement industry so severely because they wish to suppress competition on behalf of their benefactors, the pharmaceutical industry.

CONCLUSION

We covered a lot of territory in this chapter. The takeaway message is that the FDA hits Americans with a double whammy: it hinders the development and marketing of genuinely useful drugs, while at the same time giving the public a false sense of security for drugs that are quite dangerous. We are not demanding the impossible; private-sector groups have a much better track record when it comes to drug evaluation.

Finally, we made it clear in this chapter that large pharmaceutical companies are not innocent babes in the wood when it comes to the scandals of drug development. Although ultimately the power flows from the government and its giant stick, "Big Pharma" has been involved in the revolving door corruption in which industry leaders join the ranks of those regulating their former colleagues.

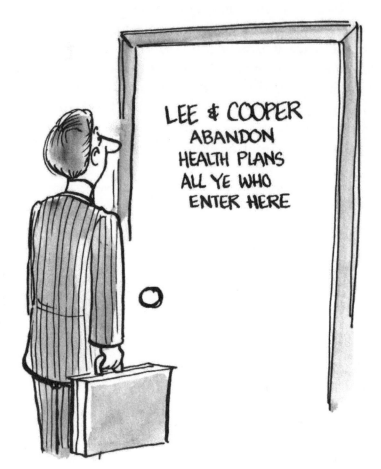

Chapter 3

THE MEDICARE
PONZI SCHEME

S o-called Ponzi schemes are illegal, at least when conducted in the private sector. The Securities and Exchange Commission (SEC) discusses them in this way:

What is a Ponzi scheme?
A Ponzi scheme is an investment fraud that involves the payment of purported returns to existing investors from funds contributed by new investors. . . . In many Ponzi schemes, the fraudsters focus on attracting new money to make promised payments to earlier-stage investors to create the false appearance that investors are profiting from a legitimate business.

Why do Ponzi schemes collapse?
With little or no legitimate earnings, Ponzi schemes require a consistent flow of money from new investors to continue. Ponzi schemes tend to collapse when it becomes difficult to recruit new investors or when a large number of investors ask to cash out.[1]

In 2009, Bernie Madoff was sentenced to 150 years in prison (the maximum sentence allowable) for running what has been called the biggest Ponzi scheme in US history, defrauding thousands of investors of many billions of dollars.[2] However, there is an even *bigger* Ponzi scheme that has been foisted on Americans: Social Security (and Medicare).

Think about it: the government taxes current workers in order to pay current retirees their Social Security and Medicare benefits. When today's workers grow old and retire, they in turn will receive their benefit payments from payroll taxes taken from *future workers*. The whole system depends on bringing in new "participants," or else it collapses. Indeed, as we will soon see, the system *is* collapsing, because of shifting demographics.

For these reasons, Social Security and Medicare are quite understandably referred to as Ponzi schemes—and not just by its critics, but even by supporters such as liberal economists Paul Samuelson and Paul Krugman.[3]

Precisely because of the Ponzi game aspect, the Social Security and Medicare programs will constitute a growing burden on the general taxpayer, as we will explain shortly. This is why analysts have been wringing their hands over "entitlement spending" for decades—they know that these programs contain the seeds of the government's fiscal destruction. Furthermore, it's not really Social Security that's the problem: it's *Medicare* that will break the bank (i.e. taxpayer) if the country remains on its historical trajectory.

Why is this relevant to us, in our discussion of US health care? The answer is that Medicare epitomizes the problems that occur when health care is paid for—and ultimately controlled by—the federal government. So long as politicians (from both parties) were handing out money to the politically active retirees, spending surged, such that Social Security and Medicare absorbed growing shares of the federal budget. Analysts kept warning that eventually this trend would make the programs crowd out defense and other spending items, ultimately bankrupting the government. But very few people in Washington really cared; they kept postponing the day of reckoning with little tweaks, which would include rising tax burdens on workers (that's what the "FICA" deductions from your paycheck are).

As we'll discuss in Part II of this book, the financial projections actually *did* improve significantly after the passage of the Affordable Care Act, but only by building in assumptions of draconian cuts to Medicare spending. As usual, the bulk of those painful projected budget cuts conveniently occur in the future, when other people will be in office.

The whole episode thus serves as a useful case study in what happens when the federal government gets a foothold in the provision of health care. Compared to their promised flow of benefits from the federal government, American seniors would have far more disposable wealth today had they never had their paychecks taxed to fund Social Security and Medicare during their working careers. Yet because Americans were allegedly too shortsighted or weak-willed to save for their own retirement and medical expenses, the federal government came in, forced participation in these "social insurance" programs, and in the process bankrupted the whole system. Note that we use the term "bankrupt" quite literally: as we will soon document, the government's own actuaries report that Social Security and Medicare are in the hole by many trillions of dollars.

Given that this is what happened with the major "social insurance" programs—one of which deals specifically with medical spending—run by the government so far, it gives us little hope for the future now that the Affordable Care Act has significantly expanded the federal government's role in US health care for *everyone*, not just seniors and the poor.

WHY DO DEMOGRAPHICS MATTER SO MUCH FOR GOVERNMENT SOCIAL INSURANCE PROGRAMS?

Before we dive into the scary numbers regarding Medicare's impact on the federal budget, it's important to first explain why demographics matter so much when it comes to Social Security and Medicare. The answer is that they are indeed Ponzi schemes, where the original "investors" are paid *not* with the genuine earnings created from the wise investment of their initial contributions, but instead with the money flowing in from the next wave of "investors." It is the Ponzi nature of government social insurance programs that makes them so vulnerable to demographic shifts, where the United States has been "growing older," meaning that over time there are fewer and fewer workers supporting each retiree.

In contrast, if the default situation were for the members of each household to take care of their own financial future, then demographic shifts would be irrelevant. For example, picture a 23-year-old who has graduated from college and is now starting his serious career. He knows that decades down the road, he may lack the ability and desire to work full-time, and he also knows that in his old age he will face much higher medical expenses. To deal with these facts of life, during his prime working years our young man faithfully puts aside a portion of his income in a growing stockpile of assets (stocks, bonds, life insurance, precious metals, real estate, etc.). When he decides to retire at age 73, he has accumulated (say) $2 million worth of assets. He then begins drawing down these holdings, selling them off in order to enjoy a pleasant lifestyle—which includes routine medical treatment for a person of his age and health status. At that point, whether the United States has more workers than retirees is an interesting bit of trivia that has virtually no bearing on the lifestyle our now-73-year-old man can enjoy, because he has provided for his own retirement.

Although it's obvious that *on paper* our hypothetical man is immune to demographic trends (because of his stockpile of financially assets), you might have a gut feeling that somehow he really is dependent on young workers to grow food, provide medical services, and so on. However, this intuition is wrong; there really *is* an important difference between a person funding his retirement and medical expenses through genuine saving, versus Ponzi-type transfer payments. The easiest way to visualize this crucial difference is to abstract away from the financial assets, and instead imagine that our hypothetical man during his working career directly invests in *physical capital* (not financial capital). In other words, imagine that over the decades our man builds up a growing stockpile of tools and equipment, which he stores in a warehouse, and which finally hits a market value of $2 million by the time he turns 73 and is ready to retire. At this point, he puts his physical capital "to work" by renting out his hammers, power saws, forklifts, etc. to the next generation of workers who have entered the labor force. His physical capital augments their raw labor power, increasing the total amount produced. The older man's "cut" of the total output, then, is what he gets to enjoy as his retirement living. In this scenario, our 73-year-old can live a comfortable lifestyle while not lifting a finger, *and* the young workers don't need to cut back their own lifestyle in any way to provide for him, because he is merely enjoying the *increment* in output that his large stockpile of tools and equipment makes physically possible. His existence isn't a burden on the rest of society; he actually *helps* the workers when he brings his warehouse of goodies to the table.

Our simplistic story captures the essence of what happens in the real world when someone saves in the present in return for a greater amount of enjoyment in the distant future. The economy simply "rebalances" its mix of output, so that it cranks out fewer movie theaters but more factories. This change in the mix of output obviously means that people *today* won't get to enjoy as many movies, but the extra factories mean that people *in the future* will be more productive, and hence have a higher standard of living because of today's discipline.

GOVERNMENT SOCIAL INSURANCE SCHEMES: THERE'S NO SAVING!

Now let's tweak our story yet again. Rather than our hypothetical 23-year-old setting aside a portion of his earnings in stocks, bonds, and other private-sector assets, instead suppose that the government confiscates some of his earnings while giving the 23-year-old its solemn promise that *the government* will fund his lifestyle and medical bills when he retires.

Now if the government took the funds and itself invested in stocks, bonds, and other assets, it would effectively be acting as a giant (and involuntary) mutual fund, and we would merely be arguing over whether the government versus citizens were better at investing for their future.

Yet in reality, the government *doesn't* invest the money it takes in payroll taxes the same way that a private individual would when saving for retirement. No; the politicians take those payroll "contributions" and *they spend them right away*. For example, they might send the money as benefit checks to *current* retirees, who can now afford to go out to more dinners and pay for medical treatment.

Thus, when the government muscles in and takes over old-age financial planning, it *greatly reduces the total amount of genuine saving and investment* that occurs. Yes, the young worker still lives below his means, because he has money taken from every paycheck that is earmarked for social insurance programs (these deductions aren't income taxes, but instead are called "FICA" or "payroll taxes"). But the government's programs then allow older people to simultaneously live *above their means*. So there is no *net* or *aggregate* saving occurring; the worker's saving is offset by the beneficiary's consumption.

Now we see why demographics matter so much for government social insurance programs. When our hypothetical man reaches age 73 and wants to retire, he doesn't possess implicit ownership claims on a stockpile of $2 million worth of physical tools and equipment. No; society *didn't have the physical resources to build those tools and equipment* over his working career, because the government squandered the man's savings on current spending each year. Therefore, our 73-year-old has nothing to bring to the table that will augment output. If he is to eat, then the young workers at that time will have give up some of the food that is actually due to their own labor efforts. Since he now really *is* "skimming off the top" of what the young people are producing, we can see why the overall ratio between retirees and workers is very significant, and how the whole system creates needless conflict between young workers and old retirees.

Later in this chapter, when we review the Trustee Report for Social Security and Medicare, we will see the absolutely shocking figures for how deep in the hole these popular programs are. The main explanation is that the benefits the government promises to retirees cannot be funded with the existing level of FICA "payroll contributions" as the ratio of retirees to workers grows. To understand just how enormous this demographic shift has been—the "aging of America"—since Social Security was created in 1935 and Medicare was created in 1965, consider the following table presented by the Social Security Administration:

Table 3-1. Ratio of Old Age, Survivors, and Disability Insurance (OASDI) Covered Workers to Beneficiaries, 1945-2090 (projections in italics)

Year	Covered Workers	Total OASDI Beneficiaries	Ratio of Workers to Beneficiaries
1945	46,390,000	1,106,000	41.9
1950	48,280,000	2,930,000	16.5
1955	65,066,000	7,564,000	8.6
1960	72,371,000	14,262,000	5.1
1965	80,539,000	20,157,000	4.0
1970	92,963,000	25,186,000	3.7
1975	100,193,000	31,123,000	3.2
1980	112,651,000	35,117,000	3.2
1985	120,238,000	36,636,000	3.3
1990	133,087,000	39,459,000	3.4
1995	140,892,000	43,096,000	3.3
2000	154,666,000	45,162,000	3.4
2005	158,848,000	48,133,000	3.3
2010	157,257,000	53,398,000	2.9
2015	*167,340,000*	*61,004,000*	*2.7*
2020	*176,941,000*	*69,921,000*	*2.5*
2030	*184,939,000*	*85,667,000*	*2.2*
2040	*194,267,000*	*93,570,000*	*2.1*
2050	*205,049,000*	*97,606,000*	*2.1*
2060	*214,295,000*	*103,864,000*	*2.1*
2070	*224,337,000*	*111,386,000*	*2.0*
2080	*235,141,000*	*118,114,000*	*2.0*
2090	*245,311,000*	*126,364,000*	*1.9*

As Table 3-1 illustrates, the demographics have moved against Social Security (and thus against Medicare) as the population distribution has skewed more heavily to older Americans. With baby boomers retiring and fertility rates seeing a general decline, the number of workers supporting each beneficiary has steadily dropped since the creation of Social Security and other government social insurance programs. As the table shows, back in 1965 there were four workers whose payroll deductions supported each beneficiary. By 2010 it had dropped to fewer than three workers per beneficiary, and in the "Intermediate" cost scenario, the government's Trustees project the number will drop to a mere two workers supporting each beneficiary by the year 2070.

To reiterate: these demographic shifts would be largely irrelevant in a private-sector voluntary framework, where the default position is for every person or household to save aside enough funds to finance the retirement years, including standard medical expenses in old age. Yet because Social Security and Medicare *spend the money as soon as workers "contribute" it from their payroll deductions*, there is no pool of savings for older Americans to draw upon when they retire. Instead, the government must pay current beneficiaries out of the payroll taxes levied upon current workers. Such a Ponzi setup, when coupled with the demographic trends outlined in Table 3-1, is a ticking time bomb—albeit one with a very long fuse.

THE FINANCIAL POSITION OF SOCIAL SECURITY AND MEDICARE, AS OF 2009

In this section we summarize the financial position of the federal government's major entitlement programs as of 2009. We chose this year to take a snapshot of how things stood before passage of the Affordable Care Act (in March 2010).

The following chart is taken from the Congressional Budget Office's (CBO) June 2009 long-term budget outlook. Specifically, this shows the "Alternative Fiscal Scenario" in which policymakers are assumed to behave as they have done historically:

Figure 3-1. CBO Long-Term Federal Budget Outlook, "Alternative Fiscal Scenario," 1962 to 2080, as of June 2009

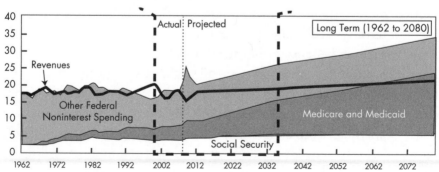

As Figure 3-1 shows, it is a bit misleading when pundits discuss the need to reform "entitlement spending." Even though Social Security is literally bankrupt, in an accounting sense—as we'll discuss shortly—it did not pose a *runaway* threat to the overall budget, the way Medicare and Medicaid did as of 2009. The analysts at the CBO predicted that Social Security spending, as a share of the total economy, would drift upward to 6 percent of GDP by the year 2035, but after that they predicted Social Security expenditures would very gently recede compared to the size of the overall economy.[4]

In contrast, the figure shows that as of 2009, CBO-projected federal spending on Medicare and Medicaid would continue an upward climb as far as the eye could see. If we include state-level spending, the CBO predicted that total spending on Medicare and Medicaid would reach a shocking 22 percent of the entire economy (15 percent for Medicare, 7 percent for Medicaid) by 2080. In the CBO forecast, health care spending on the elderly (Medicare) grows so much faster than Social Security because it suffers from a double whammy: not only does the proportion of elderly in the population grow, but health care costs in general are expected to continue expanding faster than the overall economy.

Another way of illustrating the "ticking time bomb" aspect of federal entitlement programs is to consider their share of the overall federal budget. For example, in Table 3-2 we show the CBO's forecast for the respective federal budget shares of major spending categories for the year 2050:

TABLE 3-2. CBO 2009 Forecast of Federal Spending by Category, in Year 2050, Assuming Historical Policy Trends

Spending Category	Share of Federal Budget	Share of Overall Economy
Social Security	13.5%	5.7%
Medicare	22.5%	9.5%
Medicaid	7.6%	3.2%
Interest on Debt	32.0%	13.5%
All Other Federal	24.4%	10.3%
TOTAL	100.0%	42.2%

As Table 3-2 shows, back in 2009 the CBO projected that by 2050, what is called "non-discretionary spending"—including the major entitlements and interest on the federal debt—would absorb so much of the budget that only 24 percent would be left for things like the Departments of Defense, Education, and Transportation, as well as NASA and federally funded poverty relief. Note too that this "crowding out" of federal spending by entitlements and interest payments wouldn't be due to budget austerity; by 2050 the CBO projected that total federal spending would absorb a whopping 42 percent of the entire US GDP. To get a frame of reference: federal spending was 27 percent of the economy in 2009 when the forecast came out, and that included large expenditures related to the Troubled Asset Relief Program (TARP) and the American Recovery and Reinvestment Act, also known as the "Obama stimulus package."

To be clear, nobody really expected these CBO projections to come to fruition. They merely served to underscore just how *unsustainable* the federal entitlement programs had become. Thus far, we've shown the relation of Social Security and Medicare to the federal budget and overall US economy. In the next section, we'll walk through the internal structure of the programs to show just how absurd the government's promises have been.

THE 2009 TRUSTEE REPORT: SOCIAL SECURITY AND MEDICARE ARE BANKRUPT—LITERALLY

Another way to gauge just how bankrupt—literally—the government's social insurance programs are is to quote from the official Trustee Report. Table 3.3 reproduces a portion of the Trustees' projections as of January 1, 2009:

TABLE 3-3. Trustee 2009 Present-Value Estimates of 75-Year Open-Group Obligations for Government Social Insurance Programs (trillions)

Category	HI (Hospital Insurance	SMI Supplementary Medical Insurance	OASDI (Old-Age, Survivors, and Disability Insurance	Combined
Revenues from public				
Payroll and benefit taxes	$12.0		$37.2	$49.2
Premiums		$7.2		$7.2
Other taxes and fees		$1.0		$1.0
Total revenues	$12.0	$8.2	$37.2	$57.4
Total expenditures to public	$25.8	$32.5	$44.9	$103.2
Net for Budget Perspective	**($13.8)**	**($24.3)**	**($7.7)**	**($45.8)**

The figures in this table are staggering once we understand their meaning. First we have to set the context, because there are various accounting tricks people can play with these numbers. For example, for years before the 2008 recession hit, the Social Security Administration had been running cash-flow surpluses, meaning that it was collecting more in payroll "contributions" than it paid out to beneficiaries. Unfortunately, those surpluses weren't invested in productive enterprises to generate future income for the program (the way a private retirement program would have done). Instead, the federal government spent the extra money, with the Treasury issuing IOUs to the Social Security Administration. This is the Social Security "Trust Fund"—a record of how much one part of the federal government owes to another part. As of January 1, 2009 (when the numbers here were estimated), the Social Security Trust Fund held $2.4 trillion in assets. But to repeat, those "assets" were merely pieces of paper saying that the US Treasury owed the Social Security Administration money.

Another accounting trick is that the SMI program (which includes Medicare Part B and Part D) has a formal funding requirement for any shortfall, whereas the HI and OASDI programs do not. Thus, the official figures of the "unfunded liability" of these programs exclude the $24.3 trillion shortfall that SMI faced when the previous table was compiled. But it obviously doesn't make the financial burden of Medicare any easier if we simply assert, "Congress in the future has to pay for this." The fact that its projected spending will exceed dedicated premium payments means that the general taxpayer will be on the hook to cover the shortfall.

In light of these considerations, we have chosen to highlight the "Budget Perspective" in Table 3-3, because this comes closest to what the average person has in mind when wondering, "How deep in the hole are these programs?" In the words of the Trustee Report: "From the 75-year budget perspective, the present value of the additional resources that would be needed to meet projected expenditures, at current-law levels for the three programs combined, is **$45.8 trillion**" (emphasis added).[5]

Such a gigantic number may cause your eyes to glaze over, but it's crucial to understand what it actually means. First, just to get a feel for how *enormous* the figure is, consider that in 2009, the total GDP of the United States was only $14.4 trillion—meaning that the official budget hole from the three social insurance programs was more than triple the size of the economy's entire output.

Yet it might *still* be hard to grasp just how severe the figure is. The $45.8 trillion number is a *present-value* calculation. The Trustee Report was saying that in 2009, the federal government would have needed $45.8 trillion *right then* to invest and start earning interest, so that over the next 75 years the government could draw down this side fund rather than hit up the taxpayers.

For one final clarification, the $45.8 trillion figure *assumed payroll taxes and Medicare premium payments remained at scheduled 2009 levels*. In the projections underlying Table 3-3, over the 75-year window workers still have money taken out of their paychecks, and the elderly still make premium payments for Medicare. That $45.8 trillion side fund was nonetheless needed *to cover the projected shortfall* between these dedicated revenue streams and the spending on the programs.

Thus we see that it is by no means metaphorical when critics deride the Social Security and Medicare programs as being "bankrupt." If a private company had such books for its contractually guaranteed employee retirement and health insurance programs, it clearly would be declared insolvent.

CONCLUSION

In this chapter, we have described the financial position of the government's major social insurance programs as of 2009, before the introduction of the Affordable Care Act. We explained that voluntary, private-sector planning for old age does *not* rely on favorable demographics, because each household longitudinally provides for its own future spending during a career of saving and investing.

In contrast, the government has run Social Security and Medicare as giant Ponzi schemes from their very inception, dependent on an influx of new workers to support the obligations due to those entering retirement. Rising medical costs, the aging of the baby boomers, and a decline in fertility rates placed the government's insurance programs in an untenable position. On the eve of the Affordable Care Act, the government's own analysts projected that these programs—primarily Medicare—were grossly underfunded by their dedicated mechanisms and would constitute a growing drain on the taxpayer.

As of 2009, every serious analyst knew that "something had to be done" to address the problem of Medicare and other government insurance programs. A rational response would have been, "Hmm, the government has been dabbling in providing health care to a large segment of the population—the elderly—for several decades, and it's currently run up a funding hole bigger than the entire economy. Let's try something else."

Unfortunately, the politicians took America even deeper into the abyss. After blowing up the economics of health care for the elderly, the United States government would embark on "guaranteeing" health care for the entire population.

What could go wrong . . .?

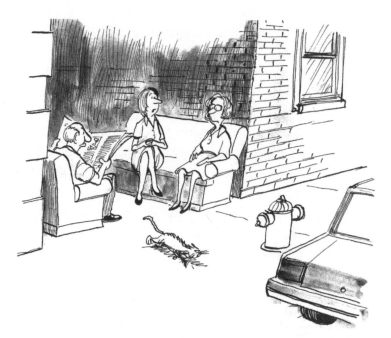

"Oh, it's a great healthcare plan...
well worth selling the house to pay for."

Chapter 4

THE PERVERSE ECONOMICS OF U.S. MEDICINE

In the first chapter, we gave a broad historical sketch of the development of US health care up through the eve of the Affordable Care Act (ACA), and then in the following two chapters we studied the FDA and Medicare in detail. In the next part of the book, we will show that the ACA won't solve the festering problems in the US health care system, but rather, will exacerbate them and hasten the degradation of the private sector.

The present chapter serves as a transition from the historical trends to the present realities of America under the ACA. In this chapter we summarize some of the major problems with the economics of health care in the United States. Once we correctly identify the problems in this fashion, you will easily see that the ACA only makes them worse. The following problems are not necessarily listed in order of importance, but taken together provide a quick summary of what the heck went wrong with America's medical care.

PROBLEM #1: CONFLATING "HEALTH CARE" WITH "HEALTH INSURANCE"

There are legitimate reasons why people associate health care with insurance, but the two concepts are quite different. If we are to make sensible decisions—regarding both government policy and personal medical options—we need to keep these concepts distinct. The popular tendency to interchange these terms inappropriately is epitomized when people refer to the Affordable Care Act, which is a massive piece of legislation dealing with *insurance*, as "health care reform."

Note that we are not merely being quibblers over grammar here. *One of the biggest problems* with the entire US health care system is the predominance of third-party payment. Thus, when people casually conflate health insurance and health care, they are unwittingly perpetuating the problem; it is impossible to fix something if your very vocabulary makes the solution impossible to articulate.

PROBLEM #2: U.S. "HEALTH INSURANCE" ISN'T REALLY INSURANCE

It is understandable that Americans conflate health care with health insurance, because *"health insurance" no longer functions as insurance.* The way insurance is *supposed* to work is that you enter into a contractual arrangement with the insurance company: you the policyholder make premium payments, and if a well-defined event occurs, the insurer sends you a specified amount of money. Note that if the event occurs and you receive a check, it's not even necessary for you to spend the money replacing or repairing the loss; the purpose of the insurance is to financially compensate you to offset the bad fortune of an unlikely event that could strike many people but happened to hit *you.*

By their very nature, "insurable events" should be expensive and *unpredictable for the specific policyholder.* It wouldn't make any sense to ask your car insurance company to reimburse you for your oil changes, because they would simply have to charge you on the front end what they knew you'd be requesting on the back end—and then they'd slap that on top of the actual *insurance* against rare-but-expensive events like a collision. However, in the unlikely event that you *do* need your car insurance company because of a serious accident, then you will typically be insured for the full value of the property.

Notice that typical health insurance in the United States operates nothing like this model. Many health insurance policies cover routine care such as office visits, the human equivalent of an oil change.[1] Moreover, if a specified "health event" occurs, the policyholder (typically) can't simply request a check for the amount listed in the contract—the way a motorist could have his new car totaled, take the insurance money, and switch to a cheaper vehicle to pocket the difference. On the contrary, with health insurance the policyholder (typically) only gets paid—with the payments very often going right to the provider—for services actually performed to address the "health event."

Another difference between health insurance and other types of insurance is that many health plans—even "good" ones offered by reputable employers—have caps on total coverage, or insist on co-pay percentages that could overwhelm the policyholder in the event of a serious illness. In his book critiquing the US health care system, economist John Goodman first quotes a news article explaining that some employers are requiring employees to pay a quarter, a third, or even more of the cost of "specialty drugs." Goodman then comments: *"Increasingly, the health plans employers offer defy all of the traditional principles of rational insurance, which require people to pay out of their own pockets for the expenses they can afford but protect them against catastrophic costs they cannot afford."*[2]

THE POLITICS OF U.S. HEALTH CARE

"In the US Medicare program, policymakers achieve through patient cost sharing what other countries achieve through the rationing of services: They punish the sick to reward the healthy. For example, although basic Medicare pays for many minor services that most seniors could easily afford to purchase out of pocket, it leaves the elderly exposed to thousands of dollars of catastrophic costs. This is exactly the opposite of how insurance is supposed to work."

—Health economist John Goodman[3]

Finally and perhaps most perverse, the health insurance company *expects you to keep paying your premiums even if a specified "health event" is triggered.* Notice that we have been using the odd phrase "health event" *not* because it is standard in the field, but precisely because it sounds so foreign. In any other area of insurance, there are well-defined *events* that trigger a payment, and that's why it makes perfect sense for the policyholder to no longer owe premium payments at that point. For example, if a man dies, his widow gets the death benefit check from the life insurance company, period; she isn't expected to continue making premium payments on the policy.[4]

Yet this isn't true with health insurance. If you are diagnosed with cancer and begin very expensive treatment, you will—at the bare minimum—need to keep making premium payments, in addition to whatever co-pays or deductibles you may owe. We do not mean to suggest that this is some sinister feature dreamed up by the health insurers; there are obvious differences between a one-off event (such as death or a car accident that takes the vehicle off the road) and a person receiving expensive medical treatment but still needing continuing health insurance for other possible expenses. Nonetheless, it is perverse that someone could have "good health insurance" to cover major illness, then *because* of that illness lose his or her ability to afford the premiums, and hence lose coverage for the continued expenses. This is particularly relevant because so many Americans have their (expensive) health insurance premiums paid directly by their employers as part of the overall compensation package—the topic of the next section.

PROBLEM #3: HEALTH INSURANCE IS PREDOMINANTLY TIED TO *EXISTING* EMPLOYER

One of the major problems with the existing health insurance market—and yet another way in which it differs from other types of insurance—is that so many Americans are reliant on their employer to provide them coverage. Indeed, during the period of 2011 to 2012, some 48 percent of Americans—almost 150 million people—received their health coverage from their employer.[5] This is inherently unusual; people don't lose their auto insurance if they get laid off.

The connection between employer and health insurance is partially responsible for the vulnerability many felt in the pre-Affordable Care Act status quo, particularly because insurance policies are not easily *portable* from one job to the next. If someone develops a serious condition while working for one employer, and then attempts to switch jobs, that employee would now bring a "pre-existing condition" with him or her to the new job.

The built-in turnover of health insurance policies, due to employment changes, greatly weakens the rationale of insurance in the first place. Consider for a moment what this would mean in the context of *life* insurance. For example, a 20-year-old breadwinner supporting a wife and two young children might take out a $1 million 30-year life insurance term policy with a fixed premium. This allows the young man to "lock in" his life insurance protection through age 50. Even if he develops a brain tumor the week after signing the contract, the young man can keep his life insurance policy in force, so long as he pays the original premium.

Now what if we tweaked this scenario and said that, for whatever reason, every three years people had to drop whatever life insurance policy they had and reapply for a new policy? In this case, our young man—and his family—would be in serious financial trouble, above and beyond the medical bills. If he should happen to survive to the third year, then at that point he would lose his existing life insurance and have to reapply. But at that point, having a brain tumor, he would be denied. (Or, if we used a less extreme example than a brain tumor, he would have to pay a much higher premium on the newly issued policy, in light of his recently diagnosed condition.) Thus we see that our hypothetical rule that forces people to drop and reapply for life insurance every three years would greatly rob life insurance of its value to society.

Something akin to our fictitious story is what happens in the real world with health insurance. People typically can't lock in long-term coverage at contractually guaranteed fixed premiums, making these policies less like genuine insurance as we know it in other fields. There are several factors driving this outcome, but a major one is—to repeat—the fact that a huge segment of the market consists of employer-based coverage, and that employees are not allowed to take their policies with them when they change jobs.

PROBLEM #4: THE PREDOMINANCE OF THIRD-PARTY PAYMENT

Throughout this book, we will be breaking this particular problem down into its root causes, but here it is definitely useful to put our finger on the fact that the vast majority of Americans do not feel as if they're *really paying* for their health care services. When they get a bill after a visit to the doctor's office or (hold onto your hat) the hospital, the numbers don't even seem real. This feeling of unreality is partly because the numbers are often outrageous and seemingly bear no relationship to the service or goods involved, but it also occurs because experience has shown that after working with the insurance company, the health care provider will end up "adjusting" the actual amount that the patient owes out of pocket. Furthermore, even after the dust settles—a process that could take months after the actual date of service—if the amount is still astronomical, then the office fully expects patient requests for lengthy installment payment plans (at 0 percent interest), and already knows the drill of how to refer a delinquent account to collections when the patient reneges on the payback plan.

Everyone who participates in this system—either on the side of suppliers or customers—knows that it's nutty. Precisely *because* Americans don't treat their doctor or hospital bills as "real" in the same way that a trip Disneyworld or a new set of tires cost "real money," they are not as conscious about price when agreeing to a battery of tests that their physician recommends. We imagine the people in your social circle know which are the priciest steakhouses in town, and whether they are "worth it," and they also have an idea of where to go when buying a new car. But do they have a similar feel for the pricing structure of the local hospitals or clinics? Probably not, which leads to our next section.

PROBLEM #5: PRICES AREN'T ALLOWED TO DO THEIR JOB

Because the actual consumers of health care in the United States care very little about the price at the "point of sale," and because the providers must try to at least break even on average by dealing with huge bureaucracies using reimbursement formulas, we observe wildly divergent prices for similar procedures. For example, Table 4-1 reproduces data from Goodman's book on the average cost of knee replacement, according to the location and type of patient:

Table 4-1. Knee Replacement Costs, Various Providers and Patients

LOCATION TYPE	AMOUNT
Asking Prices	
Hospital Gross Charge	$60,000 - $65,000
What Private Insurers Pay	
Range (Dallas)	$21,000 - $75,000
Average (Dallas)	$32,500
Medicare (Dallas)	
What Medicare Pays	$16,000 - $30,000
Cost Reported to Medicare	$14,627 - $15,148
Physician Fees	$1,400 - $1,700
Domestic Medical Tourism	
Medibid Rate (US)	$12,000
Canadian Citizen US Cash Price	$16,000 - $19,000
International Medical Tourism	
Medibid Rate (overseas)	$7,000 - $15,000
Bumrungrad (Thailand) Median Price	$14,916
US dog (Dallas)	$3,700 - $5,000

SOURCE: John Goodman, *Priceless*, Table 2.1, p. 16

Indeed, the absurdity illustrated in the table is the type of phenomenon that led Goodman to title his book *Priceless*: he is obviously making a pun relating to the lack of market pricing in health care. The pattern in this table shows up throughout the health care system. For example, LASIK eye procedures, as well as cosmetic surgery, show historical pricing trends that look more like "normal" services than "US health care." The reason isn't physiological, but *economical*: because of insurers' policies and relatively looser government regulations, these types of procedures have robust markets in which customers can walk into a "store" and pay cash, thus allowing all of the usual market forces of innovation and cost-cutting to operate.

In a market economy, prices serve to equalize the quantities produced by sellers and demanded by consumers. There tends to be a uniform price charged for "the same" good or service. Sellers constantly strive to deliver products of higher quality and lower price, while those who most urgently want items can bid them away from others by offering more money. If there is a temporary interruption in the supply— let's say the influx of crude oil is halted—then the market price shoots up. This is exactly what we *want* to happen, as the unusually high price acts as a signal that motivates other producers to scramble into the market, while it causes consumers to economize on their purchases. As Friedrich Hayek explained, market prices act as a type of communication network by which humans rapidly transmit essential information all over the globe, so that producers and consumers can constantly tweak their plans in light of new revelations about resource supplies, technology, and customer desires.

Nobody likes high prices, but they serve a definite social function— so long as they are the *correct* prices, formed on a voluntary and genuine market. When the government imposes regulations that suppress prices below their market-clearing level, it's not doing us any favors; it's only muting a vital source of information. In the wake of a natural disaster, for example, the government will often make it illegal for gas stations to "gouge" their customers with large price increases. But this merely hinders the recovery effort, taking away the incentive for neighboring communities to ship in more gas and for local motorists to only take a few gallons at the pump. With price controls on gasoline, the quantity demanded exceeds the supply, leading to long lines at the pump and more arbitrary forms of rationing—such as selling gas only to vehicles with certain letters on their license plate.

Surprise surprise, the laws of economics work in the health care sector as much as in oil and gas. If the government implements policies that limit the price suppliers receive for medical products or services, then we will observe *shortages*. In 2003, the Medicare Modernization Act (MMA) adjusted the payment formulas in Medicare Part B to limit the speed at which prices could rise on drugs. The obvious rationale here was for the government to use its "buying power" to tighten the screws on those greedy pharmaceutical companies. But by taking the existing (crazy) system as it was, and slapping on arbitrary limits for how fast drug prices could rise, the government simply assured that bottlenecks would fester. Indeed, the new drug pricing rules spawned growing supply problems from the moment they took effect on January 1, 2005: the number of newly reported drug shortages skyrocketed from 74 in 2005 to 211 in 2010.

Let's be clear what we mean: hospitals now routinely find that they simply lack *generic* drugs that their staff have been using for years. A June 2011 survey found that 82 percent of short-term care acute hospitals reported delaying treatment for patients because of a drug shortage, with 17 percent of all surveyed saying such an outcome occurred "frequently." Perhaps more alarming, 35 percent of the hospitals surveyed reported that a patient had "experienced an adverse outcome" because of the shortage.[6]

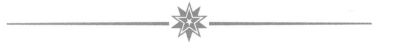

AN ER DOCTOR REPORTS FROM THE FRONT LINES . . .

"In the last few years of my practice of emergency medicine, I have noted a disturbing trend: the medicines that I have found most useful, as well as the medicines that are needed for life-saving resuscitation, have been disappearing. From 1989 to about 2006 I always had at my disposal cheap medicines that were incredibly effective, as well as any medication needed to run a major resuscitation. This was particularly true for sterile injectable medications. However, beginning around 2006 I started to notice that I would order one of these medications, only to find them unavailable and 'on national backorder.'

Initially, the shortages were infrequent and a minor nuisance. As time went by, the shortages became more and more common. The medications I relied on to manage violent or combative patients were suddenly unavailable. IV nitroglycerine for managing unstable angina or heart attacks was frequently in short supply or unavailable. Occasionally, cardiac resuscitation drugs would run out of stock in our crash carts. As it currently stands [in 2015], generic injectable sedatives, antipsychotics, and anti-nausea medications are completely unavailable. There have even been cases where my nurses and I had to hand-mix epinephrine during advanced cardiac life support. In such a situation, we have to commandeer a 1:1000 dilution used for subcutaneous allergic reactions (similar to an Epi-pen) and dilute it to the 1:10,000 dilution for IV injection. Imagine the pressure of doing this and not making a decimal point error while trying to save a dying patient! What could be the cause of all of this? My scouring of online discussions by other experts eventually led me to the government's price controls embedded in the 2003 Medicare Modernization Act."

—Co-author Doug McGuff

There are other ways that the implicit price controls in the US health care system manifest. For example, at least for patients dealing with the mass-market in-patient facilities (which rely almost exclusively on third-party payment), getting health care involves a lot of *waiting*—not only in calendar time for even routine appointments, but also *sitting in various rooms for perhaps hours on end* even during the officially designated appointment. This is not "how health care has to be." Rather, it is the predictable result of *price controls*.

If you don't believe us, try comparing the wait times you see in a "public" hospital emergency room setting versus a truly private outpatient medical clinic that doesn't accept Medicare or Medicaid patients. The difference is startling—not just in terms of the structural appearance of the buildings, but also in terms of the treatment you will receive and the speediness of the visit.

PROBLEM #6: PRICE CONTROLS AND OTHER GOVERNMENT MANDATES CREATE TWO-TIERED HEALTH CARE SYSTEM

One of the tragic ironies of the US government's footprint in medical care is that on balance *it doesn't actually help the disadvantaged*. It would be one thing if the government's massive taxes, subsidies, and mandates *actually created* a truly egalitarian society, where the rich and politically connected had no special advantages in obtaining quality and convenient health care. Then we could have an interesting debate about what we value as a society, and whether we trumpet freedom and property rights versus safety and social equality.

Yet in practice, there *is* no such trade-off; we don't have to make such hard choices. Just as the party officials in the old Soviet Union were truly members of a higher caste than the rest of their "comrades," so too do we have a "two-tiered" (at least) system of health care in the United States, even though federal and state governments have literally spent trillions of dollars over decades in the name of providing equal opportunity for all. The solution is *not* to double down and try even harder to redistribute wealth or mandate "equal treatment"; theory and history show repeatedly that these attempts *do not work*.

We will demonstrate throughout this book that "wards of the State"—especially those on Medicaid—are helpless cogs at risk of being devoured in the US health care system. But the problem goes beyond just Medicaid patients. More generally, the sick and financially needy are left out in the cold, and their plight is exacerbated by the very government policies supposedly designed to help them.

Government reimbursement formulas and mandates (such as "community rating," which we will study extensively in Part II) create a situation in which *health insurers do not want a certain type of customer*. Specifically, if you're already sick or are likely to require expensive treatment down the road, the health insurance companies want to make it as difficult as possible for you to get one of their plans. You are a ticking time bomb and the insurance companies know that they will not be able to even "break even" on you, let alone turn a profit. Paying for your medical expenses is, to them, a cost of doing business, similar to paying corporate income taxes. They'll do it to stay legal, but they will use every tool at their disposal to minimize the financial bleeding.

John Goodman shows how this insight explains the design of typical health insurance plans:

> [T]he easiest way to overprovide to the healthy is to offer services that healthy people consume: preventive care, wellness programs, free checkups, and so on. The way to underprovide to the sick is to strictly follow evidence-based protocols and to be slow to approve expensive new drugs and other therapies. Beyond that, a health plan can underprovide to the sick and discourage their enrollment by not including the best cardiologists and the best heart treatment centers in the plan's network, by not having the best oncologists and the best cancer treatment centers in the network, and so on.[7]

You may no doubt recognize the pattern Goodman has identified. However, we stress that these policies are *not* simply the result of greedy insurance executives screwing over the little guy. This behavior—outrageous as it is, especially for heart or cancer patients who thought they "had good insurance" and realize *after* being diagnosed that the best treatment in their area is "out of network"—is the unavoidable consequence of government policies that many people erroneously believe are "pro-patient."

If you walk into a diner that has an all-you-can-eat buffet, and you want some really good eggs, you obviously order them right from the menu. You know *that's* the way to get a really good serving of eggs, compared to the relative slop that they put out in the buffet. You can't explain this difference by saying the cooks are incompetent or hate their customers, because we're talking about *the exact same cooks* serving certain customers better eggs than other customers. In the case of the diner, the obvious difference is due to the pricing incentives in the buffet versus the one-off order.

The same principle carries over to health care. It makes no sense to expect hospitals, doctors, and insurance companies to provide the same quality of care to all comers regardless of payment structure. The end result is that the normal market forces of competition and innovation are crippled, resulting in massive inefficiency piled on top of the still-festering problem of the genuinely needy receiving shoddy medical care.

PROBLEM #7: REIMBURSEMENT FORMULAS AND MALPRACTICE SUITS LEAD TO ABSURDITY AND OVERTESTING

The state of US health care would be comical if it weren't such a deadly serious matter. Because of the way reimbursement formulas work, patients are often asked to schedule multiple visits to see the same doctor for different conditions. Think about how ridiculous that is: if you have a few questions for your CPA or lawyer, you can schedule a phone call (or office visit) and fire away; you are either paying them a flat fee or by the hour, so they are happy to be as efficient as possible and knock all of your issues out at once. In contrast, under Medicare's payment formula, specialists and primary care physicians typically receive either half payment or *no* additional payment for treating multiple conditions during the same office visit.[8]

Government regulations and other "best practices" standards interact with malpractice lawsuits in an insidious way. Even if a particular physician *and* his patient do not think a certain procedure is necessary, they may nonetheless be overruled by the hospital or insurance company, with the doctor being compelled to follow so-called "best practices." The reason is that if the doctor does something unorthodox and then *things go badly*, both he and the institutions behind him are especially vulnerable to a malpractice suit.

The threat of lawsuits hangs over the entire medical profession, crippling productivity and multiplying costs. In Chapter 12, we will relay anecdotes of the perversion of safety protocols (such as "time outs" before operations) that are the understandable consequence of this litigious environment. The threat of malpractice suits explains some (but not all) of the initially shocking disparity in Table 4-1 earlier, which, if you recall, showed a human hip replacement costing up to $50,000 more than that for a dog. If something goes wrong and the dog dies, that legal liability is much lower than if the same thing happens to a human patient. To be sure, some of this makes perfect sense: it *is* a bigger mistake if a human dies versus a dog, and so the resulting financial compensation (if any) *should* be larger. Yet our point here is that the overkill in regulations and corresponding "defensive" strategies is exaggerated in the human versus dog operations as well; there are far more ways to "officially" do something wrong to a human patient.

The waste and futility of unnecessarily defensive medicine is most obvious when it comes to the widespread promotion of medical screening. Later in Chapter 13, we will assess the pros and cons of mammograms, colonoscopies, and PSA testing, in each case focusing on the issue as a personal decision to be made in light of the statistics.

In this section, we will take the example of cervical cancer tests (Pap smears) and relate the quantifiable monetary expenses to the quantifiable benefit in terms of prolonged lifespan, as shown in Figure 4-1:

Figure 4-1. Cervical Cancer Tests: Cost per Year of Life Saved (Women Age 20)

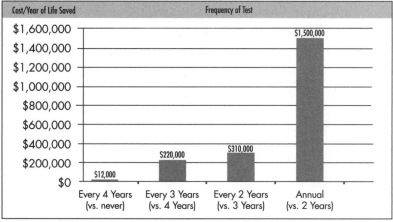

SOURCE: John Goodman, *Priceless*, Figure 2.1, p. 36

Figure 4-1 contains crucial information, but we need to explain how to interpret it. The analysis, conducted in 1995 by Tammy O. Tengs, et al., estimates the marginal cost per year of life gained at various frequencies of cervical cancer testing. For example, the first column compares the two strategies of getting a cervical cancer test every four years versus *never* getting such a test. The first strategy costs more (you have to pay for the tests), but it leads to longer lifespans, in the statistical sense that a population of 20-year-old women who are tested once every four years will benefit from the early detection of cervical cancer—and hence will tend to live longer on average—than a population of comparable women who *never* get a Pap smear. When the study divided the total cost of the testing by the increase in the number of *years of life*, it found that the cost per *year of life* saved was $12,000. (Remember, the study was conducted back in 1995.) We have been liberal with our use of italics to be sure you are reading this correctly: the study didn't find that it cost $12,000 per *life* saved, but rather per *year* gained in lifespan in the relevant population of 20-year-old women.

Now what if we increase the frequency of the cervical testing? The answer is that the cost/benefit ratio deteriorates quickly. For example, the second column in the previous chart compares the strategy of testing once every three years versus once every four years. This new strategy obviously costs more (since it involves more frequent testing), but it also enhances the benefits of early detection, leading to another incremental improvement in average lifespans among the women (in the sense we explained earlier). But when we divide the *increase* in cost by the *increase* in lifespans, we see that the *marginal* cost per year of life saved has skyrocketed to $220,000.

Finally, let's skip to the last column and interpret it. When evaluating the two possible strategies of (a) administering the Pap smears on an annual basis versus (b) administering the Pap smears every other year, the study once again found that the more frequent testing would yield an increase in lifespans among the women, but only by doubling the total cost. (The women are being tested annually rather than every other year, meaning there are twice as many Pap smears to administer.) As the fourth bar in the chart shows, the study estimated that this annual approach would cost an extra $1.5 million for every additional year of life saved from early detection.

The significance of the numbers in Figure 4-1 is not so much the absolute height. For one thing, these numbers are based on older data.

Another drawback is that they do not include the non-monetary but very real psychological costs of frequent cancer screening (which we will cover in Chapter 13).

Our reason for carefully walking through Figure 4-1 is to help open up your mind and pose questions about cost/benefit tradeoffs in medical decisions. Supposing the numbers in Figure 4-1 were roughly accurate, what frequency might you recommend for your 20-year-old daughter? Some readers might be tempted to say, "Annual testing—money is no object when it comes to my daughter's health!" but that ignores reality. If cost really is irrelevant, then why not weekly or daily testing? At *some* point it is obvious that more frequent testing "isn't worth it."

No matter *what* you do, you will eventually die. Yet beyond this truism, there is an important economic point that many people fail to grasp: there need be nothing "irrational," "selfish," or "shortsighted" in eschewing expensive measures that prolong life at a very high marginal cost. For example, suppose a woman in her early 20s is a single mother who is trying to save up money for her children's education. After reviewing the data in the prior chart, she may quite rationally, altruistically, and farsightedly decide that even getting a Pap smear every four years is not worth it, because to implicitly "spend" (in a statistical sense) $12,000 to boost her lifespan by a year is an indulgence she is not willing to make.

Our purpose in this book is not to tell readers that Pap smears are good or bad, or that they should be conducted every *x* numbers of years. Primarily we are trying to educate you on how to properly think through these important decisions. Unfortunately, the reimbursement, regulatory, and legal frameworks of US health care wildly over-promote medical screening, far beyond the point that makes any cost-versus-benefit sense.

PROBLEM #8: EXPENSIVE AND ORWELLIAN END-OF-LIFE CARE

It is unsurprising that end-of-life care is expensive, but the relative proportions can be shocking. The Centers for Medicare and Medicaid Services (CMS) reports that in a typical year, more than 25 percent of total Medicare payments go to the roughly 5 percent of beneficiaries who die that year. For example, in 2006, Medicare spent an average of $38,975 per Medicare recipient who passed away that year, compared to an average of $5,993 in Medicare benefits for those beneficiaries who survived the year. We can break it down even more finely: during the period of 1992 to 1999, Medicare spent an average of $6,620 in the final *month* of a dying beneficiary's life, versus $325 per month for those Medicare recipients who survived.[9]

Something is clearly wrong with these numbers. As with our discussion of Pap smears, here too we need to think "on the margin" as good economists. The question is not *whether* resources should be devoted to helping elderly people prolong their lives; the relevant question is, "At what point are *additional* resources *to extend life another month* not worth it?" The question is especially poignant when, in many cases, the final months are full of misery for the patient.

The issue of end-of-life care is extremely dangerous. On the one hand, figures such as the ones we've just quoted scream out that "something needs to be done." But the solution is *not* to let government officials decide who lives and who dies, all in the name of "protecting the taxpayer."

The fundamental problem is that the government has assumed the responsibility of paying for the elderly's health care, while Americans do not want to cede life and death power to that same government. The public can't have it both ways. If they want a government strong enough to take care of them, they must be willing to endure a government with the power to kill them.

In summary we note that when it comes to end-of-life care, as with just about every other problem we've discussed, the thorny issues all fade away when we restore personal financial responsibility. Few people would draw up an estate plan at age 40 and say, "I am willing to reduce my bequest by $6,620 at the time of my death so that I can live to be 82 and eight months rather than 82 and seven months." And yet, because Medicare picks up the lion's share of the expense, this is exactly the type of outcome we get.

PROBLEM #9: ASTRONOMICAL DRUG DEVELOPMENT COSTS

In Chapter 2, we studied the harmful role of the FDA in driving up drug development costs. In this section we'll provide some more specifics to show the impact of the FDA's requirements, particularly those regarding "Phase III clinical trials."

People often ask how much a pharmaceutical company had to spend on research, development, and testing for a particular drug, but that can be misleading. *Most* drugs never make it to market. In this respect, pharmaceutical companies approach drug development the way oil companies drill wells: often they will come up dry. In both industries, the companies must make so much on the drug (or well) that "hits" that they can then cover their expenses for all of the duds.

A 2012 analysis in Forbes looked at the *total* drug development expenses among major pharmaceutical companies over the period of 1997 to 2011, and then divided by the number of drugs actually approved by the FDA in this period. The staggering results are presented in Table 4-2:

Table 4-2. Drug Development Costs Among Major Companies, 1997-2011

Company	Total R&D Spending, 1997-2001, billions $	Drugs Approved by FDA	R&D Spending Per Approved Drug
AstraZeneca	$59.0 billion	5	$11.8 billion
GlaxoSmithKline	$81.7	10	$8.2
Sanofi	$63.3	8	$7.9
Roche Holding AG	$85.8	11	$7.8
Pfizer	$108.2	14	$7.7
Johnson & Johnson	$88.3	15	$5.9
Eli Lilly & Co.	$50.3	11	$4.6
Abbott Laboratories	$36.0	8	$4.5
Merck & Co. Inc.	$67.4	16	$4.2
Bristol-Myers Squibb Co.	$45.7	11	$4.2

SOURCE: Forbes[1]

As this table indicates, the expenditures to bring a new drug to market (among the companies listed) was *at least* $4 billion, and went nearly as high as $12 billion over the period in question. This fact alone sheds light on many of the distasteful practices of "Big Pharma." Besides driving up prices for patients, these staggering development costs ensure that the major companies will only invest in drugs with the chance of a large market, ignoring sufferers of "niche" conditions.

We must reiterate that the explosion in drug development costs is primarily an outgrowth of FDA regulations, particularly the more onerous requirements for Phase III clinical trials (which account for about 40 percent of the total R&D spending among pharmaceutical companies). As Avik Roy explains: "From 1999 to 2005 . . . the average length of a clinical trial increased by 70 percent; the average number of routine procedures per trial increased by 65 percent; and the average clinical trial staff work burden increased by 67 percent."[10]

Here as in other areas, there are trade-offs involved. Obviously the public would like pharmaceutical companies to engage in careful testing of their products before releasing a new drug on the market. But the explosion in cost—coupled with the poor safety record of the FDA's oversight that we have already documented—suggest that the cost/benefit dial for drug development is extremely out of whack.

CONCLUSION

In this chapter, we've crystallized our historical and in-depth treatments of the first three chapters into eight takeaway problems with US health care. By this point, we have equipped you with the analytical tools and the historical knowledge to understand why the US system was in such a shambles on the eve of the Affordable Care Act (aka ObamaCare). As we will show in detail in the following Part II of the book, the situation is only going to get worse as the various provisions of the new legislation take effect.

PART II

OBAMACARE, THE FUTILITY OF *HEALTH* REDISTRIBUTION

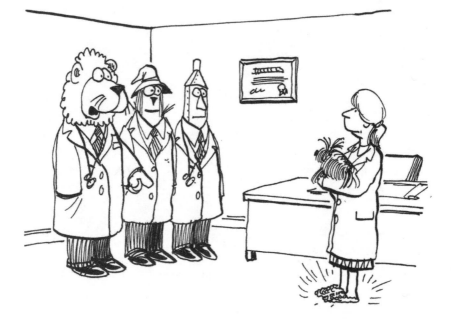

"Hey, just click your heels
and clear up healthcare."

Chapter 5

THE INNER "LOGIC" OF THE AFFORDABLE CARE ACT

On March 23, 2010, President Barack Obama signed into law the Patient Protection and Affordable Care Act. Both friends and foes wish to make the ACA (as we shall abbreviate it throughout this book) the president's signature political accomplishment: his allies want history to remember Obama's expansion of government services for Americans in line with all other advanced nations, while his Republican critics can energize their constituencies with dire predictions about the future under ObamaCare.

As our survey in Part I has demonstrated, the political debates over the ACA are detached from a larger historical context. The critics are right when they warn that the sweeping legislation will only exacerbate the problems with health care and health insurance, stifling conventional economic growth to boot. However, as you now understand, there is nothing *qualitatively* different about the ACA; it is simply an extension of trends that have been in motion for many decades.

Moreover, many of the fiercest critics of the ACA are purely political opportunists. After all, it was the 2012 Republican presidential nominee Mitt Romney himself who, as governor, ushered in a form of universal coverage in Massachusetts in 2006. What has been sarcastically dubbed "RomneyCare" adopted many of the principles of health care reform spearheaded by none other than the Heritage Foundation, one of the nation's leading conservative think tanks. In light of the excoriating attacks that Republican politicians and conservative intellectuals have lobbed against President Obama and his plan for "socialized medicine," it's interesting to look back at Mitt Romney's 2006 *Wall Street Journal* op ed in which he boasts of providing his Massachusetts constituents with health coverage. Here are some choice excerpts from that piece:

> Some of my libertarian friends balk at what looks like an individual mandate. But remember, someone has to pay for the health care that must, by law, be provided: Either the individual pays or the taxpayers pay. A free ride on government is not libertarian.

> And so, all Massachusetts citizens will have health insurance. It's a goal Democrats and Republicans share, and it has been achieved by a bipartisan effort, through market reforms.

> We have received some helpful enhancements. The Heritage Foundation helped craft a mechanism, a "connector," allowing citizens to purchase health insurance with pre-tax dollars, even if their employer makes no contribution. . . . Because small businesses may use the connector, it gives them even greater bargaining power than large companies. Finally, health insurance is on a level playing field.[1]

Beyond the hypocrisy of some of America's politicians and pundits, however, is a far graver problem: precisely because the conventional debates have been so confused, average Americans really have no idea how pervasive government had been in US health care *before* President Obama came along. Indeed, Mitt Romney himself alludes to the problem in the prior quotation when he complains that his libertarian friends are overlooking the reality that "someone has to pay for the health care that must, by law, be provided." As we covered in Part I of this book, we can see that this law—which pushed Governor Mitt Romney to take steps in Massachusetts resembling those that Barack Obama later would take with the entire nation—was the Emergency Medical Treatment and Active Labor Act (EMTALA), signed into law in 1986 by none other than Ronald Reagan. The ironic similarity between the (alleged) free-market Republican Romney and the (alleged) big-government Democrat Obama underscores the pernicious nature of government tinkering with health care and health insurance: each intervention spawns further problems, which are then cited as the rationale for *further* encroachment. This familiar historical process leads us to conclude that the ultimate destination is a "single payer" health care system in the United States, a topic we explore in Chapter 7.

In the present chapter, we lay out the basic structure of the ACA from a 30,000-foot view, as it were, so that you have a foundation upon which to place the finer details discussed in later chapters. In particular, in this chapter we'll explain the main features of the ACA:

- A mechanism to provide health insurance to (most) Americans ("universal coverage")

- Non-discriminatory pricing in health insurance premiums ("community rating")

- Minimum standards for health plans ("essential health benefits")

- A requirement that (almost) everyone obtains health insurance ("individual mandate")

- Government subsidies for the poor

- Various new taxes on "the rich" to pay for the new spending commitments

- Government guarantees for the health insurance companies

- A requirement that (some) employers provide health insurance for (some of) their employees ("employer mandate")

However, before we walk through the specifics—at least as laid out in the original legislation—for each of the features listed, we'll first explain the inner "logic" of the ACA. As we'll see, the aforementioned features are *not arbitrary*. Given that the government was going to intervene yet again into health care and try to tweak what the politicians didn't like about the system circa 2009, those features were a package deal.

ONE THING LEADS TO ANOTHER: THE INNER "LOGIC" OF THE ACA

Many Americans were dissatisfied—and understandably so—with the state of US health care delivery by the late 2000s. Few would deny the stunning technological and procedural advances in particular areas of medicine, but overall Americans were overwhelmed with the mushrooming *cost* of even routine care, let alone the price tag for extended treatments—especially those involving long hospital stays. These worries weren't merely psychological or anecdotal, either: from 1999 to 2009, the "medical care" component of the Consumer Price Index (CPI) rose almost 60 percent faster than the broader CPI itself.[2] As we reported back in Chapter 2, total US per capita expenditures on health care were a staggering $8,170 (measured in 2009 dollars) in 2009, absorbing some 17.4 percent of the total economy.[3]

What makes things even worse when it comes to health care is that not only are the average costs high, but also they are uncertain. Of course, the nature of health care expenses is precisely why there is such a large market for health *insurance*.

Yet health insurance didn't really solve the problem in health care in the way fire insurance seems to solve the problem of rare but catastrophic house fires. The reason is that health insurance itself had become very expensive, making even basic coverage unaffordable for many Americans. To give just one specific estimate of the trend, a study released by the Commonwealth Fund in 2011 reported the following pattern in health insurance costs before passage of the ACA:

> This issue brief analyzes changes in private employer-based health premiums and deductibles for all states from 2003 to 2010, and finds total premiums for family coverage [at $13,871

in 2010] increased 50 percent across states and employee annual share of premiums increased by 63 percent over these seven years. At the same time, per-person deductibles doubled in large, as well as small, firms.[4]

The study also estimated that "62 percent of the [under-65 US] population lived in states where total premiums amounted to 20 percent or more of middle incomes." In these circumstances, most heads of households could realistically only afford health insurance if it were provided through their employers. Thus, even many of those who *had* health insurance were still quite anxious, and had their job options limited for fear of a lapse in coverage.

Yet more serious still was the fate of millions who lacked coverage altogether, a situation that deteriorated over the 2000s and significantly worsened with the onset of the so-called Great Recession in late 2007, as the following Census Bureau data indicate:

Figure 5-1. Americans Lacking Health Insurance, 1999-2012
(Total number of uninsured in millions)

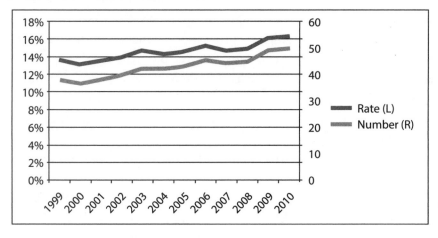

By 2010, more than 16 percent of the country had no health insurance, which translated to almost 50 million Americans. It is entirely understandable why this situation was viewed as intolerable: not only were people vulnerable, but the entire arrangement was economically untenable. For even though these 50 million people lacked formal health *insurance*, they still had access to (some) health *care*. As then-Governor Mitt Romney himself explained in the earlier quotation, it had already been decided politically that somehow every American would have basic medical care. The question was now a technical one: how to reform the system to make it sustainable.

Thus the Affordable Care Act—ObamaCare—seemed an obvious next step. Indeed, far from being the "radical move to socialism" as portrayed by its critics, in some respects the ACA was actually a relatively *conservative* package of "reforms." After all, many progressive pundits and academics were openly calling for a full-blown "single payer" system in which the US federal government would take over *all* health care payments in the nation, displacing the private sector altogether—which is how health care is delivered in some countries.

Yet that move was too bold a step and would have been politically impossible when Obama first took office. (Later on, in Chapter 7, we come back to the question of whether a single payer system lies in America's future.) Instead, proponents of yet another government "solution" to the crisis in health care sought a more modest goal: legislation to achieve **"universal coverage."** In this approach, the formal trappings of a private sector in health care provision, payment, and insurance are retained, but the government intervenes in the market in various ways to ensure that all Americans (at least in theory) are able to obtain health insurance coverage. Proponents argued that this modest goal would solve many of the undeniable problems with the US health care system as it stood in 2009.

However, as anyone with a cursory understanding of economics or history knows, government policies have unintended consequences. It would not have sufficed for the government merely to announce, "It is illegal for any US health insurance company to deny an application from a US citizen." To be sure, such a move would have lent itself to an economical Affordable Care Act—the legislation would have fit on an index card—but it hardly would have achieved the desired objective. The health insurance companies could have complied with this rule by saying, "Sure thing, we'll give coverage to anybody at all who applies.

For example, if someone with a brain tumor wants health insurance, we'll give him a policy with the same coverages we grant to a healthy applicant. It's just that we'll charge the applicant with a brain tumor a premium of $50,000 per month to keep his policy in force." It would be obvious that if such moves were permitted, then the "universal coverage" would be a farce.

To have real teeth, therefore, any legislation would need to do more than just require that insurance companies approve any and all applications. The legislation would need to go further and insist on uniformity in pricing, at least within broad demographic categories, so that insurance companies couldn't charge different premiums based on the health status of a particular applicant. In other words, the legislation would need to insist on what is called **"community rating."**

Yet we have still not solved the problem. If the legislation only insisted on universal coverage and community rating, health insurers could come back and announce, "We have revised our policies and are in compliance with the new law. From now on, we will offer the same insurance policies to all applicants, and will not discriminate in the premiums we charge: the healthy and the sick will pay the same price for the same type of policy. However, just to avoid confusion, let us be clear that from now on, none of our policies will cover any treatments relating to heart conditions or cancer. Further, all of our policies have an annual cap of $30,000 in total payments."

Once again, under such a scenario, the "universal coverage" provided by our hypothetical legislation would be a cruel joke: insurance policies would be designed to exclude expensive treatments, so that the small proportion of applicants needing extensive care could be granted coverage officially yet not pose a huge burden on the insurer. The only way to avoid such a perversity would be for the legislation to specify minimum standards for all health insurance policies, what is called **"essential health benefits."** For example, all health insurance policies would have to cover bypass surgery for patients with heart problems who needed it, and it would be illegal to offer policies with a low cap on total payments.

So far, our hypothetical reform legislation would impose burdens on the health insurance companies. Yet if we stopped here, the whole system could collapse. Faced with the requirement to offer comprehensive policies to every applicant while charging the same premium to healthy and sick alike, the insurance companies would have no choice but to "split the difference" and charge a premium that was much higher *for the young and relatively healthy* than what they used to pay. If the consumers still retained the option of buying health insurance, depending on the specifics they might roll the dice and hope that their medical expenses would be cheaper than maintaining their health insurance. Thus a "death spiral" could unfold, in which over time the pool of customers applying for health insurance got sicker and sicker (on average), meaning that the insurance companies would have to keep raising their premiums just to break even. (In the extreme, if only cancer patients and people needing major surgery wanted to buy health insurance, the resulting premiums would be so high that nobody could afford health insurance.)

To avoid this potential outcome, the new legislation would have to require that (almost) *everybody* buy health insurance. This **"individual mandate"** would thus be a new burden imposed on the general public, as opposed to the earlier measures that were targeted at the insurance companies. Whether the context is home fires or medical care, the only way *insurance* works is if a large pool of customers pay (relatively) low premiums in order to fund (relatively) large but rare payments to those unlucky customers who face unusually high expenses—because of their house burning down or because they are diagnosed with leukemia, for example. An individual mandate for health insurance thus forces the entire population into the pool of customers paying health insurance premiums, which makes it possible to keep the premiums relatively affordable.

Yet the dominoes keep falling. One reason the public clamored for the initial legislation is that so many of them found private-sector health insurance to be *too expensive*; that's partly why millions of people were uninsured. (The other reason is that the insurance companies just denied coverage to certain applicants, period.) If the government comes along and tries to "help" with new measures that will undeniably *raise* premiums and then insists that everybody *must pay them* or face government penalties, then many citizens would be worse off. They would have preferred the status quo, where they at least had the freedom to forego health insurance if they thought it made more sense to spend their limited budgets on more important items (such as rent, food, and education).

To deal with this wrinkle, our hypothetical legislative package would also include generous **government subsidies for the poor**, to help them afford the new, more expensive health insurance (which, we remember, they would now be *forced* to purchase). Yet if the government is going to commit to massive new spending programs, it will have to pay for them through higher taxes. Since it would defeat the purpose of the subsidies to the poor by enacting general tax hikes, the new legislation therefore would need **large tax hikes on the rich.**

Thus far, we have reviewed the basic features of a hypothetical piece of legislation designed to provide health insurance coverage to all Americans. Each step in the process flows naturally from the internal logic of the goal, and from understanding the *economics* of health insurance. However, we can go further and mention two additional features that would be necessary *politically*.

First, as our discussion has illustrated, health insurance "reform" of the scope under consideration would be a massive ordeal involving many moving parts. As such legislation was being crafted, there would be massive uncertainty in the health insurance industry, especially when we consider that the government could at any moment *tweak the rules* if things weren't turning out exactly as the legislators originally intended. In order to reassure their management and shareholders that they had a viable business, the government would offer generous **guarantees to the health insurance companies,** covering their losses if projections went awry and the new mandates (on plan benefits and premium structuring) ended up imposing huge financial burdens on the industry. By offering such guarantees, at least for a transition period, the government could neutralize major opposition from the insurance sector.

Finally, another complication—deriving from both the economics and the politics of health insurance—is that most Americans, on the eve of "reform," had health coverage provided by their employers, and they were largely satisfied with their plans. If the government implemented legislation that only possessed the features we've outlined, then one result would probably be that most employers dropped their employees from the now much more expensive plans. (Remember, premiums would rise because insurance companies are forced to cover everyone, and major employers aren't going to get subsidies designed for the poor.) Such an outcome would outrage many citizens, because what was sold rhetorically as "reform" to provide coverage to the small segment of the population lacking health insurance would instead completely overturn the existing system.

In order to prevent this negative outcome—which could derail political support for the new measures—our hypothetical legislation would also need to include an **"employer mandate,"** with rules dictating that (at least some) employers had to provide (at least some) of their employees with health insurance. Such a measure would minimize the disruption to the status quo, and it would also place the direct onus of the new law on the "deep pockets" of employers, rather than falling directly on the hundreds of millions of Americans who already had coverage through their employer.

You may have noticed that our quick discussion in this section has covered all of the bullet points we listed at the opening of the chapter. Starting with the goal of providing all Americans with access to affordable health care, the inner "logic" of government intervention and the response of the private sector yield a perhaps surprising list of necessary features for even a hypothetical piece of legislation. To be sure, along the way various interest groups and politicians inserted many an arbitrary detail into the finished 906-page Affordable Care Act, and they will continue to insert arbitrary and "irrational" (from a system-wide perspective) things as the many thousands of pages of accompanying *regulations* pertaining to the legislation are issued over the coming years.[5] Yet our point in this section was to show that by its very nature, legislation aimed at providing universal health coverage *had to extensively intervene into the economy by necessity.*

The massive scope of ObamaCare wasn't an accident or the result of sloppiness on the part of its designers. Once the decision was made for the government to intervene (yet again) in health care to ensure "universal coverage," it necessarily had to expand its interventions in numerous other respects. There was no way to merely "nibble at the edges" of the status quo circa 2009; any attempt at reform would have to be sweeping.

PUTTING THEORY INTO PRACTICE: SOME SPECIFICS OF THE ACA

In the previous section, we walked through the inner logic of any legislation attempting to solve the problem of increasingly expensive and—in many cases—literally unobtainable health insurance for Americans as of 2009. In this section, we'll review some of the major provisions of the actual Affordable Care Act that Barack Obama signed into law on March 23, 2010. Keep in mind that the specific details of the sweeping new law were constantly tweaked in the wake of its passage, but the following discussion is accurate concerning the ACA as originally enacted. Unless otherwise cited, the quotations that follow come from the Department of Health and Human Services website, on a page explaining the various components of the ACA as they are phased in over time.[6]

Universal coverage: Within a few months, the ACA implemented new rules to stop insurance companies from "denying coverage to children under the age of 19 due to a pre-existing condition." Specifically, the new rules applied to new plans and existing group plans beginning on or after September 23, 2010. The entire population enjoyed such protection as of January 1, 2014, at which time the law implemented "strong reforms that prohibit insurance companies from refusing to sell coverage or renew policies because of an individual's pre-existing conditions."

Community rating: As the HHS describes it, as of January 1, 2014, "in the individual and small group market, the law eliminates the ability of insurance companies to charge higher rates due to gender or health status." More specifically, as of this writing, the ACA only allows health insurers to vary their premium charges based on the applicant's (a) age, (b) geographical location, and (c) smoking status. Even here, there are limits to the insurance company's discretion: a health insurer can only charge a maximum of three times the premium for an older applicant as a younger one, and can only charge a smoker a maximum of 50 percent more for the same policy offered to an equivalent non-smoker.[7]

Essential health benefits: The ACA mandates that for health plans beginning on or after September 23, 2010, insurance companies "will be prohibited from imposing lifetime dollar limits on essential benefits" such as hospital stays. Also by this date, all new plans are required to cover mammograms, colonoscopies, and certain other preventive services "without charging a deductible, co-pay or coinsurance." By 2014, imposing annual dollar limits on essential benefits "will be banned for new plans in the individual market and all group plans."

Individual mandate: Effective January 1, 2014, with a few exceptions all Americans were required to purchase health insurance, or else owe a fine—or what the government sometimes describes in Orwellian fashion as an "individual responsibility payment"—to the IRS on the following April 15. Initially the fine is modest, but it rapidly escalates. Here is how the government explains the fee structure on its website:

The penalty in 2014 is calculated one of 2 ways. If you or your dependents don't have insurance that qualifies as minimum essential coverage you'll pay whichever of these amounts is higher:

• 1% of your yearly household income. (Only the amount of income above the tax filing threshold, $10,150 for an individual, is used to calculate the penalty.) The maximum penalty is the national average premium for a bronze plan.

$95 per person for the year ($47.50 per child under 18). The maximum penalty per family using this method is $285. ...

The penalty increases every year. In 2015 it's 2% of income or $325 per person. In 2016 and later years it's 2.5% of income or $695 per person. After that it's adjusted for inflation.[8]

The government's website also helpfully reminds the reader that if an individual ends up paying the government such fees for not having health insurance, then the individual . . . still doesn't have health insurance.

Government subsidies for the poor: Recognizing the cruelty of fining people who are too poor to afford health insurance, the ACA contains numerous exemptions from the individual mandate, as well as explicit subsidies to help poorer Americans afford their premiums. These subsidies include a large expansion of Medicaid eligibility, and the establishment of state "health insurance exchanges" or "market-places" where individuals can sign up for insurance and receive information on the assistance they will receive from the government. (We will discuss some of the details more fully in the next chapter.)

New taxes on "the rich": In order to pay for the massive new spending commitments necessary to subsidize health coverage, the ACA legislation contains numerous tax hikes, many of which were designed to fall primarily on upper-income earners. In particular, for individuals with incomes above $200,000 and married couples filing jointly with incomes above $250,000, the ACA carries a surtax of 0.9 percent on the Medicare payroll tax as well as a very misleadingly named "Medicare" surtax of 3.8 percent on investment income falling above these thresholds. Starting in 2018, there is also a *40 percent (!)* excise tax on so-called "Cadillac plans" offered by employers, which applies to the amount by which an employer's cost to provide a health plan exceeds either $10,000 for an individual or $27,500 for family coverage.

There is a host of other new taxes as well, including a 2.3 percent tax on medical device manufacturers, a 10 percent tax on indoor tanning, taxes levied on health insurers, an excise tax on charitable hospitals that fail to comply with the requirements of the ACA, and a tax on brand name drugs.[9]

It's important to note that when the Congressional Budget Office (CBO) reported—much to the delight of the legislation's fans—that the ACA would "reduce the deficit," this calculation *included all of the new tax hikes.* Also, the way the press reported the CBO's estimates for "the cost" of the ACA was often misleading, because some of the new tax hikes were rolled into the "insurance provisions" of the ACA, thus reducing its (ten-year) *gross* cost to a *net* figure about half a trillion dollars lower. In other words, the CBO's report on the budgetary impact of the ACA would make the superficial reader—which includes just about every member of the media, of course—walk away thinking that the government's new spending obligations were about $50 billion per year less than they really were.[10]

Government guarantees for health insurance companies: Inasmuch as the ACA involved a major overhaul of the market for health insurance, the companies operating in this sector were understandably very worried about their fate. What if some of the projections about enrollment, costs, and so forth were too optimistic? For this reason, the ACA contained the "Risk Corridor" program, which applies to policies issued through 2016.

Specifically, the Risk Corridor program compares theoretical "allowable costs" to a realized "target amount" in order to generate a ratio. If the ratio is greater than 1, the premium was less than what was required to cover the insurer's costs, while a ratio of less than 1 means the premium was higher than necessary. This ratio is then used to determine how much of the loss or profit the insurer must share with the Department of Health and Human Services (HHS), according to this distribution:

Figure 5-2. "Risk Corridors" for Health Insurers Under the ACA

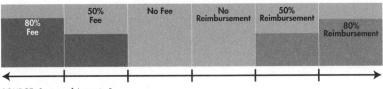

SOURCE: Society of Actuaries[2]

As Figure 5-2 illustrates, if the ratio swings 3 percent either way, then there is no transfer in any direction; the health insurance company in question either enjoys its modest profit or suffers the modest loss. However, if the ratio moves a bit further in either direction, then the insurer falls into the 50 percent corridor, where it surrenders half of its gains to the government (if it charged a higher premium than necessary) or it has half of its losses reimbursed by the government (it if charged a lower premium than necessary).

As Figure 5-2 makes clear, the federal government will pick up 80 percent of a large enough loss,[11] and for a large enough *gain*, the government will also pluck off 80 percent. Therefore, at least during the transition period applying to policies issued through 2016, the formal maintenance of private health insurance is somewhat of a fiction: the federal government is acting as a pseudo-"single payer" behind the scenes.

But that's not all. As economist Joseph Salerno explains, there is another element of the ACA that is distinct from the federal Risk Corridor Program—namely the state-based Reinsurance Program:

. . . under which large claims are capped for insurers offering individual plans under Obamacare. Insurers pay for claims up to $45,000, while the Federal government picks up 80% of the costs exceeding $45,000 up to a maximum of $250,000. This means that Obamacare is a public-private insurance scheme and that we are already half-way to the "single-payer" insurance program that Obama and his left-wing cronies so keenly pine for. Needless to say, neither President Obama nor the establishment media have publicized this provision of Obamacare.[12]

As with the federal Risk Corridor program, the state-based Reinsurance Program is (in theory) merely a transitional measure, applying only to policies issued through 2016. As the term "Reinsurance" suggests, this program involves premium payments from the insurance companies, although the ACA also funds the state-based reinsurance program with a total of $5 billion from the US Treasury through the year 2016.[13]

Employer mandate: Finally, the ACA involves stiff penalties to encourage employers to maintain coverage for their employees. The specific rules facing employers under the ACA are complicated, extending beyond the scope necessary for our discussion. But here's the big picture summary. Large employers—defined as those who have 50 or more "full time equivalent" employees, where "full time" is defined as working 30-plus hours per week (meaning two separate employees who each work 15 hours per week would count as one full-time equivalent worker)—must provide a qualifying health insurance plan to their full-time employees. If the employer does *not* provide a qualifying health insurance plan to a given full-time employee, then the employer owes the IRS an annualized fine of either $2,000 or $3,000 *for each such employee.*[14]

CONCLUSION

Many economists have noted the general pattern that whenever the government dabbles in one area, trying to "tweak" the market outcome to make things more satisfactory to government officials, this first step sets in motion a cascade of unintended consequences that require ever more rounds of government intervention.

We see the same pattern in the specific example of the Affordable Care Act, which ostensibly was "merely" trying to provide affordable health insurance for all Americans. Yet as both friends and foes agree, the ACA couldn't simply pass a new mandate on health insurance companies and have that be the end of it. No; the inner logic of so-called "health care reform" necessarily required new government regulations on numerous businesses and even individual citizens, as well as massive new spending commitments and taxes.

Yet just because the scope of the ACA's actions were (in this sense) *necessary*, that doesn't mean they were *desirable*. Now that we understand the reasoning behind the ACA's structure, in the next chapter we'll examine some of the major fallout from its features.

APPENDIX: THE CBO'S (MISLEADING) SCORECARD ON THE ACA'S FINANCES

In the political debates, one of the ACA's often-cited virtues was that it was "self-financing" and even "reduced the deficit." Although these descriptions are technically true—at least according to the celebrated report put out by the Congressional Budget Office (CBO)—defenders of the legislation often go further by suggesting that the ACA saves the taxpayers money by slowing the growth in government health care expenditures.[15] On the contrary, the only reason the ACA "paid for itself" was that it contained even bigger tax increases than the massive new government spending it entailed.

The following table comes directly from the CBO's July 2012 analysis provided to House Republicans on the budgetary effects of the ACA:

Table 5-1. July 2012 CBO Analysis of H.R. 6079, "The Repeal of ObamaCare Act"

	2013	2014	2015	2016	2017	2018	2019	2020	2021	2022	2013-2017	2013-2020
By Fiscal Year, in Billions of Dollars												
NET CHANGES IN THE DEFICIT FROM INSURANCE COVERAGE PROVISIONS[a,b]												
Effects on the Deficit	-4	-45	-95	-130	-146	146	-145	-146	-153	-160	-420	-1,171
NET CHANGES IN THE DEFICIT FROM OTHER PROVISIONS AFFECTING DIRECT SPENDING[c]												
Effect on the Deficit of Changes in Outlays	1	37	50	51	59	74	90	103	117	129	199	711
NET CHANGES IN THE DEFICIT FROM OTHER PROVISIONS AFFECTING REVENUES[d]												
Effects on the Deficit of Changes in Revenues	37	32	50	52	57	61	64	68	72	76	228	569
NET INCREASE OR DECREASE (-) IN THE DEFICIT[e]												
Effect on Deficits	34	24	6	-26	-31	-12	9	25	36	44	7	109
On-Budget	32	22	3	-32	-39	-23	-6	10	21	27	-14	14
Off-Budget[e]	2	2	3	6	8	12	14	15	16	17	21	95

SOURCE: http://www.cbo.gov/sites/default/files/cbofiles/attachments/43471-hr6079.pdf

Here's how to read Table 5-1: the CBO was explaining to John Boehner (back in July 2012) that if the government repealed the Affordable Care Act, then over the next 10 years (from Fiscal Year 2013 through 2022), the total effect on the federal budget deficit would be to *increase it* by $109 billion. That's why the press announced that repealing the ACA would worsen the deficit. More specifically, as the table indicates, the CBO reported that if the ACA were repealed, then the government would avoid $1,171 billion (i.e. $1.2 *trillion*) in spending due to "insurance coverage provisions" in the legislation, but it would also miss out on $711 billion in offsetting spending reductions and $569 billion in tax receipts.

Even at this point, we can see that the ACA is a monstrously expensive undertaking, which "reduces the deficit" only because it contains (what appears to be) $569 billion in new taxes—such as the surtax on Medicare payroll and investment income for high-income earners, and the tax on medical device manufacturers. But this is misleading. The $1,171 billion figure is a *net* figure for the ten-year cost to the federal government for "insurance coverage provisions" of the ACA. A careful reading of the 2012 CBO analysis indicates that the *gross* cost to the federal government of the ACA's "insurance coverage provisions" is actually $1,677 billion (i.e. $1.7 *trillion*) over 10 years.

So what explains this huge difference in gross versus net cost, a discrepancy on the order of $506 billion? The answer is that the ACA contains massive new taxes that are directly related to insurance coverage, and hence are rolled into the CBO's category of "insurance coverage provisions." In other words, looking just at Table 5.1, the innocent reader might think that the ACA contained "only" $569 billion in tax hikes over the ten-year period analyzed, but such a conclusion would be a vast understatement, hiding hundreds of billions in new taxes.

What specifically are these new taxes, which are directly related to "insurance coverage provisions" and hence do not appear in the revenue row in Table 5-1? Elsewhere the CBO report shows that from 2013 through 2022, the federal government is expected to collect a total of $55 billion from individuals who neglect to obtain health insurance and are fined accordingly, $106 billion from employers who neglect to provide employees with health plans and are fined accordingly, an additional $111 billion from employers (and workers)[16] for providing employees with *too generous* of a health care plan (the so-called "Cadillac plans") and are fined accordingly, $184 billion from new "contributions" to the Reinsurance and Risk Adjustment programs levied at the federal level on health insurers, and a miscellaneous $216 billion more in tax receipts flowing from existing tax provisions when the ACA causes changes in how workers are compensated.[17] Now in fairness, there are also offsetting tax *reductions* in the ACA directly related to "insurance coverage provisions": namely $222 billion in tax credits to subsidize health exchange premiums, and $20 billion in tax credits to small businesses for providing their employees with health insurance.

All told, when we disregard the somewhat arbitrary category of "insurance coverage provisions" and look at the *total impact* of the entire ACA legislation on government spending and revenue, the CBO's July 2012 analysis projected the following budgetary effects over the period of 2013 through 2022:

- A net increase in government spending of $890 billion,[18] coupled with
- A net increase in government tax receipts of $1,000 billion, i.e. $1 trillion.

So yes, the CBO reported to John Boehner in 2012, and repeated to Paul Ryan in 2013, that the ACA would "reduce the deficit" in the long run. But it achieved such a "fiscally responsible" outcome by levying a projected *one trillion dollars* in *net* tax increases over the first decade of the CBO analysis.

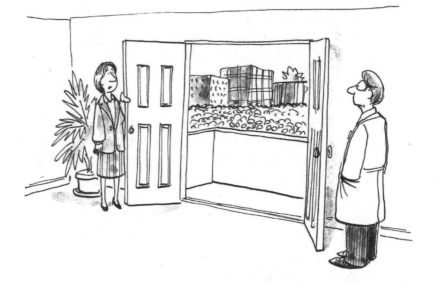

"The healthcare legislation has kicked in.
You have an appointment with the masses."

Chapter 6

FATAL FLAWS
OF THE ACA

In the previous chapter, we laid out the inner "logic" of the Affordable Care Act (ACA), showing that its basic features were integral
to the goal of providing health insurance coverage to all Americans. Once it was politically decided that new legislation would seek
"universal coverage," the dominoes began falling and it was necessary
for the ACA to include related features such as "community rating"
and an "individual mandate."

Yet just because these related features were *necessary*, it doesn't mean
the laws of economics stop working. There are obvious and inevitable
consequences flowing from each of these measures, which critics of
the legislation warned about beforehand. In this chapter we'll illustrate
some of these fatal flaws of the ACA.

"UNIVERSAL COVERAGE" FLAWED IN BOTH
PRINCIPLE AND PRACTICE

Even putting aside all of the pragmatic considerations, the very *principle* of government-guaranteed health insurance coverage is dubious.
For one thing, it reinforces the confusion between health *care* and
heath *insurance*, a conflation that itself is part of the problem. Beyond
this quibble, the more fundamental flaw with the entire premise of
the ACA is that *it is not the federal government's responsibility to provide
health care to Americans.*

The classical liberal conception of government—deriving from the political philosophy of writers such as Thomas Paine and extending up through the structure of the US Constitution—was a strictly limited institution that enforced "negative" rights. In this view, the purpose of government was to protect a sphere of autonomy for the individual within which he or she could operate, free from interference. The government, if it were to retain any legitimacy at all, could only exercise those powers that the people had the natural right to delegate in the first place. For example, individuals had the right of self-defense, and therefore they could collectively delegate the task of military defense to a government for pragmatic reasons.

This classical liberal approach is utterly incompatible with so-called *positive* rights. No individual has the natural right to force his neighbor to pay for his cancer treatments, and so by the same token (in the classical liberal view) it is illegitimate for a government to force some citizens to provide health care to others. Once the government goes down this path of "legalized plunder"—as the great nineteenth century polemicist Frédéric Bastiat described it—there is no end to the growth of a Nanny State that provides for its citizens from cradle to grave. In the race to the bottom that such a system entails, we arrive at another of Bastiat's famous dictums: "The State is the great fictitious entity by which everyone seeks to live at the expense of everyone else."[1]

To recoil from *government*-guaranteed universal coverage *is not the same thing* as opposing aid to the poor. Regarding medicine in particular, there was a long tradition for doctors and hospitals to provide care for the poor either at no charge or reduced prices. Furthermore, if Americans want to ensure that nobody dies on the street from lack of medical care, they can contribute to churches and/or secular charities that provide basic services for the truly needy. The objection that "the private sector lacks the resources" for such undertakings is unfounded: the government doesn't have any resources—to fund the ACA, for example—that it doesn't first take from the private sector. And to those who retort that "the free market was tried in health care and failed," we remind you of everything we documented in Part I of the book: the United States government has been ramping up its interventions in the health care and health insurance markets since the early 1900s. What would US history need to look like for us to conclude that *government intervention* was tried in health care—and failed?

"COMMUNITY RATING": A CLASSIC EXAMPLE OF *HEALTH* REDISTRIBUTION

Just as the progressive left in general—and President Obama in particular—are associated with *wealth* redistribution, the ACA at its core rests on *health* redistribution. That is, the very nature of the ACA seeks to erase genuine differences among the health status of individuals, and tries to force the entire health care system to treat people as if they were all "equals" in this dimension. As with economics, so with health: pretending people are the same, when in fact they are vastly different, is inherently unfair and produces undesirable consequences.

The most obvious manifestation of the ACA's reliance on health redistribution is the so-called "community rating" principle, by which the government forces health insurance companies to charge different applicants the same price for the same policy. Currently, the only four types of (limited) exceptions are pricing differentials based on age, geography, smoking status, and family size (for family versus individual plans).[2] Even here, there are limits on pricing flexibility: insurers can only charge a maximum of three times as much to older applicants as to younger ones, and they can only charge a smoker a maximum of 50 percent more for the same policy offered to a nonsmoker of the same age.

The unfairness of (mandatory) community rating is that it implicitly forces the healthy and young to subsidize the sick and the old. The point is obvious enough when it comes to people with pre-existing conditions that require expensive treatment; forcing insurers to offer coverage to a 45-year-old with a serious heart condition—while only charging the same price as they must charge all healthy 45-year-olds— clearly implies a subsidy to the heart patient and a "tax" on the healthy members of the pool.

A similar principle holds for the constraint placed on pricing differences between young and old. To repeat, the ACA only allows insurers to charge a maximum of three times as much on policies issued to older applicants versus those issued on younger ones. This too sets up an implicit subsidy, because pre-ACA, the industry norm was closer to a 5-to-1 gap. Thus, once health insurers adjust their overall premium structures in light of the new constraint, premiums for younger applicants will be higher than they otherwise would have been, while premiums for older applicants will be lower than they otherwise would have been. To illustrate the size of this effect, a 2013 study estimated that if the ACA allowed a range of 5-to-1 (rather than the actual limit of 3-to-1) in policy premiums according to age, then premiums for 21- to 27-year-olds would fall by $850 per year, while premiums for applicants aged 57 to 64 would be $1,770 higher.[3] Going the other way, then, the fact that the ACA does *not* allow a 5-to-1 range, but instead mandates a narrower 3-to-1 range, means that the younger group is charged $850 more (before considering government assistance), while the older group enjoys premiums that are $1,770 lower.

Besides the unfairness of the implicit "tax" and "subsidy" scheme involved, the principle of community rating also leads to undesirable consequences. For example, **moral hazard** refers to the problem of individuals taking bigger risks because of faulty incentives. In the context of auto insurance, the principle of moral hazard refers to the possibility that a motorist will not drive as carefully if he knows he will be indemnified for any damage to his vehicle. Obviously, the point isn't that people with auto insurance go out and *intentionally* get in car accidents, but that they tend to drive a bit more recklessly—perhaps going slightly faster, or fiddling with the radio just a little bit longer—than if they had no auto insurance and had to bear the full cost of any vehicle damage out of pocket.

In the context of health insurance—particularly when the highest premiums are being artificially suppressed—the principle of moral hazard asserts itself when individuals engage in riskier behavior that could cause health problems. By limiting the ability of insurers to charge higher premiums for higher-risk clients—including conditions that are exacerbated by lifestyle choices—the ACA fosters poorer diet and exercise decisions in the aggregate.

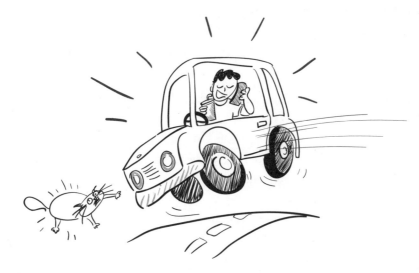

"I'm not doing much, how 'bout you?"

Besides moral hazard, economists also warn that improper pricing in insurance markets can lead to **adverse selection**. In our context, the problem is that community rating may induce young and healthy people to drop out of the insurance market altogether, raising the average health care costs of the people remaining in the pool. Depending on the numbers, this process in theory could lead to a "death spiral" in which the premiums rise so much that only the very sick remain to apply for health insurance, causing private-sector health insurance to become unviable: no insurance company can stay in business if all of its clients have serious conditions. Adverse selection shows that the principle of "community rating" isn't just a *zero*-sum game—in which the government forces young and healthy people to implicitly subsidize the older and sick—but is actually a *negative*-sum game, chasing some people out of the market altogether and leaving the remainder worse off.

The problem of adverse selection is partially addressed by the ACA's individual mandate, but as of this writing, it is still an open question whether the escalating fines will be high enough to induce enough young people to obtain health insurance, particularly as the full brunt of the ACA has yet to be implemented.

"YOU CAN KEEP YOUR PLAN": "ESSENTIAL HEALTH BENEFITS" INVITE LIES, MORE MORAL HAZARD, REDISTRIBUTION . . . AND ABSURDITY

One of the biggest PR disasters associated with the Affordable Care Act was President Obama's broken pledge that "you can keep your plan," which won PolitiFact's "Lie of the Year" award in 2013. To understand just how duplicitous President Obama and his subordinates were, it's worth quoting from PolitiFact's explanation of the award:

> It was a catchy political pitch and a chance to calm nerves about his dramatic and complicated plan to bring historic change to America's health insurance system.
>
> "If you like your health care plan, you can keep it," President Barack Obama said—many times—of his landmark new law.
>
> But the promise was impossible to keep.
>
> So this fall, as cancellation letters were going out to approximately 4 million Americans, the public realized Obama's breezy assurances were wrong. ...
>
> For all of these reasons, PolitiFact has named "If you like your health care plan, you can keep it," the Lie of the Year for 2013. ...
>
> The Affordable Care Act tried to allow existing health plans to continue under a complicated process called "grandfathering," which basically said insurance companies could keep selling [pre-ACA] plans if they followed certain rules.
>
> The problem for insurers was that the Obamacare rules were strict. If the plans deviated even a little, they would lose their grandfathered status. In practice, that meant insurers canceled plans that didn't meet new standards.

Obama's team seemed to understand that likelihood. US Health and Human Services Secretary Kathleen Sebelius announced the grandfathering rules in June 2010 and acknowledged that some plans would go away. Yet Obama repeated "if you like your health care plan, you can keep it" when seeking re-election [in 2012]. ...

But what really set everyone off was when Obama tried to rewrite his slogan, telling political supporters on Nov. 4, "Now, if you have or had one of these plans before the Affordable Care Act came into law, and you really liked that plan, what we said was you can keep it if it hasn't changed since the law passed."

Pants on Fire! PolitiFact counted 37 times when he'd included no caveats, such as a high-profile speech to the American Medical Association in 2009: "If you like your health care plan, you'll be able to keep your health care plan, period. No one will take it away, no matter what."[4]

The reason the ACA led to the cancellation of so many previously issued health insurance policies is that they were deemed too stingy. In particular, millions of people who bought their own insurance (perhaps because they were self-employed) would opt for "catastrophic" plans with high deductibles that didn't include dental or vision benefits.

Such plans are illegal under the ACA.[5] As the government's website explains:

The Affordable Care Act ensures health plans offered in the individual and small group markets . . . offer a comprehensive package of items and services, known as essential health benefits. Essential health benefits must include items and services within at least the following 10 categories: ambulatory patient services; emergency services; hospitalization; maternity and newborn care; mental health and substance use disorder services, including behavioral health treatment; prescription drugs; rehabilitative and habilitative services and devices; laboratory services; preventive and wellness services and chronic disease management; and pediatric services, including oral and vision care.[6]

The requirement of these "essential" benefits leads to absurdities such as men and post-menopausal women being forced to buy insurance plans that cover maternity leave. This is another example of the health redistribution that characterizes the ACA; policyholders who obviously won't be receiving reimbursements for maternity care are implicitly subsidizing women who (in a free market) would have chosen plans with such coverage.

Beyond the silliness and the unfairness, the requirement of essential health benefits also creates moral hazards. For example, we have to ask *why* many health insurance plans had such high deductibles, co-payments, and other "undesirable" features before passage of the ACA. One reason, of course, is that this limited the payments that the insurance company had to make for a given procedure, but this structure also provided the critical feature of *making people more conscious of their health care decisions*. Someone with a catastrophic insurance plan that had, say, a $10,000 annual deductible, high co-payments for routine care, and no dental or vision benefits, is typically going to consume a lot less in total "health care services" per year than someone with a much smaller deductible, no co-payments for preventive services, and full vision. Thus, by making such catastrophic plans illegal, the ACA ironically destroys some of the checks on excessive health care spending that the system previously had.

THE "INDIVIDUAL MANDATE" IS AN AFFRONT TO LIBERTY AND PENALIZES THE VERY PEOPLE ALLEGEDLY BEING HELPED

In the previous chapter, we explained why the logic of the ACA required an individual mandate, in which everyone (with some exceptions) is legally required to buy health insurance. Yet even though there is a perverse "logic" to the mandate, it nonetheless should offend anyone who believes in a limited role for the State. If Thomas Jefferson or James Madison were transported to our times, they would presumably be fascinated by the Internet and space travel, but they would also be shocked to learn that the US government was now forcing every citizen to buy health insurance.

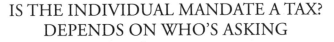

IS THE INDIVIDUAL MANDATE A TAX? DEPENDS ON WHO'S ASKING

The only way the Supreme Court could even pretend to reconcile the ACA's individual mandate with the US Constitution was by treating it as a tax (conditional on whether the taxpayer happened to have health insurance for the tax year in question).[7] Conservative critics of the ACA had a field day with the Court ruling, because proponents of the legislation—including President Obama himself—had assured Americans that the individual mandate involved a penalty, not a tax.

Beyond the abstract affront to liberty is the fact that the individual mandate fines people who consider health insurance too expensive. Remember, the penalties on individuals who commit the sin of failing to purchase health insurance become quite steep: by 2016, the penalty for an individual is 2.5 percent of income or $695 per person, whichever is more.

Now the defender of the ACA might retort that such a stiff penalty is largely for show, a mere formality as it were, because the *Affordable Care Act* will provide good options for every American, such that very few people in practice will actually *pay* that stiff fine.

Alas, that's not what the federal government itself thinks about the matter.

Table 6-1. CBO Estimate of 2016 Individual Mandate Penalties Under ACA

Estimate Distribution of Individual Mandate Penalties Under the Affordable Care Act, Calendar Year 2016				
	Individual Mandate Penalties			
Adjusted Gross Income Relative to Federal Poverty Guidelines	Total Payers (Millions)	Share of Payers (Percent)	Total Payments (Billions of dollars)	Share of Payments (Percent)
Less than 100 percent	0.2	5	0.1	3
100 percent to 199 percent	0.8	20	0.4	9
200 percent to 299 percent	1.0	25	0.6	14
300 percent to 399 percent	0.7	19	0.6	13
400 percent to 499 percent	1.2	31	2.5	61
Total	**3.9**	**100**	**4.2**	**100**

SOURCES: Congressional Budget Office; staff of the Joint Committee on Taxation.
SOURCE: CBO[2]

As Table 6-1 indicates, the CBO's latest estimate (as of this writing) projects that when the ACA's individual mandate reaches its maximum level in 2016, there still will be 3.9 million Americans who actually *pay* the fine. (More people will technically owe the fine—because they lack health insurance and are not exempt from the mandate—but simply will not pay it.) These 3.9 million Americans will pay a total of $4.2 billion to the IRS for the calendar year 2016 alone, meaning they will prefer to pay more than $1,000 on average to *not* obtain health insurance—which makes us wonder just how "affordable" it will be.

Finally, note that Table 6-1 shows that these fines are not restricted to the affluent. The CBO estimates that 200,000 people with an income *below* the federal poverty line will be assessed the penalty, along with an additional 800,000 people who make less than twice the poverty line.[8] For these *one million people*, the Affordable Care Act—according to the government's own projections—will be doing the exact opposite of what its supporters believe: these are low-income people who *still* will lack health insurance, and on top of that will pay an additional fine (of at least $695 for adults) to the IRS.

GOVERNMENT SUBSIDIES FOR THE POOR FOSTER DEPENDENCY AND DESTROY INCENTIVE TO WORK

As we explained in the previous chapter, there are various subsidies embedded within the ACA in order to (ostensibly) make insurance *affordable*. Yet along with adding more than a trillion dollars in federal spending over its first decade—spending that US taxpayers ultimately must finance—the ACA's subsidies will lead to millions more Americans who are utterly dependent on the government for health care. Furthermore, these subsidies will distort work incentives to a degree that may surprise even some of the ACA's critics.

Before relaying the size estimates of this effect on work incentives, we should spend a moment to explain how it works. Most people intuitively understand that if the government levies a high *tax rate* on additional income, then it reduces the incentive for people to work more to earn it. For an exaggerated example, if the government taxed income up to $100,000 at 10 percent, but then taxed income above $100,000 at 99 percent, then someone who originally made $90,000 probably wouldn't take a promotion to a more stressful and time-demanding position even if it paid double. That's because most of the big jump in the (pre-tax) salary would end up going into the coffers of the IRS.

There is a similar mechanism at work, but in reverse, when it comes to government *subsidies* (in the form of refundable tax credits, for example) at the low end of the income scale. Again, this effect is easiest to see if we use an exaggerated numerical example. Suppose the government pays for $5,000 in health insurance premiums for an individual who makes $15,000 or less in annual income, but gives *zero* in subsidies to anyone who makes above $15,000. Now suppose an individual starts out working part-time earning $12,000 annually, paying for his own health insurance through a government exchange and enjoying the full subsidy. Then the individual gets an offer to take a full-time position that pays $16,000 in salary, but at a small company that will not provide health insurance. It's obvious with our exaggerated numbers that it would be foolish for the man to take the new job and work more hours, because the $4,000 increase in earnings would be more than offset by the loss of the $5,000 subsidy for health insurance. Thus, in this case, our hypothetical individual would perversely be "trapped" working part-time because moderate improvements in his employment status would actually make him worse off financially—unless of course he took the pay raise and dropped his health coverage.

To be clear, this example uses the rule of a stark cutoff in a generous subsidy for health coverage above a particular income threshold; the actual subsidy structures in the ACA are more complex. Nonetheless, the obvious disincentive effect in our simple thought experiment translates to the real-world impact of the ACA: because it offers so many "generous" subsidies for health insurance coverage *tied to income level,* the ACA reduces the incentive for low-income workers to earn more money.

In its February 2014 updated forecast, the CBO shocked the pundits by more than *doubling* its estimate of the job reduction due to the ACA. Here is how the CBO report explained its new projections:

> CBO estimates that the ACA will reduce the total number of hours worked, on net, by about 1.5 percent to 2.0 percent during the period from 2017 to 2024, almost entirely because workers will choose to supply less labor—given the new taxes and other incentives they will face and the financial benefits some will receive. . . . [T]he largest declines in labor supply will probably occur among lower-wage workers. . . .
>
> The reduction in CBO's projections of hours worked represents a decline in the number of full-time-equivalent workers of about 2.0 million in 2017, rising to about 2.5 million in 2024.[9]

To repeat, this new projection (made in February 2014) of two million fewer "full-time equivalent" jobs[10] by 2017 was more than *double* the original figure of a "job cost" of 800,000 from the legislation. Most of the jump was due to the CBO's revised modeling of the disincentive effects of the ACA's subsidies on lower-income workers. When the news of the updated CBO estimate broke, naturally the *critics* of the ACA had a field day, saying "I told you so" about the devastating impact the big-government plan would have on the economy.

What *was* surprising, however, was how the defenders of the Obama Administration tried to spin the higher estimates of labor force reduction as a *good thing*, at least for the workers in question, who now could spend more time with their family or pursue other vocations because of the new options that the ACA provided to them. For example, here's how Paul Krugman tried to do damage control from his blogging perch at the *New York Times*:

> So the CBO estimates that the incentive effects of the ACA will lead to a voluntary reduction in labor supply of around 1 1/2 percent, the equivalent of 2 million full-time jobs. . . .

> [The implied drop in the size of potential economic output is] a clear overstatement of the true economic costs of the program.

> Why? Because when workers voluntarily withdraw 1 percent of their hours, it's very different from what happens when 1 percent of workers lose their jobs and become involuntarily unemployed.

> When workers lose their jobs, it's almost always a terrible experience: not only does it cause financial hardship, it eats away at the soul. . . .

> **When workers choose to work less, by contrast, they presumably do so because they gain something that is, to them, worth more than the foregone income: more time with their children, an earlier retirement, etc.** Now, in making these choices they won't take into account the spillovers to the rest of society that come from their paying less in taxes or receiving more in benefits; so you probably don't want to think of the reduction in labor supply as a net economic good. But it's surely a smaller cost than the headline effect on GDP.[11]

We have selected Krugman's attempt at damage control because he—as a Nobel Prize-winning economist—gave the CBO bombshell the most adequate pushback possible. In addition to Krugman's nuanced defense, there were plenty of lesser pundits and Obama spokespeople who were uttering abject nonsense, trying to convince gullible Americans that the news was somehow another feather in the cap of the new legislation and that the long-run reduction in the workforce of 2 percent was actually a *good thing* for the country.

These attempted spins of the CBO's bombshell fail. First let's explain what's wrong—or at least very misleading—about the argument that these worker withdrawals from the labor force are "voluntary" and hence must be good, at least for the low-income workers in question.

The crucial fallacy here, as economist David R. Henderson pointed out when the CBO story broke,[12] is to focus *only* on the subsidies for low-income people in the ACA, while ignoring the individual mandate and other restrictions. Krugman and other apologists were correct in saying that the subsidies gave options to low-income workers and thus were good *compared to the rest of the ACA without any subsidies*, but that's an entirely different claim from saying *the ACA as a whole package* helped low-income workers compared to the situation *without the ACA at all*.

Henderson clarified the point with an analogy about cars, which we'll slightly adapt here. Suppose the government forced every citizen to buy a new car with a price tag of $15,000, but recognizing that this would be a large burden to some citizens, the government simultaneously offered to pay the full cost of the new car for anybody making less than the federal poverty line. We can easily imagine in this (contrived) scenario that there would be hundreds of thousands of Americans who originally worked at jobs that paid a little bit above the poverty line, and who drove a beat-up old car or perhaps took the bus. Then, facing the new situation of being mandated to buy a new $15,000 car and having a full subsidy conditional on being in poverty, these hundreds of thousands of low-income workers could quite rationally choose to cut back their hours in order to reduce their income and hence qualify for the subsidy. When the dust settled, these low-income workers would be driving a new car and earning below the poverty line, rather than the original scenario of taking the bus and making an income above the poverty line. It's not obvious that every single one of these hypothetical workers would be better off in the new scenario, even though their narrow choice of choosing to reduce their hours was "voluntary." *Some* probably would be quite happy with the new arrangement, but we can easily imagine that others would be miserable—for example, a guy who used to drive a beat-up car but worked at a job that placed him $8,000 *above* the poverty line.

In his article, Henderson pointed out that the situation facing low-income workers after passage of the ACA parallels our hypothetical car scenario. Workers who originally chose not to carry insurance (because it was too expensive), or who had catastrophic plans with no bells and whistles, are now being forced by the ACA to buy plans that are far more expensive than what they would have chosen on their own. In order to receive means-tested federal subsidies to pay for these expensive (and mandatory) policies, some low-income workers are now "voluntarily" reducing how much they work and earn. As in our hypothetical car scenario, here too we can admit that *some* low-income workers may prefer the new arrangement, but many may have preferred the pre-ACA status quo—when they worked more hours to earn a higher income, and had the option of buying a cheaper, no-frills health insurance policy or even to go without health insurance at all.

So we see that, arguments over "voluntary" work reductions notwithstanding, it's unclear how many recipients of these subsidies are actually better off after passage of the ACA. But besides these technical quibbles, there is the overarching absurdity in the debate that *none of the ACA's champions ever mentioned the big drop in the workforce* before the legislation was passed. All of these problems surfaced only *after* the ACA had become law.

This point was made in biting fashion by Casey Mulligan, a Chicago School economist whose work on the disincentive effects contained in the ACA was one of the chief reasons that the CBO changed its forecast. After the CBO bombshell, and the ensuing efforts at damage control by the Obama Administration and its allies, the *Wall Street Journal* interviewed Mulligan and asked for his reaction to this development in the policy debate:

A job, Mr. Mulligan explains, "is a transaction between buyers and sellers. When a transaction doesn't happen, it doesn't happen. We know that it doesn't matter on which side of the market you put the disincentives, the results are the same. . . . In this case you're putting an implicit tax on work for households, and employers aren't willing to compensate the households enough so they'll still work." Jobs can be destroyed by sellers (workers) as much as buyers (businesses).

He adds: **"I can understand something like cigarettes and people believe that there's too much smoking, so we put a tax on cigarettes, so people smoke less, and we say that's a good thing. OK. But are we saying we were working too much before? Is that the new argument? I mean make up your mind. We've been complaining for six years now that there's not enough work being done. . . . Even before the recession there was too little work in the economy. Now all of a sudden we wake up and say we're glad that people are working less? We're pursuing our dreams?"**

The larger betrayal, Mr. Mulligan argues, is that the same economists now praising the great shrinking workforce used to claim that ObamaCare would expand the labor market.

He points to a 2011 letter . . . signed by dozens of left-leaning economists including Nobel laureates, stating "our strong conclusion" that ObamaCare will strengthen the economy and create 250,000 to 400,000 jobs annually. . . .

"Why didn't they say, no, we didn't mean the labor market's going to get bigger. We mean it's going to get smaller in a good way," Mr. Mulligan wonders. [Bold added.][13]

In summary, the ACA's enormous subsidies to defray the cost of health insurance for low-income Americans are problematic not only because they involve a redistribution from the taxpayers, but also because they reduce the incentive to work. This is not a controversial point; even the ACA's staunchest defenders, such as economics Nobel laureate Paul Krugman, admit it—though it would have been nice if they had admitted it *before* the ACA was passed into law.

THE ACA HIKES TAXES ON MORE THAN JUST "THE RICH"

In the previous chapter, we explained that the ACA was estimated to carry with it some *trillion dollars* in net tax revenue increases over the first decade. The defenders of the legislation of course portray this as mere nibbling at the crumbs falling from the tables of the super rich. For example, Paul Krugman—in a post ironically titled "Beyond the Lies"—described the redistribution in the ACA in this way:

> [T]he attack on Obamacare depended almost entirely on lies, and those lies are becoming unsustainable now that the law is actually working. No, there aren't any death panels; no, huge numbers of Americans aren't losing coverage or finding their health costs soaring; no, jobs aren't being killed in vast numbers. **A few relatively affluent, healthy people are paying more for coverage; a few high-income taxpayers are paying more in taxes;** a much larger number of Americans are getting coverage that was previously unavailable and/or unaffordable; and most people are seeing no difference at all, except that they no longer have to fear what happens if they lose their current coverage.[14]

Needless to say, Krugman's description stretches the truth to a degree that would impress a yoga instructor. When Krugman says "a *few* high-income taxpayers are paying more in taxes," he presumably is referring to the individuals making above $200,000 (and married couples more than $250,000) who now pay an additional 0.9 percent on the Medicare payroll tax as well as a very misleadingly named "Medicare" surtax of 3.8 percent on investment income. Far from being "a few" people, IRS data indicate that (in 2012) there were more than *5.2 million* taxable returns with adjusted gross income higher than $200,000.[15] Furthermore, Krugman's breezy discussion completely ignores the *one million* Americans making less than double the federal poverty line, whom the CBO anticipates will pay a fine for not having health insurance in 2016.[16]

Yet there is a far more insidious problem with the ACA's new revenue streams, of which even the fiercest critics of the Obama Administration seem unaware. Although the *explicit* tax rate increases embedded in the ACA legislation are indeed limited to "the rich," nonetheless hundreds of billions of dollars in extra revenue are projected to occur *from the ACA's effects working through the pre-existing tax code.*

What can happen is this: through various mechanisms, the ACA will cause some employers to reduce the quality (and expense) of the insurance plan they provide to their employees (particularly because of the 40 percent excise tax on so-called "Cadillac" plans), and it will cause some employers who are currently offering health insurance to simply abandon the practice altogether, so that their employees obtain insurance themselves—perhaps through the government exchanges. This change won't translate to a *complete* loss for the workers involved; the force of competition in the labor market will lead the employers to offer higher wages in lieu of paying for health insurance. However, under the current tax code, when an employer spends money on health insurance premiums for an employee, that is *not* taxable income for the employee. But if the employer reduces (or eliminates altogether) spending on the employee's insurance, and increases monetary compensation instead, then the extra wages *are* taxable income. Therefore, even though the ACA doesn't contain explicit income tax rate hikes for all workers, the government nonetheless anticipates that it will derive large revenues from all types of workers, not just "the rich."

To get a sense of just how big this effect may be, let us quote from the CBO's April 2014 updated estimates. In the excerpts that follow, note that the CBO breaks up the effect as due to the so-called tax on "Cadillac" plans specifically, versus the more miscellaneous effect resulting from the rest of the ACA's provisions:

> According to CBO and JCT's [Joint Committee on Taxation] estimates, federal revenues will increase by $120 billion over the 2015–2024 period because of the excise tax on high-premium insurance plans. Roughly one-quarter of that increase stems from excise tax receipts, and **roughly three-quarters is from the effects on revenues of changes in employees' taxable compensation. . . . In particular, CBO and JCT anticipate that many employers and workers will shift to health plans with premiums that are below the specified thresholds to avoid paying the tax, resulting generally in higher taxable wages for affected workers.**
>
> . . .
>
> The ACA also will affect federal tax revenues because fewer people will have employment-based health insurance and thus more of their income will take the form of taxable wages. **CBO and JCT project that, as a result of the ACA, between 7 million and 8 million fewer people will have employment-based insurance each year from 2016 through 2024** than would have been the case in the absence of the ACA. . . .
>
> . . .
>
> Because of the net reduction in employment-based coverage, **the share of workers' pay that takes the form of nontaxable benefits (such as health insurance premiums) will be smaller—and the share that takes the form of taxable wages will be larger—than would otherwise have been the case.** That shift in compensation will boost federal tax receipts. Partially offsetting those added receipts will be an estimated $7 billion increase in Social Security benefits that will arise from the higher wages paid to workers. **All told, CBO and JCT project, those effects will reduce federal budget deficits by $152 billion over the 2015–2024 period.** [Bold added.][17]

According to these estimates, the ACA will yield the government some *$240 billion* in extra tax receipts over a ten-year period *paid by workers* because their compensation packages will reduce or eliminate health coverage and will increase wage or salary.

To reiterate, these modeling effects and revenue estimates aren't coming from the Heritage Foundation or another group hostile to the Obama Administration. On the contrary, these figures come from the Congressional Budget Office, and indeed form about one-quarter of the means by which the ACA "pays for itself." Yet we sure don't remember any of its cheerleaders stressing these particular effects when they proudly announced the CBO's verdict that the ACA would "reduce the deficit."

GOVERNMENT GUARANTEES FOR HEALTH INSURERS FOSTERS CRONYISM AND HIDES FULL IMPACT OF ACA

In the previous chapter, we outlined some of the major provisions through which the government shared the risk with the health insurance companies for policies issued during the first few years of the new ACA regime. This aspect of the new legislation is dangerous for a few reasons.

In the first place, as with every other element of the ACA, it violates the principle of limited government. Just as the federal authorities have no business ordering citizens to buy health insurance, Uncle Sam shouldn't act as a giant reinsurer for the major health insurance companies, putting taxpayers on the hook in case the claims come in higher than expected.

There is also the serious matter of corruption. With many billions of dollars flowing around, surely decisions have been and will continue to be made behind closed doors that have little to do with providing quality care to the poor. Indeed, many progressive voters—who initially had such high hopes for the new President—became disillusioned at the backroom dealing that characterized the drafting of the ACA itself, rather than the "most transparent Administration in history" that Senator Obama had promised on the campaign trail.

Finally, the hidden taxpayer bailouts of the health insurance companies serve to mask the true economic distortions of the Affordable Care Act—a topic we will explore more fully in the next section. Simply put, if the federal government had not stepped in as a "backstop" to the health insurers for (at least) the transition period as the ACA's provisions were phased in, then some of the insurance companies may have exited the market altogether, or at least increased their premiums more aggressively in response to the legislation.

For example, the CBO estimated that **"reinsurance payments scheduled for insurance provided in 2014 are large enough to have reduced exchange premiums this year by approximately 10 percent** relative to what they would have been without the program".[18] By transferring some of the actual cost of the ACA away from the health insurance companies (and their customers) to the taxpayers in the first few years, the hidden bailouts will make it harder for the voters to diagnose what's happening. In particular, had premiums increased to fully reflect the new legislation in 2014 when the individual mandate went into effect, more Americans would have realized just how burdensome the ACA would prove to be. As it is, the defenders of the ACA are running victory laps over how "surprisingly affordable" the exchange-provided policies are.

EMPLOYER MANDATE
DISTORTS THE LABOR MARKET

As we have seen, various measures of the ACA will ultimately cause employers to *reduce* the health insurance coverage they offer to their employees, with some seven to eight million fewer workers having employer-provided coverage through 2024, according to a CBO estimate.[19] Yet as we explained in the previous chapter, the architects of the ACA wanted to minimize the number of employees who were kicked off of their employers' plans, for obvious political reasons. Therefore, the ACA contains an "employer mandate," with stiff fines for certain employers who choose not to offer coverage for full-time employees.

To review from our last chapter: the ACA mandates that large employers—defined as those who have 50 or more "full time equivalent" employees, where "full time" is defined as working 30 or more hours in a week—provide a qualifying health insurance plan to their full-time employees. If the employer does *not* provide a qualifying health insurance plan to a given full-time employee, then the employer owes the IRS an annualized fine of either $2,000 or $3,000 *for each such employee.*[20]

These fines for employers are quite hefty. If the health insurance provided by the ACA were indeed "affordable," one would expect that relatively few employers would decide to deny coverage and pay the fine. Yet as with the individual mandate, here too it will be very instructive to look at *the government's own estimates* of how many employers will in fact choose to pay either a $2,000 or $3,000 fine per applicable employee, rather than paying for the "affordable" coverage.

Specifically, the latest CBO report estimates that from 2015 through 2024, employers will pay *$139 billion* in penalty payments to the government for failing to provide their employees with qualifying health insurance. As with the other revenue streams, it is once again worth noting that this is yet another large chunk of the roughly trillion dollars necessary for the ACA to "pay for itself," and yet is not what most Americans probably have in mind when chalking up the needed revenue to "tax hikes on the rich."

It is worth dwelling on this astounding figure to grasp its full significance. When the government expects employers to decide it is more profitable to pay either a $2,000 or $3,000 fine and *not* offer health insurance to millions of their employees, this is very revealing as to how expensive these plans will be. The comparison is *not* "pay $2,000 as a fine, or pay a little more for health insurance for my employee." When an employer pays a fine to the government, that payment in no way benefits the employee who isn't being offered health insurance. In contrast, if an employer *does* spend, say, $5,000 on a health insurance policy, then that expenditure makes the position more desirable and can attract a higher quality candidate.

Therefore, in the same way that it should be shocking that millions of Americans will choose to pay a stiff fine and *not* have health insurance, it is also shocking that many employers will pay large fines and *not* include health insurance as part of their compensation packages for millions of employees. If these projections were coming from scholars who had a political ax to grind, they might be dismissed as paranoid criticisms of Obama. But to repeat, these projections come *from the government's own estimates of how much revenue the ACA will bring in.*

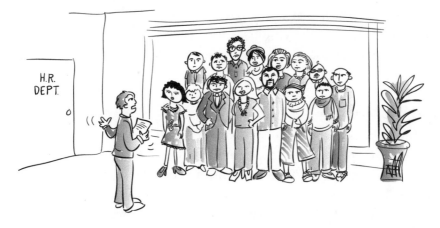

*"Sorry, but it's cheaper for us to pay a $3,000 fine
for each of you than to give you adequate health insurance.
But we have free donuts every Friday!"*

Besides the tax hike on employers, the employer mandate has another perverse effect: it provides a very large incentive for small firms to remain small, and for large firms to keep their workers part-time rather than full-time. These observations don't require a PhD in economics; the employer mandate only applies to firms with 50 or more full-time equivalent employees, and even for those employers, the fine is only applied for full-time employees.[21]

A naïve inspection of the employment data certainly seems to confirm the worst fears about this consequence of the mandate, because the proportion of part-time workers in the overall labor force has indeed risen dramatically with passage of the ACA. However, it is difficult to disentangle the effect of the ACA itself from the deep recession that began in late 2007. (It is normal for part-time employment to rise during recessions, as employers do not wish to commit themselves to the bigger responsibility of hiring a full-time worker.) On the other hand, the employer mandate aspect of the ACA has been pushed back at least twice due to complaints from business that the requirement is too onerous to be implemented while the economy is still weak. (Even major labor leaders sent an open letter to Democratic leaders warning that the ACA as originally passed could "destroy the foundation of the 40-hour work week that is the backbone of the middle class."[22]) It's therefore likely that the employer mandate's full effect on part-time versus full-time employment has not yet manifested itself.

CONCLUSION

In the previous chapter, we showed that by its very nature, the government's desire to legislate universal health insurance coverage also required several other interventions, including community rating, essential health benefits, an individual mandate, government subsidies for the poor, tax hikes (especially on "the rich"), government guarantees for the health insurers, and an employer mandate.

In this chapter, we showed that each component of these additional (yet necessary) features of the Affordable Care Act carries its own specific and undesirable consequences. The combination of universal coverage, community rating, and essential health benefits will yield a massive *health* redistribution by which the young and healthy implicitly subsidize the old and those using extensive care. This arrangement distorts incentives in the market for health insurance, weakening the motivation for people to monitor their health care expenditures and reducing personal financial consequences of health conditions that are not merely the result of genetics or uncontrollable circumstances, but can be influenced through lifestyle choices. Furthermore, by "overcharging" the healthy and frugal while "undercharging" those responsible for most of the health care spending, the framework also encourages relatively healthy individuals to drop out of the insurance pool altogether, raising premiums for those who remain.

The individual mandate adds insult to injury for what may be millions of Americans who will *still* lack health insurance but will pay stiff penalties on top of it, along with those who obtain coverage but will be forced to buy more expensive policies than they would have voluntarily selected. The combination of massive subsidies for low-income individuals to receive coverage, higher tax rates, and the employer mandate will—among other things—grossly distort the labor market. These influences lead to a "voluntary" reduction in labor effort, both by the relatively poor in order to qualify for the subsidies and by the relatively affluent to minimize their tax liability, as well as an effort of employers to substitute part-time workers for full-time. Finally, the hidden government bailouts for the health insurance companies will foster corruption and mask the true economic impact of the ACA for several years, making repeal that much more difficult.

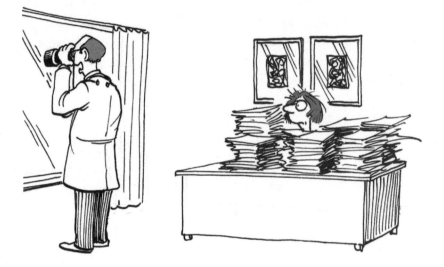

"Get ready!
The next wave of legislation is rolling in."

Chapter 7

PAVING THE WAY
FOR "SINGLE PAYER"

In Chapter 5 we explained the "inner logic" of the Affordable Care Act, showing that the desire to legislate universal coverage necessarily carried with it a string of further features, such as community rating and the individual mandate. Then in Chapter 6 we outlined some of the immediate consequences of each of these features, using simple economic logic to explain why the ACA would backfire, and drawing on the government's own estimates to get a sense of how bad the fallout would be.

Relying on the material developed in the prior two chapters as our foundation, in this chapter we look ahead to provide a qualitative sketch of what is likely to unfold in the US markets for health insurance and health care over the next few decades. To anticipate our prognosis: the current framework is utterly unsustainable. The perverse incentives inherent in the system *before* passage of the ACA have only been exacerbated by the massive burst of new legislation. Over time, the problems spawned by the ACA will continue to grow, while its ostensible benefits will remain elusive.

At some point in the not-too-distant future, Americans will realize that they must make another momentous decision when it comes to the provision of health care and health insurance. One path would be a massive rollback of the federal government's interventions into these markets.

Unfortunately, if history is any guide, the pundits and politicians will probably convince enough of the public to "finish the reform" initiated by Barack Obama, and move the United States to a "single payer" system in which the government pushes those pesky private sector insurance companies out of the picture and directly pays for all major health care in the country. It is necessary to understand the urgency of the situation in order to appreciate the strategies outlined later in this book, which will guide Americans through what appears to be an inevitably approaching storm.

PREMIUM HIKES: STICKER SHOCK OR PLEASANT SURPRISE?

The most obvious impact of the ACA worth closely monitoring was the increase in health insurance premiums that most Americans would experience. Readers who followed the pundits and political debates may recognize a feeling of two parallel universes, as conservative media outlets trumpeted studies showing enormous projected rate hikes—particularly for young people in states that previously had little regulation of the health insurance market—while liberal media outlets published reports showing the "good news" that health care spending was growing more slowly than anybody had expected.[1] The average American could understandably feel helpless in parsing through the analyses, since the experts in the two partisan camps—those who were demonizing the Obama Administration versus those who defended it—seemed to be making completely opposite claims. Was one side in the debate simply fabricating figures?

As with most things involving economics and statistics, neither side was necessarily lying; they didn't need to. By carefully choosing modeling assumptions, the group of individuals being examined, and the relevant baseline, an analyst could truthfully paint a picture of the ACA either sharply increasing premiums *or* making health insurance much more affordable. In this section we'll explain some of the biggest sources of confusion.

When considering the impact of the ACA on health insurance premiums, the most important thing to keep straight is whether we're looking at premium hikes *for a given person* or premium hikes *for a given type of policy*. It is precisely this ambiguity that allows friends and foes of Obama to point at the exact same study and claim, "We told you so!"

This distinction between people and policies is crucial because the ACA—with its requirement of a suite of "essential health benefits"—forces people to buy insurance plans that are more generous than what these people may have wanted to buy voluntarily. To return to a car analogy: if the government forces everybody to buy a Ferrari, people who previously drove Toyotas are going to face a huge increase in their car payments, even if the model 2015 Ferrari is only modestly more expensive than the model 2014 Ferrari.

To see the importance of picking a baseline, consider a 2009 CBO analysis on the impact of proposed legislation on 2016 premiums. Ironically, this CBO estimate gave *both* groups the talking points they wanted to say that ObamaCare was either awful or wonderful.

Table 7-1. CBO Estimate (Made in 2009) of ACA's Impact on 2016 Premiums

Effect of Senate Proposal on Average Premiums for Health Insurance in 2016			
	Percentage, by Market		
	Nongroup[a]	Small Group[b]	Large Group[c]
Distribution of Nonelderly Population Insured in These Markets Under Proposal	17	13	70
Differences in Average Permiums Relative to Current Law Due to:			
Difference in Amount of Insurance Coverage	+27 to +30	0 to +3	Negligible
Difference in Price of a Given Amount of Insurance Coverage for a Given Group of Enrollees	-7 to -10	-1 to -4	Negligible
Difference in Types of People with Insurance Coverage	-7 to -10	-1 to +2	0 to -3
Total Difference Before Accounting for Subsidies	+10 to +13	+1 to -2	0 to -3

The CBO estimate in Table 7-1 was made back in 2009, so for our purposes the specific numbers in the table aren't as important as the various factors that the CBO analysis so clearly delineates. The top row shows the distribution of the US population into various types of insurance offerings; for example, the CBO projected the biggest impacts on premiums in the nongroup market, which only affected 17 percent of the population. For these people, the effect of *having to buy more generous insurance plans* was quite large, increasing premiums by

27 to 30 percent. However, even within this segment of the market, the *total* projected effect on premiums was a more modest 10 to 13 percent hike. That's because the CBO estimated that the ACA would reduce the premiums necessary *to provide a given insurance policy*, since (among other things) the individual mandate would force young and relatively healthy people into the insurance pool who might otherwise not buy coverage. Notice also that the CBO report projected modest overall impacts on (small and large) group insurance. Here, the effect of the "essential health benefits" requirements in the ACA is less significant than for the nongroup segment, because existing employer plans typically were in or near compliance with the standards.

Thus we see that the 2009 CBO forecast of the legislation's impact on premiums offered something for everyone: Obama's critics could highlight the top left figure of a 27 to 30 percent increase, while Obama's allies could claim that most people would see a slight drop in premiums. Relying on the 2009 forecast, neither side would be lying, but it would be hard for an average member of the public to parse the claims to understand the true situation.

In addition to the 2009 forecast, we can see other, more recent examples of different groups using the same data to reach (seemingly) opposite conclusions about the ACA. In September 2013, the Department of Health and Human Services (HHS) issued a slender report discussing the premiums that individuals would face once the new exchanges opened. (Recall that the Healthcare.gov website officially launched—with dramatic problems—on October 1, 2013.) The Abstract of the HHS report concluded on this cheerful note: "[N]early all consumers (about 95%) live in states with average premiums below earlier estimates."[2]

That sounds like great news, right? The problem is, the HHS report was comparing the 2014 premiums to *earlier estimates of 2014 premiums*. That's not what most people had in mind when they wondered, "How much is ObamaCare going to cost me?" Indeed, former CBO director Douglas Holtz-Eakin said this of the HHS report: "There are literally no comparisons to current rates. That is, HHS has chosen to dodge the question of whose rates are going up, and how much."

To get a better sense of what was really in store for most Americans, scholars at the Manhattan Institute used the very same data compiled by the HHS, but this time asked the question: what are some pre-ACA and post-ACA apples-to-apples premium comparisons for various demographic groups? There were many permutations in the analysis, but here we can reproduce some of their key findings.[3] When looking at the cheapest insurance plans for 27-year-olds in 2013 compared to the cheapest plans that had just been announced for the ACA exchanges, the Manhattan Institute analysts found that on average (across states) rates went up 97 percent for men and 55 percent for women. (In Nebraska the sticker shock was the worst, with rates for the cheapest policy available to 27-year-old men increasing *279 percent*.) Perhaps surprisingly, the Manhattan Institute analysts found a similar pattern even for 40-year-olds, with men on average seeing the cheapest available plan increasing 99 percent in price while women faced a hike of 62 percent.

Now to be sure, this technique *overstates* the impact of the ACA for those people in 2013 who weren't buying the cheapest health insurance policy available. (Specifically, people who had health insurance that was already in compliance with the ACA's "essential health benefits" requirements would not see such drastic premium hikes.) On the other hand, what of the young and healthy people who originally chose not to buy health insurance because they had more important things to do with their limited budgets? Now that the ACA is forcing many of them to spend large amounts on health insurance, these particular Americans have seen an *infinite* percentage increase in their premiums (or fines, if they choose to pay the IRS the penalty). Keep that in mind when you see estimates of the "average" (and finite!) effects of the ACA on premiums: this group of Americans (which could be millions of people) is obviously not having their percentage hike entering the computation.

To get an estimate of the increase in premiums across the population as a whole, we can look to Yale University's Amanda E. Kowalski: she developed a full-blown model with all the bells and whistles, which weighted premiums by enrollment size. In a study for the Brookings Institution, she concluded:

In the vast majority of states, in the first quarter of 2014 premiums rose relative to state seasonally adjusted trends. Health insurance premiums almost always go up, but it is striking that they went up so much relative to trend…[P]remiums increased relative to seasonally adjusted trends in the first half of 2014 in the four most populous states. Across all states, from before the reform to the first half of 2014, enrollment-weighted premiums in the individual health insurance market increased by 24.4 percent beyond what they would have had they simply followed state-level seasonally adjusted trends.[4]

It is important to note that Kowalski's estimates refer to the *unsubsidized* premium amount, meaning what health insurers are actually receiving for policies as opposed to the out-of-pocket payments made by individuals. This is yet another crucial "switch" that can be flipped on or off in the arguments over the impact of the ACA. In a typical unfolding of the current political debate, the critic of the ACA will argue that it is grossly inefficient, driving up premiums across the board. The defender will then argue that the statistics involved only look at the market rates; once we take into account the help various individuals will get from the government, then all of a sudden ObamaCare should seem like a good deal to lots of people. Whether or not this is true—we'll see in a minute that we strongly disagree—forcing some people to subsidize the premiums of others doesn't change the fact that multiple features of the legislation make health insurance far more expensive than it needs to be.

As of this writing, the simple truth is that *we really don't know* the full impact of the ACA on typical premiums. Several elements of the original legislation were designed to ease Americans into the new regime, rather than "shocking" them upfront and giving a chance for people to demand repeal. For example, the screws don't really tighten on the individual mandate until 2016. This feature of the ACA is supposed to force enough young and healthy people to enter the risk pool and thereby curb average costs. Insurers may be holding off on major rate hikes, waiting to see the composition of their enrollment pool once the individual mandate is at full blast.

Second, remember that the ACA contains various measures by which the federal government temporarily shares the risk of unexpectedly high claims with the insurance companies. For example, in its April 2014 analysis, the CBO wrote:

> **. . . CBO and JCT expect that reinsurance payments scheduled for insurance provided in 2014 are large enough to have reduced exchange premiums this year by approximately 10 percent relative to what they would have been without the program.** However, such payments will be significantly smaller for 2015 and 2016, and they will not occur for the years following. Therefore, that program is expected to have resulted in lower premiums in 2014, to reduce premiums by smaller amounts in 2015 and 2016 than in 2014, and to have no direct effect thereafter.[5]

We should emphasize that a *10 percent* suppression of premiums in 2014 is a very large effect. This factor alone would have been enough to force many pro-ACA pundits to abandon the claim that "ObamaCare proved the worrywarts wrong."

For a third example, the tax on employer-provided "Cadillac plans" isn't even scheduled to go into effect until 2018. This 40 percent (!) surtax on high-premium plans could have an enormous impact on the health insurance market for group plans. Until then, current talk of the ACA's ultimate impact on private health insurance, and the fate of the taxpayer, is quite premature.

So far, we've outlined three major wild cards in the *legislated* unfolding of the ACA. But in addition to the *designed* delay, the Obama Administration has also postponed the application of onerous provisions through Executive fiat. For example, in response to the outrage over the millions of plan cancellations, the Administration (as of this writing) has twice extended the grace period for non-compliant plans—meaning that people can "keep their plan if they like it" through September 2017.[6] It is not surprising that some of the critics' worst fears have not yet been realized, since the Obama Administration postponed several of the most onerous portions of the new legislation.

TREND TOWARD MORE DEPENDENCE ON GOVERNMENT FOR HEALTH INSURANCE

It is undeniable that a key result of the ACA will be a huge expansion of the number of Americans who are dependent on the federal government for their health care, either directly (through Medicare, Medicaid, Veterans Administration, etc.) or indirectly (through generous subsidies for otherwise unaffordable "private" health insurance). As usual, we can use the government's own estimates to demonstrate our claim.

First let's consider Medicaid, the federal government's program (acting in cooperation with state governments) for providing health care financing to low-income Americans. For those who supported passage of the ACA, one of the most obvious "gains" it achieved was expanding Medicaid eligibility and federal funding for the program. The CBO estimates that by 2018, the ACA will place an additional 13 million people on Medicaid and CHIP (the Children's Health Insurance Program), and that "the added costs to the federal government for Medicaid and CHIP attributable to the ACA will be $20 billion in 2014 and will total $792 billion for the 2015–2024 period."[7]

Second, besides expanding existing government programs (i.e. Medicaid and CHIP), the ACA obviously will foster an enormous population dependent on large government subsidies of policies offered through the "exchanges." Again relying on the latest CBO report, the government projects that 25 million Americans will receive their health insurance through the exchanges by the year 2017. Of these 25 million, 19 million (76 percent) will be subsidized, while only 6 million (24 percent) will pay the full "market" price. Thus there will be three subsidized people for every one person paying full freight for insurance purchased through the individual marketplaces.

Also note that the *size* of these subsidies will be quite large: "CBO and JCT project that the average subsidy [per subsidized enrollee] will be \$4,410 in 2014, that it will decline to \$4,250 in 2015, and that it will then rise each year to reach \$7,170 in 2024."[8] Let's be sure we understand what that figure means: the CBO is saying that if you add up all of the money the federal government will use (either in direct spending or through tax credits) to subsidize exchange premiums in a given year, divided by the total number of subsidized individuals it expects to buy coverage through the exchanges, then the result will be \$4,250 in 2015 and \$7,170 by 2024.

It should thus be crystal clear that the millions of people added to Medicaid, CHIP, and the ACA exchanges will generally be utterly dependent on the federal government for their health care.[9] At the same time, various measures of the ACA are projected to significantly *reduce* the incentives for employers to offer coverage to their employees.

The following table is the CBO's snapshot (as of April 2014) of the various trends in sources of health insurance coverage attributable to the ACA:

Table 7-2. CBO Estimate (April 2014) of ACA's Impact on Sources of Insurance Coverage

Effects of the Affordable Care Act on Health Insurance Coverage

(Millions of nonelderly people, by calendar year)	2014	2015	2016	2017	2018	2019	2020	2021	2022	2023	2024
Insurance Coverage Without the ACA[a]											
Medicaid and CHIP	35	35	34	33	33	34	34	34	35	35	35
Employment-based coverage	156	158	160	163	164	165	165	165	166	166	166
Nongroup and other coverage[b]	24	24	25	25	26	26	26	26	27	27	27
Uninsured[c]	54	55	55	55	55	55	56	56	56	57	57
Total	270	272	274	277	278	280	281	282	283	284	285
Change in Insurance Coverage Under the ACA											
Insurance exchanges	6	13	24	25	25	25	25	25	25	25	25
Medicaid and CHIP	7	11	12	12	13	12	13	13	13	13	13
Employment-based coverage[d]	*	-2	-7	-7	-8	-8	-8	-8	-7	-7	-7
Nongroup and other coverage[b]	-1	-3	-4	-4	-4	-4	-4	-4	-4	-5	-5
Uninsured[c]	-12	-19	-25	-26	-26	-26	-26	-26	-26	-26	-26

SOURCE: CBO, "Updated Estimates of the Effects of the Insurance Coverage Provisions of the Affordable Care Act," Table 2, p.4.

Regarding Table 7-2, we will walk through the column for the year 2018, because the numbers have leveled off at this point and are fairly representative of the medium-term impact. The numbers in the bottom group show the CBO's projections for the *change* in insurance coverage (by various sources) due to the ACA; the numbers in the top group show the baseline, if the ACA had never been passed.

The table shows that in 2018, the CBO projects an additional 13 million Americans will have Medicaid and CHIP coverage—an increase of about 40 percent from the baseline of 33 million, for a total of 46 million people getting their health care expenses paid through these programs. The CBO also projects that 25 million Americans will be covered through exchanges, an "infinite" percentage increase relative to the (non-existent) baseline. In contrast, employer-based coverage will fall by 8 million employees, about a 5 percent drop from a baseline of 164 million. Nongroup and other coverage will fall by 4 million, about a 15 percent drop relative to the baseline of 26 million.

Added together, the CBO projects that in 2018, the exchanges, Medicaid, and CHIP will have picked up 38 million people, while employer-based and individual coverage (outside of the exchanges) will have dropped 12 million, for a net fall in the ranks of the uninsured by 26 million. It is worth emphasizing that this projected *net* drop in 26 million uninsured people occurs because of a *gross* increase of 38 million people getting their coverage from the government-facilitated programs, with the 12 million-person discrepancy due to a shrinking of insurance coverage through non-governmental sources.

But wait: we need to make an adjustment to the figures we've been using. You see, the CBO reports are very nice and tidy—the authors do a great job spelling out the assumptions they used to generate the numbers that come out the other end—but typically they analyze the ACA from the perspective of the "nonelderly population." In other words, the enrollment projections in Table 7-2 *completely ignore Medicare*, as well as the millions of elderly people on Medi*caid*.

Using projections from the Centers for Medicare and Medicaid Services (CMS), in Table 7-3 we give a fuller picture of the *total* number of Americans who will receive their health insurance through various channels by the year 2018:[10]

Table 7-3. Government Estimates of Sources of Health Insurance in Year 2018

SOURCE OF HEALTH INSURANCE	Millions of Americans in 2018	% of U.S. Population
ACA Exchanges	25	8%
Medicare	59	18%
Medicaid	76	23%
CHIP	3	1%
Employer	173	52%
Nongroup, Nonexchange Insurance	7	2%
Uninsured	24	7%
Total U.S. Population	330	
NOTE: Categories sum to more than total population because of overlap.		

SOURCES: CBO, CMS

As Table 7-3 indicates, the central warning of this chapter—that the US is headed toward an explicitly "single payer" framework in which the government directly pays for everyone's health care—will be significantly closer by 2018, using the government's own figures. According to this particular forecast, out of a projected 330 million Americans total, fully 126 million—almost 40 percent—will receive their health insurance through government channels, with the vast majority getting explicit payments from the government.

If the government's own projections admit such a future, imagine what will *actually* happen as the economy limps along, with more employers kicking workers off their company plans and the "unintended consequences" of the ACA making truly private health insurance increasingly unrealistic. If the ACA remains intact for even just one decade, the United States will be much closer to a *de facto* single payer system than most people expect.

ACA WILL FAIL IN ITS MISSION OF "UNIVERSAL COVERAGE," AND WILL LEAD TO (EVEN MORE) RATIONED CARE

So far in this chapter, we've shown that premiums may be a ticking time bomb, that major elements of the ACA have yet to fully kick in and wreak havoc on the system, and that the government's own projections show an *additional* 38 million people getting their insurance through government channels in the near future.

Now we are ready to explain why we can expect massive public dissatisfaction with this new state of affairs. The "solution" supposedly offered by the ACA will turn out to be like all of the previous health care "fixes" of the twentieth century: the government will massively expand its power and spending, and the public will be glad to see some apparent improvements in a few important criteria, but eventually it will become clear to the pundits and political officials that the "free market system" is still broken and the government "needs" to intervene yet again.

The overarching problem with the ACA is that it promises the economically impossible: it seeks to (1) massively *increase the demand* for medical services while (2) *containing the growth in medical prices*, and yet (3) not sacrifice the *quality* or *availability* of medical services to the public. Absent other major reforms that would massively increase the *supply* of medical personnel (such as an unexpected advance in robotics, special immigration waivers to bring in foreign doctors, or a rollback of government licensing requirements), this combination of features is truly impossible.

In practice, the government will play "whack a mole" with all three objectives, opting to partially satisfy each of them—which means it will *fully* satisfy *none* of them. Yes, the feds have expanded the demand for health care services, but they won't actually achieve the original goal of "universal coverage." And yes, the government will probably "bend the cost curve" and push out the day when its major entitlement programs officially run out of money, but the enormous "savings" that are built into the ACA's rosy budget accounting will prove politically impossible to push through: future legislators will realize that cutting back so sharply on reimbursement rates for various medical services will simply make them unavailable to anyone relying on the government system. Finally, Americans will notice the overall system become increasingly bureaucratic, impersonalized, and sluggish, with barebones one-size-fits-all service rationed out in diluted form by an overworked core of frazzled "health care providers."

We realize we are painting a bleak vision of the not-too-distant future, but it's important to fully understand the situation. Let us buttress our bold claims with some numbers.

• "Universal" coverage? Hardly!

The government's own projections of health care coverage from the ACA have been consistently scaled back as time has passed. Table 7-4 draws on a five different CBO reports, issued from March 2010 through April 2014, to show the consistent drop in expectations regarding "universal coverage":

Table 7-4. Government Reduces Projections of Coverage Over Time

CBO Estimate as of...	Increase in nonelderly coverage in 2016	Increase in nonelderly coverage in 2019	% of nonelderly legal residents with coverage 2019	Nonelderly Americans WITHOUT Coverage in 2019
March 2010	30 million	32 million	94%	23 million
March 2011	32 million	33 million	95%	22 million
July 2012	26 million	29 million	92%	29 million
February 2013	26 million	27 million	92%	29 million
April 2014	25 million	26 million	92%	30 million

SOURCE: Various CBO reports[4]

As Table 7-4 shows, the forecast for approximating universal coverage slightly improved from March 2010 to March 2011. But from that point forward, every year the CBO became *more* pessimistic on some dimension. Over the four-year period (from the first report in March 2010 through the April 2014 report), the CBO scaled back its estimates of 2019 coverage by *seven million* people. Note that the most recent estimate has the CBO projecting that even by 2019, there will still be 8 percent of nonelderly *legal residents* who lack coverage, and 11 percent of the *total* nonelderly population if we include illegal immigrants (not shown).

Here's another way of looking at the situation. That latest CBO forecast also says (not shown in the previous table) that *without* passage of the ACA, in 2019 the US would have had 56 million uninsured people among the nonelderly. But because the ACA was passed, the CBO is projecting that only 30 million will lack coverage. That change of "26 million" also shows up in the bottom row of the third column in Table 7-4. That means the ACA won't even cut the problem of uninsured Americans in *half*, let alone solve it. And this is for the year 2019, a full decade after the ACA was passed. Would anybody have supported President Obama if he had announced in 2010, "I am going to sign this legislation that over the next ten years will add a trillion dollars in new taxes, will cause millions of you to get kicked off your existing insurance plans, and when all is said and done will leave us with 30 million Americans who still lack health insurance. Now who's with me?"

• ACA only "reduces the deficit" via massive cuts to Medicare reimbursements

You may remember that back in Chapter 3, when discussing the Ponzi schemes of Social Security and Medicare, we summarized their literal bankruptcy *as of 2009*. That's because that passage of the ACA did indeed dramatically improve—at least on paper—the solvency of Medicare. (To be sure, normal accounting still says it's bankrupt, just not *as* bankrupt.) In his own book indicting the US health care system, economist John Goodman emphasized just how dramatically the ACA affected the Medicare spending projections with the following table:

Table 7-5. Impact of the ACA on Long-Term Medicare Unfunded Obligations

	As of 2009	As of 2010	Change Due to ACA
Medicare Part A	$36.7 trillion	($0.3 trillion)	($37.0 trillion)
Medicare Part B	$37.0 trillion	$21.2 trillion	($15.8 trillion)
Medicare Part D	$15.6 trillion	$15.8 trillion	$0.2 trillion
Total Medicare	$89.3 trillion	$36.7 trillion	($52.6 trillion)

NOTE: Figures use "infinite time horizon" accounting.
SOURCE: John Goodman, *Priceless*, Table 14.1 (p. 222)

We'll let Goodman explain the meaning of these figures, and why they should make us very concerned about the future of US health care delivery:

> **. . . [T]he Affordable Care Act uses cuts in Medicare to pay for more than half the cost of expanding health insurance for young people, but it contains no serious plan for making Medicare more efficient. All it really proposes to do is pay less to doctors and hospitals**. That's why the Medicare actuaries are predicting greatly reduced access to care for the elderly and the disabled.
>
> Most serious people inside the Washington, DC beltway believe these cuts will never take place. The reason: our experience with similar cuts in Medicare under previous legislation. If Congress has been unwilling to allow reductions in doctor fees for nine straight years under previous legislation, how likely is it to allow the even greater spending reductions called for under ACA?[11]

We realize that the incomprehensibly gigantic figures of Medicare's long-run unfunded liabilities may not resonate with you. Consider instead Table 7-6, which is also adapted from Goodman's book. It summarizes a National Center for Policy Analysis study that estimated the impact the ACA would have on Medicare recipients, broken up by age:

Table 7-6. Lifetime Medicare Benefits versus Payments, Before and After ACA

As of Year...	Category	Medicare Lifetime Value for someone who turns...		
		65 in 2011	65 in 2020	65 in 2030
2009 (Before ACA)	Value of Lifetime Benefits	$192,421	$254,900	$345,237
	Value of Lifetime Taxes and Premiums	**($132,305)**	**($200,651)**	**($298,362)**
	Lifetime Net Medicare Benefits	$60,116	$54,249	$46,875
2010 (After ACA)	Value of Lifetime Benefits	$156,833	$192,585	$240,233
	Value of Lifetime Taxes and Premiums	**($124,027)**	**($181,358)**	**($251,660)**
	Lifetime Net Medicare Benefits	$32,806	$11,227	($11,427)
	Reduction in Lifetime Net Medicare Benefits Due to ACA	$27,310	$43,022	$58,302

SOURCE: John Goodman, *Priceless*, Table 14.2 (p. 223)[3]

Table 7-6 shows us that the passage of the ACA—with its built-in cuts to Medicare expenditures—instantly changed the expected value of the entitlement program. Moreover, the changes do not hit all Americans equally, but instead tighten the screws as time passes. For people who turned 65 when the analysis was published (in 2011), the ACA was responsible for a reduction of $27,310 in *their* lifetime net benefits (using discount rates to compare dollars in different years of life) of the Medicare program. But for people who will turn 65 in 2030, the ACA causes more than double the hit, reducing *their* lifetime net benefits by more than $58,000. Indeed, for these people, Medicare is a *losing* proposition, considered as an investment vehicle: over their lifetimes, they can expect to pay $251,660 in a combination of payroll taxes while working and then health insurance premiums when retired, but will only draw out $240,233 in medical reimbursements after "going on Medicare."

Our point in reproducing these Medicare projections isn't to pine for a continuation of the program as it stood on the eve of the ACA's passage. Rather, we are simply warning the reader that *a massive financial crunch in the health care sector is coming.* The government is going to drastically scale back its reimbursements to hospitals and doctors through Medicare, and to the extent that some of these projected cuts are postponed—perhaps because the collapse in care for Medicare patients becomes too intolerable politically—then all of the rosy fiscal analyses of the ACA go out the window.

• The expansion of government-provided health insurance, combined with watered-down employer plans, will lead to longer waits and cattle-car care

It is inevitable that hospitals, doctors' offices, and health insurance companies will adopt more bureaucratic and penny-pinching measures in response to the ACA's overhaul. We've already shown the farce of the promise of "universal coverage," but even those people who *have* health insurance—particularly if they are dependent on the government to pay the bills—will learn the important difference between health *insur-*

ance and health *care*. Navigating through the health care system will become more Kafkaesque as the years pass.

In his book *Priceless* John Goodman gives many anecdotes and statistics to demonstrate that having "guaranteed" health coverage is not at all the same thing as having *actual access* to medical care. For example, almost one-third of US doctors refuse to accept Medicaid patients, period, and even those who *do* accept them will often take on only a limited number. Medicaid patients in Denver had to endure six- to eight-month waits for appointments at specialty clinics.[12]

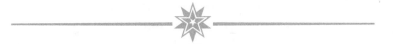

HEALTH "COVERAGE" DOESN'T NECESSARILY EQUAL HEALTH *CARE*

A nonprofit group tried to enroll people in the "free" health insurance offered through "Medi-Cal," California's Medicaid program, and this is what happened:

"Of the 50 calls made over a three-month period, only 15 calls were answered and addressed. The remaining 35 calls were met by a recording that stated, "Due to an unexpected volume of callers, all of our representatives are currently helping other people. Please try you call again later," followed by a busy signal and the inability to leave a voice message. For the 15 answered calls, the average hold time was 22 minutes with the longest hold time being 32 minutes."[13]

The problems of rationed, cattle-car care are not limited to Medicaid. Consider the *other* major vehicle for expanding health insurance coverage, namely the exchanges or "marketplaces." In early 2014, after seeing the exchanges in operation, the CBO revised *downward* its forecasts for exchange premiums, since they were coming in cheaper than it had expected. Naturally, this was welcome news to fans of President Obama. But it's interesting to read the April 2014 CBO discussion of *why* it was revamping its estimates:

> A crucial factor in the current revision [of forecasted exchange premiums] was an analysis of the characteristics of plans offered through the exchanges in 2014. Previously, CBO and JCT had expected that those plans' characteristics would closely resemble the characteristics of employment-based plans throughout the projection period. **However, the plans being offered through the exchanges this year appear to have, in general, lower payment rates for providers, narrower networks of providers, and tighter management of their subscribers' use of health care than employment-based plans do.**[14]

We should also expect employer-based plans to become more bureaucratic and mediocre. Remember that the whole point of the ACA's whopping 40 percent surtax on employer-provided health plans that are too expensive—so-called "Cadillac plans"—is to *convince employers to stop giving their employees such generous plans.*

Note the irony here. On the one hand, the "essential health benefits" aspect of the ACA forces health insurance plans to meet *minimum* standards, while the looming 2018 surtax on Cadillac plans effectively enacts *maximum* standards. Thus the ACA surrounds its enemy, attacking from two fronts—where the "enemy" in this case is product variety in a market, giving consumers a choice among options with different prices and features.

All in all, the ACA's projected shift of millions of people into government channels for their health insurance, combined with the dilution of the quality of existing employer-based plans, will lead to growing dissatisfaction among the public. As wait times increase, quality suffers, premiums and out-of-pocket payments continue to rise, and millions of people are fined for not being able to afford health insurance, Americans will become *angry*. They will realize that the "Affordable Care Act" is a cruel joke, and they will demand that the politicians in DC fix what they broke. Ironically, that is exactly what many of the ACA's proponents secretly welcome.

INTERVENTIONISTS WILL BE OH-SO SURE: THE "FREE MARKET" DOESN'T WORK IN HEALTH CARE

As we hope our analysis in this book so far has made clear, the ACA will simply exacerbate the problems in US health care and insurance that existed circa 2009, when President Obama took office. Most Americans are going to experience a massive shock over the next few years as the provisions of the ACA fully kick in.

The tragedy of all of this is that *most people will misunderstand what's happening*. In particular, they will survey the slow-motion train wreck and conclude, "Yep, that's the free market for ya. We need more government to fix this." This reaction will be understandable, because Americans are going to directly experience frustration with "private sector" institutions, not realizing the various government interventions are what spawn such outcomes.

For example, one of the popular provisions of the ACA that went into effect a few months after passage (in the fall of 2010) was that children (under certain conditions) would be allowed to stay on their parents' health insurance plan until age 26, which was an extension compared to many plans at the time.[15] Another aspect of the ACA that went into effect in 2010 forbid insurance companies from denying coverage to children for pre-existing conditions. This set up a scenario where a family might strategically *not* buy health insurance for the children, because if they later got sick they could at that time be added.

These two provisions of the ACA taken together perversely gave an insurance company an incentive to simply *drop coverage for children altogether*, since the law technically only said that a health plan needed to cover children through age 26 *if it covered them at all*. And in fact, that is precisely what happened. Yet the blame wasn't put on the perverse incentives of the ACA. Let us quote from a news article in *The Hill* to show how all of this played out *politically* as it went down:

> Health plans in at least four states have announced they're dropping children's coverage just days ahead of new rules created by the healthcare reform law, according to the liberal grassroots group Health Care for America Now (HCAN). . . .
>
> "We're just days away from a new era when insurance companies must stop denying coverage to kids just because they are sick, and now some of the biggest changed their minds and decided to refuse to sell child-only coverage," HCAN Executive Director Ethan Rome said in a statement. **"The latest announcement by the insurance companies that they won't cover kids is immoral, and to blame their appalling behavior on the new law is patently dishonest.**
>
> . . . This offensive behavior by the insurance companies is yet another reminder of why the new law is so important and why the Republicans' call for repeal is so misguided."[16]

This episode epitomizes the dynamic in government intervention in health care: a sweeping new measure tries to transform good intentions into a better world, without even a cursory consideration of the actual *effects* it will have on the decisions of the major players involved. Then when the initial intervention results in a predictable, undesirable consequence, its supporters get mad at reality and double down on their stance.

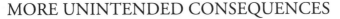

MORE UNINTENDED CONSEQUENCES

Despite the official protections that the ACA gives to those with pre-existing conditions, nonetheless the health insurers have found ways to discourage HIV+ customers from enrolling. From a story five months after the ACA's "exchanges" went into effect:

"Four Florida insurance companies offering Affordable Care Act policies are discriminating against people with HIV or AIDS, according to two health-rights organizations that plan to file a formal complaint with the federal government Thursday. . . .

'Not only did the companies place HIV/AIDS drugs in the plans' highest formulary tiers — even generic drugs — they required prior authorization for any HIV/AIDS medication,' said Wayne Turner, the National Health Law Program staff attorney who drafted the complaint. Turner said he could find no justification for such a benefit design. **'From our reading, the companies were looking for a way around the ACA's protections to discourage people with HIV/AIDS from enrolling in their plans.'"**[17]

The end limit of this process is a "single payer" system, in which the federal government brushes those pesky private-sector insurance companies out of the way and directly handles medical expenses for all Americans. Think of it as Medicare *starting at birth*, rather than at age 65. For example, remember the debacle when Healthcare.gov was first rolled out in October 2013, and hardly anybody could even sign up? Here's how Paul Krugman tried to do damage control a few weeks later:

Obamacare isn't complicated because government social insurance programs have to be complicated: neither Social Security nor Medicare are complex in structure. **It's complicated because political constraints made a straightforward single-payer system unachievable. It's been clear all along that the Affordable Care Act sets up a sort of Rube Goldberg device, a complicated system that in the end is supposed to more or less simulate the results of single-payer, but keeping private insurance companies in the mix** and holding down the headline amount of government outlays through means-testing. . .

So [Mike] Konczal is right to say that **the implementation problems aren't revealing problems with the idea of social insurance; they're revealing the price we pay for insisting on keeping insurance companies in the mix, when they serve little useful purpose.**[18]

So there you have it: a monumental flaw in the implementation of the ACA so comical that nobody would have put it into a fictional story—even the harshest conservative critics of the ACA weren't predicting that *the government's website wouldn't work*—and the ACA's Nobel Prize-winning cheerleader tries to spin it as the fault of keeping private health insurance companies in America. That is why we can be so sure that when the ACA fails to solve the problems in US health care and insurance, these same "experts" will come back with just the solution: *more* government intervention and *less* freedom.

PATIENT CHOICE: "LESS IS MORE" ACCORDING TO FANS OF THE ACA

To provide yet more evidence of the pattern we've described, it will be instructive in this section to examine the topic of restrictions on patient choice. As we explained earlier in this chapter, the insurance plans offered through the ACA-established exchanges (or marketplaces) typically have much narrower "provider networks." This is one of the ways insurers keep down costs and avoid massive sticker shock, given the other mandates in the ACA.

As we have warned earlier, Americans should get used to this treatment: they are going to see their freedoms and choices chipped away on various margins in the coming years, in health care as in other areas of life. Although the shriller supporters of bigger government will no doubt use the restricted choice to blame the private sector—who can forget Helen Hunt's famous indictment of "f***ing HMO bastard pieces of sh**!" from *As Good As It Gets?*—the pro-ObamaCare website Vox has been buttering up its readers to the idea of restricted patient choice being a necessary evil for health "reform." For example, in an article with the headline "Limited doctor choice plans don't mean worse care," Vox contributor Sarah Kliff explains:

> **Narrow networks are common on Obamacare's new exchanges**, as health insurers try to hold down premium prices by contracting with fewer doctors. McKinsey and Co. estimates that **more than a third of the plans sold on the new marketplaces left out 70 percent of the region's large hospitals**. This unsurprisingly led to a barrage of negative headlines about insurers leaving well-known hospitals out of network.
>
> But narrow networks aren't all bad. Health economists actually tend to be quite fond of these products, as they help hold down spending. The potential for savings is big: **limited choice plans can reduce patient spending by as much as a third, new research** from economists Jon Gruber and Robin McKnight finds.[19]

The ostensibly good news from the Gruber/McKnight study is that an experiment in Massachusetts showed that limited choice plans not only save money (which is unsurprising) but also apparently had no adverse consequences on patient health. Specifically, in 2011 the state government of Massachusetts offered large financial incentives—paying three months of the insurance premiums—to some of the state's employees to switch to a limited choice plan. The Gruber/McKnight study then looked at the employees who took the plan and those who kept the original plan, both a year before and a year after the switch (i.e. in 2010 and then in 2012). We'll quote from the Vox article's summary of their findings:

1. With the three-month premium holiday, lots of people switched to the narrow network plan . . .

2. Health spending fell by one-third for those who switched . . .

3. Patients used more primary care—and got fewer specialty services. . . While urgent care clinics and emergency room travel didn't change, **trips to the hospital became much longer, by as much as 40 miles.**

4. The narrow network hospitals provided just as good care. . . . Gruber and McKnight look at a typical panel of health indicators, like how many heart attack patients die within a month and re-admission rates where the hospital messed up the first time.

    They find that hospitals in and outside of the narrow plans look pretty similar; there's no significant difference in quality. "Enrollment in limited network plans is not associated with any change in the quality of accessible inpatient hospital care," Gruber and McKnight conclude.

    Gruber and McKnight were unable in this particular study to look at the health outcomes of patients — to explore whether limited network enrollees fared better, worse, or the same in the care of a smaller handful of providers.

Did you catch the magic trick that Gruber and McKnight—and the Vox writer summarizing their research—pulled off in this excerpt?

Note the last sentence we put in bold: because they said they lacked precise enough data, the researchers *didn't actually take a stand on whether the Massachusetts employees who enrolled in the narrow plan did better or worse than their peers who had remained in the original plan.* And yet, that was the whole point of the Vox article; remember, its title was, "Limited doctor choice plans don't mean worse care."

We can illustrate the enormous potential problem here with an analogy. Suppose the New York City branch of Goldman Sachs thought its executives were abusing their travel budgets. In order to weed out the frivolous flights, Goldman thus institutes a new policy: Any New York-based executive who agrees to *only* fly in and out of Reagan airport—located in Washington, DC—will get a $5,000 bonus. Executives who wish to retain the option of being reimbursed for their work flights using JFK or LaGuardia may continue to do so, but they forfeit the $5,000 bonus.

Now what would happen if we checked on the groups who did and did not take the bonus money a year after the new policy had been implemented at Goldman Sachs? We would presumably find that the executives who took the money ended up requesting much less in travel reimbursements. After all, if they wanted to fly somewhere for work, they would have to book the flights through DC, meaning they would need to take Amtrak or some other mode of transport down to that airport, rather than the much more convenient NYC-based airports. This is why executives opting for the restricted-choice air plan would end up making fewer trips to the airport than their peers who had *not* joined the (voluntary) Goldman program.

It is no surprise that our hypothetical restricted-airport plan could hold down travel expenses for the Goldman employees who opted to participate in the program. However, Goldman management would also want to know whether the program had any adverse effect on employee satisfaction and firm productivity. To this end, imagine that they hired outside researchers to conduct a study, asking them to quantify not merely the cost savings on travel expenses (which would be obvious) but also to gauge the *downsides* of the program.

The most obvious comparisons would look at the actual executives split into two groups: those who opted into the restricted-airport plan and those who didn't, examining what their work performance was like before and after the program was implemented. If the group that opted into the plan saw a reduction in productivity relative to the control group (perhaps because they spent some of their time traveling to the DC airports, or because they opted for a conference call when a face-to-face meeting would have sealed the business deal), then Goldman could compare the savings on travel expenses with the reduction in employee output—thus determining whether, on net, the restricted-airport plan made financial sense for the company.

Ah, but what if the researchers said that they lacked the data to make such assessments? Rather than report on the outcomes of *the actual Goldman employees involved with the new plan*, instead the researchers looked at various metrics relating to the general users of the NYC versus DC airports. For example, the researchers reported statistics showing that flight delays, emergency landings and crashes, lost luggage, and so forth, were not significantly different when looking at passengers flying out of DC versus NYC airports. Armed with this research, the people at Goldman Sachs who had always been in favor of the new policy happily announced at the next meeting, "Limited airport-choice executive travel plans don't mean worse air travel. We have hard evidence showing that our plan has saved the company hundreds of thousands of dollars without hurting the quality of accessible air travel for our employees." Then these proponents of the plan make a move to *mandate* it for *all* executives, since the voluntary test-run showed that there were no quantifiable downsides to the program.

We hope our silly analogy helps illuminate the serious flaw in the Gruber/McKnight health care study: it is hardly consolation to know that one's health insurance plan has a "good hospital" in network *when that hospital is an extra 40 miles away*. Nonetheless, pro-ACA media outlets trumpeted the study as showing limited-choice plans don't hurt participants, when the authors themselves said quite explicitly that they had not been able to perform that measurement.

It is no coincidence that the biggest supporters of the ACA are preparing the public to accept restrictions on choosing their doctors and hospitals: this is our inevitable future. It is economically impossible to let Americans treat the health care sector as an all-you-can-eat buffet that comes with a flat and reasonable fee. That might work for (moderate quality) Chinese food, but not for state-of-the-art medicine. If Americans really want to follow the political promises of "free and universal" coverage, they necessarily will have shortages, bureaucracy, and rationing in their future.

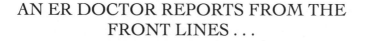

AN ER DOCTOR REPORTS FROM THE FRONT LINES . . .

"One of the major quality improvements touted by ACA proponents is the decreased hospital readmission rates following implementation of new CMS [Centers for Medicare and Medicaid Services] rules under the ACA. Beginning in 2013, CMS began denying payment to hospitals or physicians for any patient discharged from a hospital and then readmitted within 30 days. If a patient "bounced back" and required readmission, then CMS would not reimburse for any care administered during the readmission. The rationale was that this would encourage higher quality care during the initial hospital stay, which would therefore prevent the need for a repeat admission within 30 days. Driving this rule change was the assumption that before the ACA, patients only "bounced back" because doctors and hospitals had been cutting corners during the initial admission.

What this assumption ignores is that readmissions within 30 days can be a very necessary component of caring for sicker patients, particularly those with chronic diseases. For example, a COPD [chronic obstructive pulmonary disease] patient who gets admitted for pneumonia during flu season, and discharged when well enough that hospitalization offers no further benefit, still runs a very high risk of needing readmission within 30 days. The patient may continue to smoke. The disease is more active when such a patient has to use home heat, which dehumidifies the air, and the patient may come into contact with others carrying flu or other viruses. In summary, such a patient may bounce back for reasons that have nothing to do with the quality of care at the first visit.

Another consideration is that CMS incentives on the front-end of a hospital admission may actually drive decisions to discharge patients home prematurely. The DRG [diagnosis related group] system generates fixed payments that only cover a limited amount of time in the hospital. Hospital-based physicians are thus under intense pressure from their hospital administrators to discharge patients in a timely manner so the expenses of providing care do not exceed the fixed fee provided for the patient's primary diagnosis. While it is doubtful that anyone is deliberately discharging patients home prematurely, when you consider the pressures exerted through CMS rules, then transmitted by hospital administrators down to those who provide the care (and whose jobs may be at risk if they push back), it is not hard to see that it does happen. I myself have not provided inpatient care since residency, but I cannot recall ever being able to treat and discharge a patient within the time frames that are expected today.

My actual experience is that the number of bounce-backs is not decreasing and may actually be increasing. The number of readmissions, however, is decreasing. Due to the financial pressures of this new ruling, hospitals are finding other venues of care for patients who return within 30 days of hospital discharge, legitimately needing readmission. Some of these patients are readmitted and the hospital and doctors just take the financial hit. However, many times an alternative disposition is found. For example, case managers may arrange for home health to visit and provide care at home. Other times, the patient may be directed to "short-term rehab" in a nursing home or assisted care facility. Another possibility is that *a patient will be directed to hospice for comfort care. It is not uncommon for an elderly person with pneumonia to be discharged home and then return, having decompensated. Rather than being admitted for IV antibiotics and further care, the patient and family may be nudged toward hospice care and succumb from the illness. Some may argue for the appropriateness of this approach, but at times it can be a bit fuzzy.*

What is disturbing is that ACA and CMS officials are touting the 30-day rule as an indicator for improved quality of care because statistics show that fewer patients are being readmitted. My personal experience is that decreased readmissions are just a response to economic incentives put in place by CMS, and that the number of bounce-backs has not decreased at all. My fear is that there may be some dead bodies hidden within those decreased readmission numbers. There could be people who could have been saved by a readmission but are instead dying at home, at a nursing home, or at hospice. I suspect it is happening but may never be discovered, and will be represented as a quality improvement when it is, in fact, a way of sweeping the new system's failures under the rug."

—Co-author Doug McGuff

IS OUR PROGNOSIS "PARANOID"?

We realize that our description of the country's trajectory is alarming. However, we have not been throwing out idle speculation; we have explained the logic of our projections and backed our claims with examples and data. To further defend ourselves from charges of "paranoia," in this final section of the chapter we will show that *fans* of the ACA are making similar forecasts.

The single best "smoking gun" for this issue is the first-hand testimony of Nevada Senator Harry Reid, one of the major forces behind the Affordable Care Act. In August 2013, Reid participated in a PBS show called *Nevada Week in Review*, in which the discussion turned to health care reform.[20] The following (lightly edited for readability) excerpt of the interview between the Las Vegas Review-Journal's Steve Sebelius and Reid is on the long side, but it confirms exactly what we have been warning:

SEBELIUS: . . . The system is better than it was when President Obama started his reform. But every problem that Mitch and Rick have identified, relate to the fact this was really health *insurance* reform not health *care* reform. If we had gone to a single payer system, none of these problems would have come up . . .

REID: My liberal friend, it's nice of you to say that. . . . Don't think we didn't have a tremendous number of people who wanted a single-payer system. . . . Well, you have to get a majority of the votes, we weren't able to do that. . . .

SEBELIUS: . . . From what the public saw, the public option notwithstanding, there wasn't even an attempt to get—

REID: Oh sure there was. Sure there was. We had a number of different iterations at health care. . . . We had a real good run at the public option. We thought we had of way of doing that. We couldn't get it done . . .

SEBELIUS: Last question on this topic: Do you think that the health insurance model that started in World War II as a benefit when the wage-and-price controls were imposed, do you think that that is going to continue into the future, as the American model of health care delivery, or do you think eventually we'll have—

REID: I think we have to work our way past that. Prior to World War II, there were no health benefits from your employer, it didn't exist. Wage-and-price controls came into effect, and so the Big Three . . . got into fringe benefits: health care, vacation time, retirement time, all this kind of stuff. That's where the model started, and we've never been able to work our way out of that. What we've done here with ObamaCare is a step in the right direction, but we're far from having something that's going to work.

SEBELIUS: So eventually though you think we'll work beyond the insurance—?

REID: Yes, absolutely, yes.

Another bugaboo in the debate over the ACA is the notion of "death panels." Conservative critics of the Obama Administration warned Americans that eventually bureaucrats would have the power to make life or death decisions. The pro-Obama pundits rolled their eyes at the "paranoid" rantings of Sarah Palin and the like.

Our purpose here is not to defend every specific complaint that any person on FOX ever launched against the ACA. Yet consider the following excerpt from a public talk that Paul Krugman gave in February of 2013. After fielding a question about whether a particular level of government debt would lead to a crisis, in the course of his answer Krugman said:

There is this question, how are we going to pay for the programs? In the year 2025, 2030, something is going to have to give, right?... Surely it will require some middle class taxes as well, so we won't be able to pay for the kind of government as a society we want, without some increases in taxes—not a huge one—but some increases in taxes on the middle class taxes, maybe a Value Added Tax. **And we're also going to have to do, really, make decisions about health care, and not pay for health care that has no demonstrated medical benefits.** And so, you know, the snarky version I use—which I shouldn't even say because it will get me in trouble—is **death panels and sales taxes is how we do this**. But it's not that hard.[22]

Now to be sure, Krugman was "just joking" with his use of the term "death panel," but as they say: it's funny because it's true! If Krugman had been discussing, say, government funding for new schools or a mission to Mars, then labeling it "death panels" wouldn't have made any sense. But because Krugman was talking about the *government* ultimately protecting its financial position by refusing to pay for health care that "has no demonstrated medical benefits," that's why the "death panel" joke worked. If everyone's health care is paid for by everyone else as a taxpayer, then it won't suffice to let individuals choose to run up huge medical bills in the last year of life.

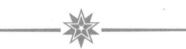

IF HISTORY IS OUR GUIDE . . .

If all of our talk still sounds paranoid, we can also look to the past to see precedents for what happens when the government has power over someone's treatment. Those with a strong stomach are encouraged to Google the 1946 *Life* magazine article by Albert Maisel titled, "Bedlam 1946."[22] The piece was a shocking exposé on the horrid condition of many state-run psychiatric hospitals. The anecdotes and grisly photos reveal what can happen even here in America.

For a recent example of the dangers of government health care, we can look at the unfolding scandal with the abysmal treatment and subsequent cover-ups in Veterans Health Administration (VHA) hospitals. On April 30, 2014, CNN relied on whistleblowers in a report that at least 40 veterans had died while waiting for care at the Phoenix VHA facilities. By June 5, 2014, VA internal investigations confirmed that at least 35 veterans in the Phoenix area had indeed died while awaiting treatment.[23] A broader investigation began, implicating more VHA hospitals around the country, while the VHA's top health official, Dr. Robert Petzel, as well as the Secretary of Veterans Affairs Eric Shinseki, eventually both resigned. The ultimate fallout from the VA scandal is not yet clear, but what *is* certain is that the dangers in government health management are still very real.

PART III
SAVE YOURSELF

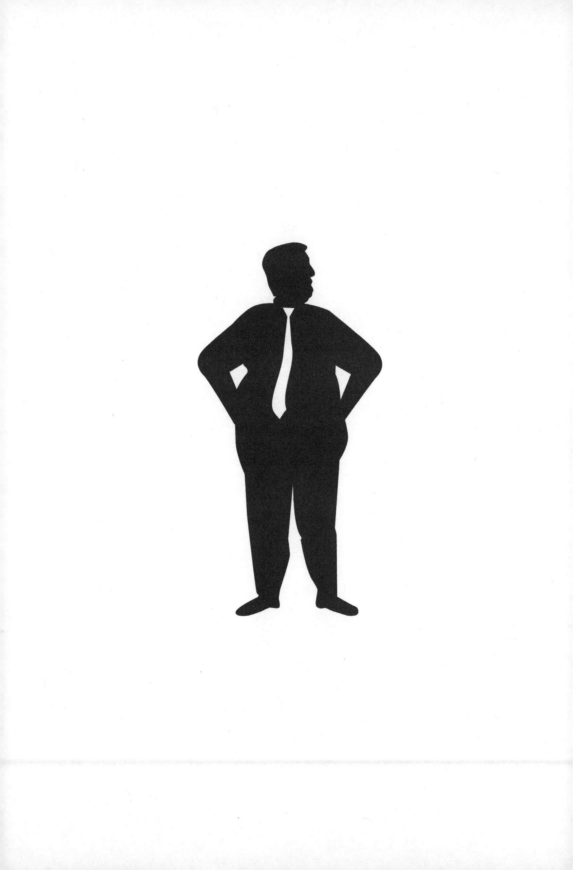

Chapter 8

KEN KORG
BATTLES THE BEAST

We realize that in the first two parts of this book, we threw a lot of information at you, the beleaguered reader. We thought it important to explain why the US health care and insurance markets are in such a dismal state, so that you could understand where they're heading.

Now that we've established our foundation, in Part III we are ready to explain how you can save yourself from falling into the trap that threatens to engulf so many Americans. As a transition from our historical and economic analyses in the previous parts to the individualized how-to manual here in Part III, this chapter offers a parable of Ken Korg, a middle-aged American husband and father who is about to have a dreadful experience with the US health system—one that will only become more typical as the years go on.

Readers of the *The Primal Blueprint* by Mark Sisson will recognize the name "Korg" as the mirror image of "Grok," the ancestral human whose diet and exercise habits offer clues for regaining our health today. When we first meet Ken Korg, he is the opposite of his forefather Grok. As we'll soon see, Ken Korg has fallen into the self-destructive diet and lifestyle patterns that plague so many modern Americans. Yet because Ken lacks the historical, economic, and medical insights that we have already discussed in the first two parts of this book, he is initially completely unprepared for the challenges he will encounter.

Keep reading to learn Ken's fate, so you don't have to repeat his experience.

KEN KORG FALLS INTO
THE BELLY OF THE BEAST

Ken had been feeling run down for some time. Life had been unusually hectic lately, and despite a downturn in the economy, Ken had landed a promotion. In an attempt to prove himself worthy (and out of fear of being let go), he was working 60 to 70 hours per week. The kids were older now, but being understanding of Mom and Dad's stressors was not one of their advancements. Everything they desired was more expensive, they were involved in even more activities, and their school (the best that could be afforded) was 40 minutes from the house. Mrs. Korg was also preoccupied with her business, and it was all they could do to keep up. Family meals were a rarity, as everyone was late or in a hurry getting where they had to be (and trying to beat the traffic).

Ken wondered how long he could continue this way. In the morning he was almost too exhausted to function, and in the evening—after checking email and surfing the Internet—he was "wired but tired," unable to fall asleep until after 1 a.m.

It was during one of these sleepless nights that he realized he had been feeling even worse than usual over the past few days. He had been in a fog, his vision was blurry, and was battling a vague, persistent sense of nausea. It was the kind of nausea that made him feel like he needed to eat something, but whenever he did, it only added a sense of bloating on top of the queasiness.

As Ken lay in bed thinking about it, he became more worried and felt the nausea rise up in a wave. He got up and tried to calm himself. He ate a spoonful of peanut butter and blasted some whipped cream into his mouth. This seemed to settle him down, and he transiently felt a wave of sleepiness, so he went back to bed. As he crawled into the cool sheets, Ken thought, "If I can fall asleep right now, I can get five solid hours of sleep."

And then it hit him. A sudden, sharp, stabbing pain in his right flank that was so severe that he thought an intruder had stabbed him.

As he jumped out of bed from the most intense pain he ever experienced, something unexpected happened: it got even worse. The pain brought him to his knees and was accompanied by sudden and profuse sweating, as well as a massive wave of nausea that culminated in a fountain of vomit so forceful that it actually came out his mouth and nose simultaneously.

Mrs. Korg awoke to the commotion to find Ken writhing on the floor in the disgusting mixture of his evening meal and the recently consumed peanut butter and whipped cream. She asked Ken what was wrong, and he honestly replied, "I don't know, but I think I am about to die."

Just then, Ken was hit by another wave of pain. This one was even more intense, and the location of the pain had changed: it was very low in his abdomen and radiated into his right groin. It literally felt like his right testicle was being crushed with a pair of vice grips. He immediately crumpled to the floor.

Mrs. Korg called EMS.

* * *

It was about 1:45 a.m. when Ken was wheeled through the ambulance entrance of the ER. Still writhing in pain, he thought, "At least at this hour, the place will be desolate and I will be seen immediately and get something for this pain." What Ken saw instead looked like a disaster zone. The place was completely packed; every room was full, and stretchers with sick and injured people lined the halls. The paramedics stopped in the middle of the hall with Ken, waiting to be acknowledged.

He continued to writhe and vomit until finally the paramedic got the attention of one of the nurses. The nurse interrupted the ER doctor, who appeared to be arguing with someone on the phone. The doctor quickly listened to the nurse, turned toward the paramedics with a look of "just shoot me" on his face, and said, "Give us a minute to find another stretcher and we will make a hall bed for you."

Ken was moved from the ambulance stretcher to another small stretcher against the wall of the hallway. On either side of him were other patients in hall beds. One was a large man with an orange jumpsuit, handcuffs, ankle cuffs, and a large gash in his forehead. Every time someone walked past, he would scream obscenities and try to fling blood at the passerby. The other patient was an elderly man, weighing all of 80 pounds, who appeared to be actively dying, with slow, feeble, gasping breaths. Between waves of pain, Ken heard one of the nurses say, "Yeah, he was on home hospice, but when he started to die, the family freaked out, revoked hospice, and called the ambulance." Intermittently, a nurse or doctor would come by and stroke the man's hair and give him something through his IV.

After what seemed like an eternity (actually about 15 minutes), one of the doctors walked up to Ken with a touchpad and said, "Hi, I'm Dr. Leslie." Without asking a single question or laying a hand, he continued, "Looks like you're passing a kidney stone; have you done this before?"

Ken responded "no" while the doctor briefly poked his belly and then gave a gentle thump to his right flank with his fist. This thump mysteriously sent a wave of pain from his flank, around his side, into his lower abdomen, and then finally concentrating in his testicle, accompanied by a brief episode of dry heaving. The doctor ordered some IV pain and nausea medicine (Toradol, Morphine, and Zofran), along with a urinalysis and a CT scan. The nurse was at the bedside with the medicine even as the doctor was ordering it; apparently they had done this before.

As the drugs were given, Ken had almost immediate and complete relief from his pain. Ken thought silently, "Thank God for modern medicine." As the nurse withdrew the syringe from the IV port, she commented, "Your blood pressure was really high; we'll recheck it after your pain is controlled."

The remainder of the ER visit went fairly smoothly. Ken provided a urine sample (which came out the color of iced tea), and returned with lots of blood cells but no infection. The nurse rechecked Ken's blood pressure and found it high at 182/94, but much improved from the 205/110 reading when he first arrived. The nurse suggested he get it rechecked at his family doctor (which he didn't have), as it may just be "white coat hypertension" or the chaotic environment in the ER.

The doctor came by and told him the CT scan showed a 3 mm kidney stone lodged at the entrance to the bladder. Apparently the stone passed through the kidney into the tube that connects to the bladder. It was the movement of the stone through this very small passageway that caused all his pain. Currently it was stuck at the entrance to the bladder, which is the smallest portion of the ureter. The doctor felt it should pass without complication and offered to provide medicine to relax this passageway, along with prescriptions for pain and nausea medicine.

By this point, the ER had actually started to clear out and the doctor was able to take more time with patients. He pulled up a rolling stool to speak some more to Ken. Mrs. Korg and the kids, who had ridden in the family car while the ambulance wheeled Ken away, were finally allowed to come back, as the crowds had cleared enough to not have to worry about violating any federal privacy laws.

The doctor informed Mr. and Mrs. Korg that in addition to the kidney stone, there were some incidental findings that would need follow-up. The doctor inquired about Ken's use of alcohol, because the CT scan showed evidence of fatty liver. Ken said he only had a couple of beers or glasses of wine a week, but the doctor seemed skeptical because the condition is most commonly seen in alcoholics. In addition, the CT uncovered the presence of some gallstones in his gallbladder, but there was no evidence of inflammation. Nonetheless, Dr. Leslie was providing referral to a surgeon. Along with the gallstones, Ken was to also have the surgeon comment on the incidental finding of a 1 cm nodule on the tail of his pancreas. This was likely nothing, but it would need to be "evaluated" because there was some chance of this being cancerous.

When Ken received his discharge instructions, he was told to follow up with his family doctor to recheck his blood pressure and to begin a workup of his fatty liver. In addition, he had a referral to the urologist for the kidney stone and a general surgeon for the gallstones and the nodule on his pancreas.

Ken was happy to be out of pain, but he found himself wondering how he was going to fit all this into his already overburdened life.

Further, he tried to remember the particulars of his insurance policy, as he handed over a credit card for a $500.00 "co-pay" that the discharge clerk told him his policy required. Ken wondered what other surprises would be coming in the mail and how he would afford it.

On the way home, they swung through the drive-through pharmacy and ended up paying $180.00 for the prescriptions because they were not covered by his insurance plan. The Korgs got home just before the sun came up. Mrs. Korg called Ken's boss and let him know he would not be at work today. Ken crawled into bed and fell asleep, unaware that his adventures were just beginning . . . unaware that he had fallen into the belly of the beast.

NAVIGATING INSIDE THE BEAST

Ken awoke around 1:30 p.m. to the ringing of the doorbell. Apparently, his wife had called the carpet cleaning service to come over and steam clean the vomit out of the bedroom floor. Ken got up and served himself some coffee, adding a splash of non-dairy creamer and a packet of artificial sweetener. As he shook off the cobwebs from the night before, he began to look through the Yellow Pages for a primary care doctor. It was assumed at the ER that he had a primary care doctor, but that wasn't the case. The kids had their pediatrician and Mrs. Korg relied on her OB/GYN for most of her medical needs, but Ken had not had any medical needs up until now.

Ken began by calling the offices that were geographically closest to home. For the first office, the phone rang about seven times before it connected to a voice menu. The menu offered nine different choices that did not fit Ken's need. The last choice was for those seeking to become new patients. Ken pressed "0" and was connected to some horrible background music and a pleasant voice that assured Ken, "We value your time and appreciate your patience." Ken held on line for about 20 minutes before he gave up and went to the next office in the Yellow Pages.

It took two more identical attempts before he connected with a real human at the fourth office he called. The receptionist seemed to be caught off guard, and was curt and irritated. Ken surmised that she had picked up the wrong flashing line by mistake. She asked if Ken could hold, but Ken immediately responded "NO!", and the receptionist realized she would have to see this one through. She asked Ken what health insurance he had. Up until the previous night, Ken would not have known offhand, but after answering that question a dozen times by this point, he was able to immediately answer with the name of his provider. The receptionist, seemingly relieved, informed Ken that their office did not participate with his insurance.

Ken asked what this meant, and the receptionist explained that as out-of-network providers, they could still see Ken as a patient, but his out-of-pocket costs would be much higher and he would have to file all insurance paperwork himself. The receptionist recommended against this as she jokingly told Ken that in their office's experience, his particular company was notorious for providing shoddy customer service. Ken empathized.

He thanked the receptionist, but asked her advice for how to find a primary care doctor who would take his insurance. She told Ken to check with his HR representative at work; they could tell him which providers were "empaneled" with his company's insurance. Ken thanked her and hung up.

Ken then decided to try to contact the offices of the urologist and the surgeon that the ER had referred him to for follow-up. Again, there was more hold music, reassurances about the value of his time, and a long phone menu. This time there was no option that fit Ken's needs, but a reminder that a proper referral from a primary care provider or the ER was required, and a warning that if you are having trouble to go to the ER or call 911. Ken continued to try to get through several more times that afternoon, until finally the phone menu connected Ken to an answering service; apparently the office had closed. Ken thought he may have found an end-around to the byzantine phone service, but was disappointed when the operator could only contact the on-call doctor if Ken was a current patient of the practice. Ken hung up on the operator in disgust.

Just then he felt a twinge of pain in his groin. Not wanting to experience pain like the day before, Ken took one of his prescribed Lortab 10 tablets and waited for relief.

* * *

With the evening setting in and Ken's pain subsiding in a narcotic fog, he and Mrs. Korg and the kids hopped in the car to get some dinner at McDonald's. As they were eating, Ken noticed a pharmacy next door. He decided to check his blood pressure on the machine at the front of the store. Maybe now that things had settled down, his blood pressure may have normalized.

After the cuff finished deflating, Ken stared at the red numbers on the screen: 186/94. He decided to buy a home monitoring blood pressure machine so that he could keep an eye on things until he could see a doctor. Maybe the machine at the drug store just needed calibrating.

As Ken searched the shelves for a blood pressure monitor, he felt the familiar sensation of heartburn after his meal of chicken nuggets and fries. He purchased some Prilosec-OTC along with his blood pressure machine and then went back out to the car where Mrs. Korg and the kids were waiting. Mrs. Korg, seeing the package, asked, "What is that?" Ken answered, "You don't want to know."

That evening, Ken set up his home blood pressure machine and took several readings before bed. Most readings were in the 180s/90s, but two were around 190/110. Ken decided to do a little Internet research on blood pressure before going to bed. He read about the long-term risks of hypertension, but most sources reassured him that if he was asymptomatic there was no need for emergency evaluation. As Ken felt another twinge of pain from his kidney stone, he reminded himself that pain (or just having a kidney stone) may be driving his blood pressure up. He went to bed around 11:30, resolving to visit the urologist's and surgeon's office in person (thereby avoiding the phone labyrinth) to arrange his follow-up. He would also drop into HR to get a list of "preferred providers" so he could establish a family doctor.

Unfortunately, Ken could not fall asleep until after 1 a.m. Unbeknownst to him, the bright blue spectrum light from his computer screen had disrupted his melatonin secretion, which made it nearly impossible to fall asleep.

Ken woke to the sound of the alarm on his iPhone at 6 a.m. He felt hung-over and groggy. He popped a dark roast coffee into the Keurig. When it was done brewing, he threw in some non-dairy creamer and poured in a couple of packets of sweetener. As he drank it, he experienced a little rush of euphoria and felt the cobwebs dissipate. He made another cup in a travel mug and left early for work, without breakfast.

As he drove, he checked his email and calendar on his iPhone. He was excited to see that a two-hour meeting for later in the morning had been cancelled. Ken decided to use this time to drop into the offices of the urologist and the surgeon to arrange his appointments. This would dovetail nicely into lunch. Ken got to work and arranged an appointment with his HR rep at 1:15 p.m. He would be able to get his appointments, have lunch, and line up a family doctor all in one swoop.

Ken's morning went fairly smoothly and was topped off by the likely passage of his kidney stone. As he was getting ready to leave for the urologist, he felt a sharp twinge in his testicle and thought, "Oh no!" He went to the bathroom in case he got sick. He attempted to pee, and felt the pain increase and then suddenly release. As he began to pee, he noted that he was peeing almost pure blood. Then it turned the color of iced tea, and then turned pale yellow. As he finished, he felt some burning and a tiny black speck came out and stuck to the side of the urinal. Ken surmised that this was his kidney stone. He could not believe this tiny thing that looked like a speck of pepper had caused him so much misery. He thought about trying to retrieve it, but decide that was too disgusting and flushed it down the urinal. Ken muttered "good riddance" as it swirled away.

Ken left the building with a new lease on life, knowing that his tormenter was gone.

Ken's first stop was the urologist's office. After a dizzying attempt to navigate the medical center's many parking lots, ambiguous signage, and multiple directories that gave no hint of which way to turn for a given room, he finally made his way into the correct office. Inside, the waiting area was full and a queue of people hovered near the receptionist's window. As he dutifully waited his turn, he looked around the room and noted that the patients waiting seemed bored and annoyed. Old magazines were strewn about and the TV was playing the Dr. Oz show.

Once Ken reached the front of the line, he noticed the receptionist seemed to be ignoring him: she was preoccupied with her computer screen, tapping it repeatedly. After a few minutes, she seemed to complete her task and finally looked up at the exact moment he was glancing at his watch. She registered a look of contempt.

Ken relayed his situation, explaining that he needed to schedule an appointment. The receptionist asked Ken why he had not called to make an appointment. Ken, now irritated, pointed to the bank of flashing phone lines and stated that he had tried for an entire day, but could not get through. The receptionist stared for a moment, and then opened up another window on her computer. She pushed a clipboard filled with forms towards Ken and instructed him to "get to work filling these out" while she began to search for an appointment. Ken could detect a sense of urgency in her voice.

It was almost lunchtime when Ken completed the forms—a lengthy "Notice of Privacy Practices," a slew of insurance questions, and a very small section requesting his clinical information. She smiled and told Ken that the next available appointment was in six months. Ken expressed his disbelief while the receptionist glanced over the forms he had filled out. She seemed relieved as she looked at them, tapped some more on her computer screen, and announced that she could fit him in six weeks. It seemed that the urologist was an in-network provider.

As Ken left the office, he realized his last similar experience was at the DMV. Nonetheless, he felt a sense of victory as he walked toward the elevator towards his next appointment at the surgeon's office.

* * *

It was 12:30 by the time Ken left the medical center, feeling famished. Realizing that he was not going to have time for the drive-through, he stopped at the nearest convenience store to grab a meal bar and a diet soda.

Ken unwrapped the meal bar as he drove off for his meeting at HR. Ken arrived a few minutes early, so he read an old copy of *Men's Health* while he waited to be called in. He perused articles advising him how to get "shredded" in six weeks, how to drive his wife crazy in bed, how to relate to his kids, and how to fine-tune his retirement portfolio. Ken felt inadequate. He rolled his eyes and thought, "I can't even get a damn doctor's appointment in six weeks, much less get ripped."

Ken was called into the HR manager's office. Ken briefly explained his situation and the difficulty he had trying to find a family doctor. Ken told the HR rep that he thought having health insurance meant that his medical bills would be covered, and consequently, finding a doctor would not be a problem. The HR rep simultaneously closed his eyes and rolled them upward. He apparently had heard this before.

He explained that in order to keep their health care costs down, the company sought bids from competing insurance companies. The company selected the bid that provided them the lowest premium costs possible. The insurance company used the low bid to entice most of the employers in the region into contracting with them. Having secured most of the "covered lives" in the region, the insurance company then used their market share in negotiations with the hospitals and doctors in the region. Since the insurance company had captured almost all of the people in the region who were likely to pay their bills, they were able to negotiate rates that were barely above the hospital's and doctor's cost of providing care. Those who could not (or refused to) operate on such a tight margin were the out-of-network providers. If Ken selected someone in network, his insurance would pay the total bill after he paid a co-pay that varied based on the situation (routine visit, emergency care, or preventive care). If Ken selected someone "out of network," the co-pay still applied, but in the case of his policy, only 80 percent of the in network rate would be paid, and Ken would be responsible for the rest.

Ken's head was spinning.

The HR rep handed Ken a list of providers that looked like a Chinese restaurant menu. There was a long listing of in-network providers and a much shorter listing of out-of-network providers. Ken scanned the list. It showed the name of the practice, the name of the doctor (or doctors), the address/phone number, the insurance accepted, and finally the amount of time one would have to wait for an appointment. More than half of the practices listed were followed by the statement "not accepting new patients." The remaining practices all specified that they did not accept Medicaid and were not accepting new Medicare patients. The few practices that took Ken's insurance had a wait time of four to six months. The out-of-network providers showed wait times of four to six weeks.

Ken asked the HR rep why he shouldn't just schedule with an out-of-network provider, saying "paying 20 percent of the bill wouldn't be too bad." The HR rep reminded Ken that the 80 percent that was paid was 80 percent of the discounted amount that in-network providers had agreed upon, and that this amount was barely above operating costs. The bill from the out-of-network practice would be much higher, so Ken would not just be paying the 20 percent, he would also be paying the difference between the discounted and actual rate charge by that practice. Further, most practices required that he pay this on an up-front basis, or on the day of service. The HR rep explained that the practices that simply filed insurance and then later "balance-billed" the patient found that those bills rarely got paid. Most patients just assumed that insurance was covering their visit and were perplexed when a large bill arrived many weeks later.

Furthering the confusion was the fact that both the insurance and the practice sent a statement of what was paid and what was owed, and it was very hard to interpret what was a statement, what was a bill, and how much was paid or owed. The HR rep showed Ken that most of his remaining appointments were with employees who were turned to collections by medical practices because the ensuing confusion had resulted in the balance of their bill not being paid. A couple of employees were having trouble securing a home loan because of being reported to credit agencies showing up on their credit report. The HR rep strongly recommended Ken select an in-network provider just to avoid this kind of headache.

Ken explained that he had issues with high blood pressure and fatty liver and didn't know if it was safe to wait that long. The HR rep suggested Ken secure an appointment and perhaps go see a doctor at the urgent care or ER in the meantime. Ken mentally performed a face-palm as he took the list and shuffled out of the HR rep's office.

Ken got back to his office with about 20 minutes to spare before his next meeting. He looked over the list of practices he got from HR. He thought about the advice he was given about staying in network and decided to start calling some offices on the in network column. He looked them over and started with the office closest to home. The phone rang several times, and then connected to the familiar menu and the pleasant voice assuring him that his time was valuable. He "pressed 5" on the phone menu to schedule a new patient appointment. The mailbox was full and could not accept more messages. Ken returned to the phone menu and "pressed 0" to wait for an actual human. After 10 minutes, Ken had to give up to make it to his meeting.

Ken was preoccupied throughout his meeting. He could not believe that all of his efforts resulted in an appointment with a urologist in six weeks for a kidney stone he had already passed, and an appointment with a surgeon to see about gallstones and a spot on his pancreas that he never even knew he had. Furthermore, he still had not secured a family doctor to address the more basic problems of high blood pressure and the mystery of his fatty liver.

At more than one point, Ken was asked by the chairman of the meeting, "Ken, is this boring you?" Ken was dying to answer honestly, but instead he said, "No sir, I'm sorry."

By the time Ken got out of the meeting and was packing up to go home, he felt so agitated that he realized that this was probably driving up his already high blood pressure. Ken resolved to put it out of his mind for now. Realizing that any help with these issues was going to be weeks or months away, Ken also resolved to take things into his own hands. He needed to lose weight and to eat healthier.

On the way home Ken ran by the grocery store to peruse some of the low-fat, low-sodium microwave dinners. Perhaps he could use these as a first step to lowering his weight, getting the fat out of his liver, lowering his blood pressure, and perhaps even making his gallstones go away. He looked over his options and chose a couple of weeks' worth of sub-500 calorie, low-fat, low-sodium entrées that were approved by the American Heart Association.

* * *

Ken awoke the next morning in his usual groggy state. He decided to check his blood pressure on his home monitor. He tried to perform some deep breathing and relaxation before he actually pressed the button to start the machine. Once he reached his "moment of Zen," he pressed the button and awaited the reading. He looked at the results on the LED readout. The numbers 178/92 were staring back at him. Ken became determined to get an appointment with a family doctor today.

When he got to work and settled at his desk, he dialed the first practice on his list. Again, he waited patiently as he listened to the voice menu. Eventually he "pressed 5" to be put in the queue to schedule a new appointment. Knowing that this would not be answered quickly, he put the phone in speaker mode and went about his tasks.

Ken was feeling quite productive and had almost forgotten about the hold music that was providing the background noise for his morning's work. He had even forgotten that he had been holding most of the morning, but was abruptly reminded when the repetitive music was interrupted by a voice that said, "Sunnyvale Family Practice, can you hold?" Ken snatched the phone off the receiver and yelled, "NO! I've been holding all morning." It was too late: the hold music was back on before he could finish his sentence.

He must have been heard, however, because the woman's voice came back on line in about 30 seconds. Ken explained his situation and his need to establish a family doctor. Silence. About 10 seconds later, the woman on the other end asked Ken about his insurance. Now a veteran, Ken was quick to respond as he already had his insurance card laid out on the desk in front of him. Ken gave the name and policy number, and heard the tapping of keys in the background. Ken inferred he had finally given some information that this person cared about.

After about three minutes of key tapping, the receptionist announced that she could get Ken a new patient appointment in six weeks. Knowing that this was as good as he could hope for, Ken pounced on the appointment. He was reminded to bring all of his insurance information and to fast after midnight the night before in case his provider needed to order any blood work. Ken was thrilled and thanked the receptionist, who in turn flatly thanked Ken and said, equally as flatly, to have a nice day. Ken hung up the phone and thrust both fists in the air in triumph.

But his sense of victory faded quickly as the thought entered his head: "How messed up is it that I am this excited to get an appointment six weeks away for what could be a serious problem?" Ken still felt good. He had done the right thing. He would be getting proper health care.

* * *

It was six weeks later, and the night before the appointment was tough. Starting around 1 a.m. Ken was restless and hungry. He was also "wired and tired" as usual. He very much wanted a few tablespoons of peanut butter and a blast of whipped cream, but he was supposed to be fasting. As a result, he was unable to fall asleep. He was worried about what the doctor would say and if anything serious was going on. He tossed and turned until Mrs. Korg kicked him out onto the couch.

The alarm on his iPhone went off at 5:30 a.m. Instinctively, Ken swiped the face of the phone and shut off the offensively cheerful marimba tone of the alarm. He felt absolutely hammered . . . and hungry. Despite the instructions not to eat or drink anything before his lab work, Ken rationalized if he did not have a cup or two of coffee he would likely fall asleep at the wheel. Ken threw a breakfast blend into the Kuerig and added some Coffee-mate and Splenda to the cup.

Ken arrived at the hospital and came into the front entrance. It was a beautiful lobby with hardwood floors, lined with vibrant paintings of local landmarks on the walls. He asked the very nice retired lady at the volunteer desk for directions. To his surprise, she actually walked him down the corridor and around the corner and said, "Just beyond that row of planters to the right."

Ken felt upbeat as he headed down the hall, but as he approached the row of planters his heart sank. In the waiting area were at least 40 bored and angry-looking people. When he reached the front of the line for the reception desk, he gave his name and birthdate, and was strapped with a wristband before being handed the familiar privacy papers and consent-for-treatment papers he had signed at the other offices. He then looked for an open seat that was not too close to anyone that appeared contagious.

As he sat watching CNN and flipping through outdated copies of "O" magazine with Dr. Oz on the cover, Ken realized, to his relief, that this was a shared waiting area for the laboratory and the radiology department. Ken was called back fairly quickly. A heavyset girl asked him to take a seat in what looked like an old school desk. She snapped a blue rubber tourniquet around his arm, pushed on a vein in the crook of his elbow, and swabbed it with an alcohol prep. Ken's heart raced as he prepared for a needle poke. She approached the area with a plastic tube with a needle on the end. Ken turned his head. Suddenly he felt . . . nothing! Damn, this girl was good! She shoved glass tubes inside the plastic tube and they rapidly filled with his blood. She snapped the tourniquet loose and taped a cotton ball over the puncture site. She said, "You're good to go, the results will be at your doctor's office in about an hour or so." Ken glanced at his watch. Plenty of time to drop by Starbucks.

After scarfing down a grande latte and a large blueberry scone, Ken drove to the doctor's office holding his iPhone on the steering wheel, watching the blue dot that represented his car until it met up with the red pin that represented his destination. The building was in a small complex of doctors' offices. The parking spaces were almost all full and the landscaping was untended and overgrown with weeds. Ken found a parking space and walked to the door marked "Sunnyvale Family Practice."

Ken walked through the door into the waiting area. Everything looked familiar. There were about six people in the waiting area. The way they were seated suggested only three patients, each with a family member. The office was filled with old chairs arranged in groups of three or four with beat-up end tables. On the tables were even older magazines: *WebMD,* *"O,"* and *Prevention* seemed to dominate. Two-thirds of the magazines had pictures of Dr. Oz on them. The TV was playing (you guessed it) the Dr. Oz show.

Once it was his turn, the nurse led Ken into a cubby where she took his temperature, weight, and blood pressure. She shook her head at him and made a "tsk tsk" noise when the LED readout showed 183/94. Ken explained that was why he was here, along with the fatty liver. The nurse tried to make Ken feel better by suggesting he might have white coat hypertension. He didn't bother to tell her he was getting similar readings on his home BP monitor. From there she escorted Ken to an exam room and asked him to strip down to his underwear bottoms and place the gown on with the opening to the back, and that his provider would be in shortly.

Thirty minutes passed and Ken was getting uncomfortable on his perch at the end of the exam table. After 45 minutes, Ken decided to get up and study the anatomy chart hanging on the back of the exam room door. Sure enough, as soon as Ken got close enough to read the lettering on the anatomy chart, the door burst open and nearly hit him in the face.

Ken jumped backwards and felt the cold air rush up the back of his gown. The young lady that opened the door looked visibly irritated that Ken was not on the exam table. Ken shuffled back to his proper place, being careful not to expose his boxers in the process. Once Ken was seated, the young lady introduced herself as Nancy Jones, the nurse practitioner. She explained that she would be performing his initial history and physical exam and that she would be managing his care with input from the doctor. Ken was tempted to say that he had expected an appointment with the doctor, but did not want to rock the boat or insult the nurse practitioner.

The nurse practitioner pulled what she called a "cow" (computer on wheels) up to the exam table and began to ask questions. Ken watched as she ticked off boxes on the computer screen. She did not look up as she asked questions in a rapid-fire manner; most of the questions were of the yes-no variety, and there was not much opportunity to really tell his story. He had a fairly clear view of the screen that she was working on, and found himself disturbed that she was filling in elements of the physical exam even though she had not yet laid a hand on him.

When she was done tapping on the computer screen, she began her exam. She briefly looked in his eyes with an ophthalmoscope and then used her stethoscope to listen on either side of his neck, and then briefly on the front of his chest. Ken found it odd that she had tapped on the body diagram on the computer screen in areas that were not examined. She had entered information on the abdomen, back, and extremities but did not actually end up examining him in these areas. Ken decided to shrug it off.

She then pulled up the results of Ken's lab work and clicked on what he presumed were the abnormal results. When she finished, she told Ken that his blood potassium was a little low, and that his blood sugar was moderately high. His total cholesterol was elevated, as was his LDL and triglycerides. She also said his HDL or "good" cholesterol was not as high as she would like. She explained that he would need to be started on medication for his blood pressure and his cholesterol, and that his fatty liver was due to his elevated cholesterol.

The nurse decided to start Ken on Prinivil (Lisinopril) to lower his blood pressure and Lipitor to lower his cholesterol, and gave him a pamphlet to guide him on the dietary changes needed to improve his blood sugar and cholesterol. The pamphlet looked familiar and included a shopping list that matched what he was already attempting (including the Healthy Choice and Lean Cuisine microwave meals he had already suffered through). She then abruptly got up, shook Ken's hand, and left the room, stating that the nurse would be back shortly with his papers and to help him arrange a follow-up in four to six weeks. She told Ken he could go ahead and get dressed.

Just as Ken got his pants up, the nurse returned with his prescriptions and some computer-generated instructions about hypertension, elevated cholesterol, and the low-fat diet. She had already arranged an appointment date in four weeks. Ken didn't even bother to check his schedule to see if the date was compatible, as he was fearful of losing his appointment. As Ken was leaving, he ran into the doctor in the hallway. He was dressed in jeans and a bright red Hawaiian shirt. He sported a ponytail and an earring. He was friendly and shook Ken's hand, welcoming him to Sunnyvale Family Practice.

SIDE EFFECTS

In the weeks that followed, Ken was feeling a little bit more upbeat. He began taking his blood pressure and cholesterol medicine and was doing fairly well with his low-fat diet. His enthusiasm to get better made him able to surf the waves of hunger that hit him throughout the day. Instructions he received during his kidney stone follow-up revealed that his new diet—low in sodium and fat—already put him on the right track for preventing future kidney stones, and that he didn't need to do anything different. His blood pressure was also trending down nicely, measuring 122/73 at his latest check on his home monitor. Ken finally felt like he was getting on top of his health, and might actually get to see the kids grow up, get married, and have children of their own.

While Ken was pleased with his progress, and his numbers looked better on his home blood pressure monitor, he couldn't help but notice that he just did not feel that good. His muscles ached as if they had been beaten with hammers, and he felt quite weak, especially in his hips and thighs. It was hard to stand up out of a chair without the assistance of his arms. Ken was also having bouts of weakness and shakiness combined with the sweats. It felt like his blood sugar was dropping. Ken was very disciplined with his low-fat diet, and these spells represented the only times Ken was falling off the wagon. When Ken had these spells, the only thing that seemed to help was to scarf down something sweet. These spells were not particularly severe, but their frequency seemed to be increasing.

The other thing Ken noticed was that his libido was gone. Recently, Mrs. Korg, happy that Ken was taking charge of his health, announced that she was feeling amorous. Ken was pleased to oblige, but found himself completely unable to do so. They shrugged it off to fatigue from work and all of the scrambling around to meet appointments, but Ken secretly worried that he would be back at the doctor's office begging for a prescription for a certain little blue pill.

A few mornings after Ken's epic fail in the bedroom, he awoke with a funny sensation of tingling in his lips and tongue. Ken crawled out of bed and went into the bathroom. When he looked in the mirror Ken could not believe the image staring back at him. His lips were massively swollen, and his swollen tongue was protruding between them. He screamed to his wife: "Dit in heah!" Mrs. Korg walked into the bathroom and, oddly, her first reaction was to laugh because Ken looked so ridiculous. It did not take long for her to stop laughing and to become concerned. She asked Ken if he could breathe OK. Ken replied that he was having no problem breathing, he just couldn't talk right. They both realized that if the swelling got much worse, breathing might become a real problem. Mrs. Korg called the Sunnyvale Family Practice on his behalf, since Ken's tongue was interfering with his enunciation. She surfed the automated phone menu (which started off with "if this is an emergency, hang up and dial 911") for five minutes and then held for 10 minutes. When she got through, she explained the situation to the receptionist and asked to speak to the doctor. The receptionist advised her that the doctor was unavailable and that she needed to go directly to the ER or dial 911.

Once they arrived at the ER and walked up to the registration desk, the clerk's eyes bugged out almost as big as Ken's lips. She immediately called the triage nurse to the front. Ken became more concerned when the battle-weary nurse's eyes also bugged out and she immediately walked him back into the ER. Ken was surprised at how many patients were in the back and how much activity was going on, since the parking lot and waiting area had been almost empty. As the nurse walked past the central workstation, she tapped on the glass and pointed at Ken's face. One of the doctors looked up from the computer that he was engrossed in and immediately jumped up. Now Ken was *really* worried.

Ken was brought into a large room and told to sit on the bed. The nurse and an ER tech quickly pulled Ken's shirt over his head and applied three sticky pads to his chest. The tech hooked a red, black, and white wire to the sticky pads and put oxygen on his nose while the nurse put an IV in the crook of his left elbow. Ken could not believe the size of the IV needle, and clamped his butt cheeks together as the nurse forced what felt like a pencil through Ken's skin.

The doctor was standing at the foot of the bed and called out to the nurse which medications he wanted. The nurse seemed to ignore him, and it was evident to Ken that she was already three steps ahead of the doctor. The orders seemed like just a formality. The doctor introduced himself as Dr. Leslie, and Ken tried to lisp that they had met before when he had his kidney stone. The doctor ignored Ken's attempts to speak and tried to use a tongue depressor to look in the back of his mouth.

The doctor asked the nurse to bring a "Krike Tray" and a "4 Shiley" to the bedside and he pulled out a Sharpie pen. The doctor touched Ken's neck, tracing his index finger from the notch of his Adam's apple and then down a short distance to his windpipe. He then took the Sharpie and marked the skin where his index finger was resting.

Dr. Leslie explained that he had just marked the cricothyroid membrane that resides between the Adam's apple and trachea. If Ken's swelling suddenly increased, and they had to perform an emergency procedure to secure his airway, the precise location for the incision would be marked ahead of time.

The nurse opened a large surgical tray next to him. Ken's heart raced as he looked at the scalpel and surgical instruments. As the doctor explained that he was having an allergic reaction called "angioedema," the nurse poked him in the arm with a shot of epinephrine while another nurse pushed a steroid called Decadron, along with Benadryl and Pepcid, through his IV. The doctor explained that this allergic reaction would most likely not respond to the medicines they had just given, but they still give them on the off chance they may help.

Ken's head was spinning, and he tried to think of what he may have eaten or come in contact with that could have caused this. Just then Dr. Leslie asked him, "Are you on any medicines whose names end in 'pril'?" Ken thought for a moment and then realized that his blood pressure medicine was Lisinopril.

When Ken told the doctor, he stated that this was far and away the most likely cause of his angioedema. Dr. Leslie explained that his airway was already quite swollen and that they would be watching it very closely. Dr. Leslie said that if the swelling got any worse in the next half hour, he would recommend an elective intubation—a procedure where he would receive sedation, an instrument would be used to expose his vocal cords, and a plastic tube would be placed in his trachea; he would be on a ventilator until the swelling went down. Dr. Leslie also explained that the swelling of the tongue and lips makes this procedure much more difficult than usual, and this is why the cricothyrotomy tray was sitting next to him. If things worsened and they could not get the breathing tube in, they would make a surgical incision in his neck in order to get his airway secured by that route.

Dr. Leslie tried to be reassuring by telling Ken that these were all just preparations for a worst-case scenario, and that in most cases the swelling would just subside on its own. Ken was not feeling that reassured.

Over the next two hours, Ken sat in the gurney and stared at the cardiac monitor. Mrs. Korg sat in a chair next to the surgical tray that was covered with a green towel. Ken was scared that his heart rate never dropped below 120 on the monitor. Every 15 minutes or so, the doctor would come in and look at his airway. Ken watched through the door as the ER descended into chaos. Paramedics passed by with stretcher after stretcher of some of the sketchiest looking people he had ever seen. It looked like everyone came straight from the "people of Walmart" website.

After two hours, Ken's lips and tongue started to shrink. The doctor was pleased, but wanted to watch Ken longer to make sure he didn't rebound. Within another hour and a half, Ken's lips and tongue were back to their normal size.

Dr. Leslie had already paged the on-call doctor for Sunnyvale and told them what had happened. It had been decided that Ken would be taken off the Lisinopril, and that he would be listed as allergic to ACE inhibitors. In its place, Ken would be started on HCTZ (hydrochlorothiazide) along with a low-dose potassium supplement. Dr. Leslie wrote for a one-month supply of Ken's new medicines and had already arranged a follow-up for recheck at Sunnyvale in three weeks. Ken was disconnected from everything and discharged home. On the drive home, Ken was picking the monitor pads off of his chest when he realized his appointment with the surgeon was tomorrow morning.

Ken went home and had a Healthy Choice microwave dinner while the kids chowed down on the Chick-Fil-A they had picked up on the way home. It took all of Ken's willpower to eat the rubbery green beans while smelling the delectable odor of French fries and fried chicken strips.

By the time Ken finished scanning the Internet about pancreatic nodules that night, he was terrified and struggled to fall asleep.

* * *

Ken was dreaming about his appointment with his surgeon when the marimba tone went off on his iPhone alarm in the morning. He dreamed he was told he had pancreatic cancer and had months to live. As he slowly woke up, he worried that he might be like Randy Pausch of "The Last Lecture" fame. Ken tried to put it out of his mind as he went through the motions of getting ready.

At the surgeon's office, Ken had barely gotten situated on the exam table when the door burst open and a tall, elegant gentleman in a white coat walked up with an outstretched hand saying, "Hi, I'm Dr. Parker." Ken shook hands, and silently worried why he was seeing the doctor instead of a nurse practitioner. Did this mean that something serious was afoot that warranted actual contact with the doctor?

Dr. Parker explained that he had looked at his CT scan and had seen that he does have some calcium-containing gallstones, but the gallbladder showed no signs of inflammation. As he talked, he simultaneously laid Ken back on the table and poked and prodded his belly. Dr. Parker went on to explain that he also saw the nodule on the tail of his pancreas. His voice registered an air of embellished concern that spiked a rush of fear in Ken.

Dr. Parker pulled Ken back to a sitting position and seated himself on a rolling stool at the foot of the exam table. Ken was sitting above Dr. Parker, looking down on him. The meaning of this positioning was almost palpable. Dr. Parker started with some reassurance, stating that it was unusual for pancreatic cancer to appear in this location and that the nodule did not have a typical appearance for pancreatic cancer. Dr. Parker had assumed (correctly) that Ken knew the gravity of that diagnosis. He went on to explain that it may be a benign incidental finding, but it could also represent other types of cancer such as lymphoma.

Finally, Dr. Parker noted that this had been discovered incidentally on a renal stone CT scan that images in 5 mm slices. The fact that the slices were so big creates an opportunity for the computer to misinterpret as it reconstructs the data into two-dimensional images. He therefore suggested repeating a CT scan on a machine with more imaging detectors and with thinner slices of 1 mm. Dr. Parker also recommended that Ken get his study done at an outpatient imaging center rather than at the hospital. He felt their equipment was superior, and the cost was much less than what the hospital would charge.

Dr. Parker walked Ken to the front desk and signed a request form, telling the receptionist to schedule Ken's CT scan. The receptionist asked what times were best for Ken while she was waiting for the phone to pick up at the imaging center. Within a few minutes, Ken was scheduled for his CT scan for the next day and for a follow-up appointment with Dr. Parker in one week. She said that Dr. Parker would have the results called to him, and that he would call Ken with results and any further instructions.

Ken left the office concerned, but impressed with how smoothly everything went. He got the distinct impression that the surgeon was used to getting things his way. The response from the outpatient imaging center was much more like Nordstrom's compared to what he experienced trying to arrange his appointments. His upbeat mood faded, however, when he began to notice the aching in all of his muscles and how generally fatigued he was. Ken reflected on the fact that, while he was not feeling well when this all started, he actually felt better when his blood pressure was high and his cholesterol was untreated.

When Ken got to work, the first thing he did was rearrange his schedule to allow for his CT scan the following morning. His boss and the secretary were visibly irritated. It was clear everyone was getting tired of Ken's medical issues. Ken silently worried that his promotion, or perhaps even his job, might be in danger. But the possibility of pancreatic cancer weighed heavy on Ken's mind, and he realized that he had to do whatever it took to get this issue resolved. Ken dragged through the rest of his work day, distracted by what tomorrow would bring.

THE FINAL STRAW

Ken showed up at Valley View Imaging Center at 9 a.m. He was expecting the usual waiting room and registration process. However, when he walked in, he almost wondered if he was in the wrong place. The interior looked much more like a high-end law firm that you see in the movies. The floor was a beautiful hardwood, and the furniture looked like it belonged in a mansion. Gone were the rows of Office Depot chairs and out-of-date magazines. Instead there were leather couches and chairs with glass-top coffee tables and end tables. There was an incredible selection of up-to-date magazines ranging from *Sports Illustrated* to *Architectural Digest*, none of which had Dr. Oz's face on the cover. The TV was a gigantic flat screen hanging on the front wall. There were several aquariums with exotic fish. Ken walked up to the desk and was immediately greeted by a well-dressed receptionist. The only disappointment Ken had was being handed the usual privacy disclosure and insurance forms.

Ken sat down and quickly filled out the papers. He did not have much time to enjoy the luxury, as he was called back within a couple of minutes. The radiologist briefly introduced himself as Dr. Harvey and explained the procedure. He told Ken that an IV would be started to give contrast that would make the blood vessels and blood flow easier to visualize. He asked if Ken had any allergies, especially to iodine or seafood. Ken stated that his only allergy was to ACE inhibitors and recounted what had happened to him. The radiologist stated that this should not be a problem, especially since this was a known side effect of the medicine and not necessarily a true allergy. He asked if Ken had any questions, but after his renal stone CT at the ER, he felt like he knew the drill and he told Dr. Harvey, "Nope, let's go."

Ken lay down on the CT scan table and the technician started an IV in the crook of his left elbow. It was minimally uncomfortable. The tech hooked a coiled tube to his IV that led to a large plastic bottle and plunger apparatus that looked like a giant syringe. Ken was then shuttled back and forth on the sliding table, while the gantry on the giant donut he were sliding through spun in circles. Ken felt as if he was being prepared for time travel.

After the technician got all of the necessary coordinates, she warned Ken that he was about to receive a "test bolus" of the IV dye. The coiled tubing shook a little and Ken felt a warm flush at the IV site running up his arm, followed by a metallic taste in his mouth. The tech asked Ken if he felt OK, to which Ken answered "yes."

The tech told Ken that the scan would now commence. A computerized voice said, "Hold. Your. Breath," while a Pac-Man-like icon on top of the passageway into the donut appeared holding its breath. The coil of tubing shook and Ken felt an intense fluttering at the IV site. He then felt the warm flush of the contrast run up his arm, then into his neck and chest. He got a more intense metallic taste than he experienced on the test dose. As the full contents of the giant glass syringe emptied into his body, he slid through the donut hole on the table. The warm flush of the contrast spread throughout his body, tracing the blood vessels along the way, finally culminating in Ken's groin with a sensation as if he had just peed his pants. As the warmth of the IV contrast faded, the table slid back out of the donut hole and the test was over.

The tech told Ken, "Just relax a minute while I check the quality of the images." Ken lay quietly on the table, hoping that the test would bring good news. Just as the tech walked in to ask how Ken was feeling, Ken got the intense sensation of ants stinging his scalp. Before Ken could assess what was happening, the sensation spread into his neck, as well as the bend of his knees and elbows. By the time the tech arrived at the side of the scanner, Ken felt an intense burning and itching all over his body and he felt like a boa constrictor was around his chest. Ken looked up at the tech, and was alarmed when the tech actually said out loud, "Oh shit!"

At this point, Ken felt his windpipe suddenly narrow down to the size of a coffee swizzle stick. Between the weight of his chest and the narrowing in his trachea, Ken could barely breathe. He looked over at the technician, who had stumbled backwards and was frantically hitting a large red button on the wall. Ken could not talk, but looked at the technician with eyes that pleaded "please don't let me die." The tech's eyes were as wide as saucers, and they in turn pleaded "please don't let him die."

Ken turned all of his attention inward. His total being was focused on moving air in and out. He did not think of Mrs. Korg. He did not think of the kids. All he could think about was moving air back and forth through a tiny passageway. The radiologist came into the room and announced that 911 had already been called. The tech opened a small Tupperware box and drew up a dose of Benadryl and gave it through Ken's IV. Ken started to develop tunnel vision, and all of the commotion became a distant noise, as if he were hearing it all from underwater. Ken could feel his life slipping away. Flashes of his past went through his consciousness like a highlight reel, and he felt as if he were floating up out of his body.

Ken's vantage point for the entire drama unfolding vacillated between lying on the CT table and floating in the corner of the room. He watched with a now detached interest as the paramedics came into the room. They felt for a pulse in his neck and noted it was barely palpable. They argued briefly about whether to give the epinephrine through the IV or IM. They immediately decided to give it IM and go to IV dosing if it didn't work. They then rapidly gave an IV steroid (solumedrol), put on an oxygen mask, and started another IV. Two large bags of IV fluids were attached and each paramedic squeezed a bag to increase the flow of fluids into Ken's body.

The first thing Ken noted was that his attitude was no longer detached. He now cared about the outcome. Even before re-entering his body, Ken decided then and there that if he got through this, he was never again going to engage the medical system. Just as he began to wonder if he was in the bargaining stage of death and dying, he felt his consciousness being sucked back into his body. Suddenly everything was integrated again and the commotion rose to full volume. Ken took his first deep breath in what felt like an eternity, and everything around him seemed to be in a state of relief. One of the paramedics announced that his blood pressure was 100/56 and his pulse oximetry was now 95 percent. The other paramedic listened to his lungs and noted the wheezing, though still present, was much improved.

Ken was moved from the CT table to the ambulance stretcher, carried hammock-style in the sheet he was lying on. The radiologist and the tech walked out to the ambulance with Ken and the paramedics. Dr. Harvey told Ken that his wife had already been contacted and was on the way to the ER; Mrs. Korg apparently had reassured Dr.

Harvey she knew the route there. As Ken was pushed into the back of the ambulance, he made another decision. Not only would he never enter the belly of the medical beast again, he was going to take charge of his own health. He didn't know exactly how, but he new that he would find a way. He had done a test because he was worried he might be dead in a year, but nearly died today. He had gone into the abyss and came back, and he thought to himself: "I'm done with this shit."

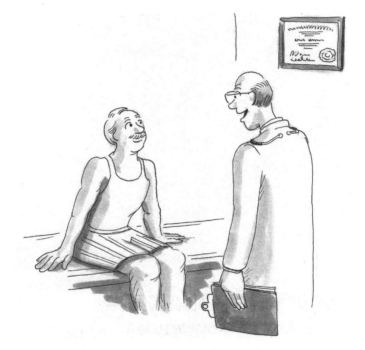

"If everyone was as healthy as you
I'd be out of business."

Chapter 9

LEAD BY YOUR (PRIMAL) EXAMPLE

"[H]ealth policy experts know that we see at best only weak aggregate relations between health and medicine, in contrast to apparently strong aggregate relations between health and many other factors, such as exercise, diet, sleep, smoking, pollution, climate, and social status. . . .For example, [one study] found large and significant lifespan effects: a three year loss for smoking, a six year gain for rural living, a ten year loss for being underweight, and about fifteen year losses each for low income and low physical activity (in addition to the usual effects of age and gender)."
—George Mason University economist Robin Hanson[1]

"The only field more self-confidently but just as regularly wrong as economics is nutrition, whose recommendations to shun butter/margarine or red meat/carbohydrates regularly reverse themselves."
—Physicist and Goldman Sachs "quant" Emanuel Derman[2]

Although we are presenting views in this book that some might describe as "radical," our mission is educational. We don't want you to go "do something" except to take steps to promote your own health and that of your family. If you are concerned about the direction of the country, as you should be, then the single best thing you can do for its future is to make sure your household is healthy.

For the vast majority of Americans, staying healthy is far more important than timing the stock market or inflation-proofing your portfolio. Your most productive asset is your body: especially in a sluggish economy, a debilitating sickness is not only expensive directly, but also in terms of lost wages and career advancement. Of course, there are many problems the country faces besides its crippled health care delivery, but if you or your loved ones fall ill, that's going to dwarf everything else. As we're constantly reminded in the safety review before a flight, in the event of an emergency, you need to first take care of yourself so that you are able to help others.

In light of the very depressing narrative we gave in the first two parts of this book, we're happy to report that there is an answer. We can return to a way of eating and living in which we're genetically, physically, and mentally adapted to thrive. In particular, we're trumpeting the "primal" lifestyle developed by Mark Sisson, whose work combines modern science with our ancient roots to create a powerfully health-promoting way of living. The tenets of a primal lifestyle—which include centering your diet on the nutrient-rich plants and animals we are evolutionarily adapted to consume, engaging in both low-intensity and high-intensity activity, lifting heavy things, and getting adequate sleep and sunlight—will help safeguard you against preventable illness and modern disease, reducing your chance of needing medical care in the first place.

Ever since the "evolutionary discordance" hypothesis was proposed 25 years ago, randomized controlled trials have begun to confirm the value of hunter-gatherer diets as protective against disease, even as compared to diets routinely recommended by the medical establishment.[3] The sheer value of this information for your health cannot be overstated. While nearly all of us will someday require medical care due to forces largely beyond our control—such as infections, car accidents, or unexpected injury—the reality remains that for many Americans, health care is mostly a matter of "chronic disease care." In modern times, a full 75 percent of the nation's health care costs stem directly from chronic conditions, with three of the most expensive being heart disease, cancer, and mental disorders.[4] To avoid the disease-stricken fate so many will succumb to is to grant yourself freedom from a lifetime of needless pain and expense.

For a full discussion of the primal lifestyle (and guidance for implementing its principles), we refer you to Mark Sisson's website www.marksdailyapple.com along with his bestselling book, *The Primal Blueprint*. Although we will be touching upon the most salient parts of primal living as they relate to health care and disease prevention, these resources offer a far more detailed exploration of the primal laws than we can provide in these pages, particularly for readers seeking a clear-cut starting point for their journey to medical independence.

For our purposes here, we will focus on the ways in which health care costs can be substantially reduced—both on an individual and national level—through the adoption of primal diet and lifestyle practices. Furthermore, by protecting yourself and your family from the biggest chronic diseases in the Western world, you can minimize the hours, days, and even years you might otherwise spend entangled in our unwieldy and inefficient medical system. The simple act of eating and living in accordance with your genes can thus save you a resource even more valuable than money: your time.

You may have heard the argument that the "costs" of healthy living—paying more for higher-quality food, purchasing a gym membership or exercise equipment, taking nutritional supplements, investing in a water filter, and so forth—will be offset by having fewer health care expenses later down the road. While true, few discussions put an actual sticker price on these savings. We will use this chapter to examine the most pervasive diet- and lifestyle-related diseases in America, discussing their cost upon the nation and revealing the ways in which primal living may be better "health insurance" than anything you or your employer could ever purchase.

THE TEN PRIMAL BLUEPRINT LAWS

The foundation of getting out and staying out of the belly of the health care beast is rooted in Mark Sisson's book, *The Primal Blueprint* (and elaborated on in his follow-up book, *The Primal Connection*). This approach offers a collection of ten "laws" that you can incorporate in your day-to-day life to optimize the signals you send to your genes, allowing you to live as vibrantly and healthfully as possible. Although we won't ask you to walk around with a club and loincloth to reenact the lives of your distant ancestors, we encourage you to see the wisdom of viewing our modern health care crisis from an ancestral and evolutionary lens, which clarifies both the problems we face and the solutions we can choose. A summary of the ten Primal Blueprint laws is as follows.

1. Eat Lots of Plants and Animals. Across the globe, our early ancestors ate diverse diets influenced by their particular climate, geographic location, available plants and animals, and cultural traditions. Although there many combinations of foods and macronutrients could fall under the umbrella of primal eating, a diet based on "single ingredient" vegetables, grass-fed meats, seafood, tubers, fruit, full-fat dairy, nuts, and seeds will provide the fuel necessary for optimizing your health.

2. Avoid Poisonous Things. Some of the substances that are truly harmful to the human body are not found under the kitchen sink, but exist directly in our food supply. In modern times, the toxic items worth avoiding are mostly man-made and include things like soda, candy, and other sugar-laden or heavily processed foods. Others are chemically altered fats used for frying. Less obvious are the things that have been marketed to us as healthy but are anything but—including grains, even in their whole form. Exploring **www.marksdailyapple.com** will provide more background on how grains and other foods touted by "conventional wisdom" can contribute to modern disease.

3. Move Frequently at a Slow Pace. Anthropological evidence suggests that ancient man spent a lot of time at leisure, but this does not mean he was sedentary. Instead, he moved around a lot, but at a very low level of intensity that most of us would not consider exercise or exertion. This backdrop of activity seems to be a prerequisite for the signaling that leads to ideal body composition and the prevention of chronic disease.

4. Lift Heavy Things. Our ancient past featured plenty of lifting, hauling, carrying, and climbing as part of basic day-to-day survival. For men and women alike, the benefits of strength training are no less powerful now than they were back then: brief, intense muscle contractions help trigger beneficial hormones, increase muscle size and strength, improve insulin sensitivity, and protect against a spectrum of modern diseases.

5. Sprint Once in Awhile. Our early ancestors did not have the luxury of hopping in a car to outrun a threat or chase down their prey: sporadic bouts of sprinting were a normal part of life. Incorporating sprints into your routine—while running, bicycling, rowing, swimming, or doing any other form of exercise that allows for rapid acceleration—can boost fat oxidation (the burning of body fat) and provide neurohormonal benefits.

6. Get Adequate Sleep. We evolved in an environment where our sleep/wake cycles were guided by the rise and fall of the sun. We are forever tied to our circadian heritage. Sleep obtained in accordance with this ancient rhythm promotes the release of hormones and neurochemicals critical to repair and rejuvenation; much of the body's cellular repair occurs during sleep.

7. Play. Both ancient humans and modern hunter-gatherers generally work fewer hours than the average American and spend more time "playing"—a form of social interaction that encourages physical movement, problem solving, interpersonal skills, and bonding. Engaging in play can help counteract the stress of work by triggering the release of feel-good chemicals called endorphins.

8. Get Adequate Sunlight. Sun exposure is a major part of our nutrition, especially our acquisition of vitamin D, which has powerful hormonal and immunological effects. While vitamin D supplementation can be helpful, there is a growing body of evidence showing that a given vitamin D level acquired by sunlight provides benefits that a given level of vitamin D acquired by supplementation cannot. Exposure to sunlight will improve your immune system and decrease your risk for cancer and cardiovascular disease, helping to shield you from the problems we have discussed in the US health care system.

9. Avoid Stupid Mistakes. Just as many early humans "weeded themselves out of the gene pool" by engaging in risky behavior and dying young, modern humans, too, can end up with severe injury or worse by making what we will call "stupid mistakes." In modern times, these include texting while driving, diving into pools of water of unknown depth, cutting down trees with a chainsaw when you are not a trained professional, getting on your roof to hang Christmas lights, driving while intoxicated, and a long scroll of other activities that could cause needless harm.

10. Use Your Brain. A hallmark of the human species is our large, hungry, and active brain, and just because we've arrived at the top of the food chain doesn't mean we should stop using it. Parallel to Law 2 of "Avoid Poisonous Things," we should strive to ration the time spent passively absorbing information from social media, advertising, the Internet, television, the news, and other sources of largely superficial content. We should instead be defending our mental space for meaningful thought, focus, and deeper self-awareness.

TYPE II DIABETES

In 2012, *Diabetes Care* published a truly alarming report entitled "Economic Costs of Diabetes in the US in 2012."[5] Between 2007 and 2012, the national cost of diabetes skyrocketed from $174 billion to $245 billion, with $176 billion of the more recent figure coming from direct medical expenses such as office visits, antidiabetic agents and supplies, hospital inpatient care, and prescription medications to treat complications of the disease. Over 29 million Americans currently have diabetes, and the harsh reality for upcoming generations is that an estimated one in three people will have developed the condition by the year 2050. If you become diabetic, you can expect to add an average of $7,900 to your annual medical expenses.[6]

Although these numbers may seem dismal, a primal diet and lifestyle assaults type II diabetes on multiple fronts and can help eliminate what is truly an unnecessary and preventable disease. A major benefit is the avoidance of refined carbohydrates, which include the breads, pastas, cereals, pastries, sodas, and processed sweeteners comprising much of the modern American diet. Our method of processing grains by crushing them into digestible powder creates a rapidly absorbed form of carbohydrate, in turn overwhelming our carbohydrate-storing capacity and causing an overproduction of free fatty acids. This, combined with our modern lifestyle of chronic energy surplus and sedentary living, makes insulin less effective and forces the body to secrete more of it. Insulin spikes and chronically elevated insulin levels are very foreign to our genes, and result in a signal of energy storage that causes us to be very efficient at fat storage and simultaneously unable to use it for energy. Along with its contribution to obesity (a major diabetes risk factor), this process can progress to type II diabetes for those who are genetically susceptible, with a gradual loss of beta cell function in the pancreas contributing to worsening glucose tolerance. By removing these highly digestible carbohydrates and replacing them with primal sources of slow-digesting starches, protein, and natural fats, you will be abolishing one of the key ingredients in the development of this disease.

Another primal tenet—moving frequently at a slow pace—also has a direct effect on diabetes risk. There is mounting evidence that walking improves insulin sensitivity above and beyond what can be achieved with diet. Researchers demonstrated this by comparing diet alone to diet plus daily walking in patients with adult onset (type II) diabetes. They found that metabolic clearance of glucose, a marker of insulin sensitivity, was improved in the group that incorporated walking but not in the group that relied on diet alone.[7]

The impact of a primal lifestyle upon diabetes has been corroborated by multiple scientific trials. As early as 1984, a study of diabetic Australian Aborigines showed significant improvements in glucose control, fasting blood sugar, and triglycerides after participants moved from a standard Western diet to a traditional hunter-gatherer way of life.[8] More recently, trials on type II diabetics have confirmed that paleo-style diets can elicit improvements in glycemic control and cardiovascular risk factors associated with diabetes.[9]

Imagine the impact upon the health care system and individual well being if the $245 billion currently syphoned into diabetes care was absolved by simply returning to a lifestyle compatible with our genes.

CARDIOVASCULAR DISEASE

Cardiovascular diseases—including heart disease, stroke, and hypertension (high blood pressure)—represent the leading cause of death in America for both men and women. As of 2010, the CDC reports that cardiovascular diseases contribute to $444 billion of the nation's annual health care costs, and that treatment for these diseases amounts to almost 17 percent of total health care spending.[10] As a greater proportion of the population ages, those numbers will only climb higher and place an increasingly heavy burden upon the public.

On an individual level, the numbers are equally alarming: in 2011, the average cost of a coronary bypass graft—used to treat severe heart disease—was approaching $40,000; pacemaker insertion or replacement was over $35,000; and heart valve procedures were approximately $52,000.[11] Add to this the cost of statins, doctors visits, heart scans, blood work, and blood thinning or hypotensive medications and it becomes clear that developing heart disease (and managing it through mainstream medicine) is expensive on many fronts.

As with diabetes, cardiovascular diseases are largely a result of diet and lifestyle factors within our own control. You may be familiar with the conventional wisdom stating that heart disease is a product of high cholesterol, and that lowering your levels to within "officially defined" limits—either by eating a low-fat, high carbohydrate diet or by accepting a lifelong course of statins—is the way to treat it. This outdated model fails to incorporate other significant steps in heart disease etiology, such as inflammation and oxidation, that happen to be vastly improved by the application of primal principles.

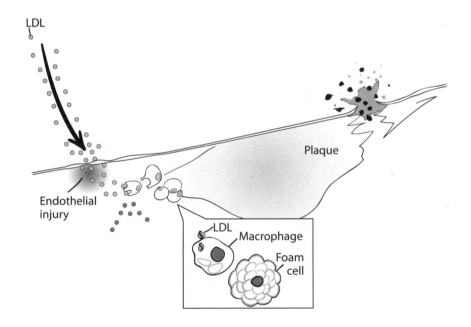

Generally, LDL (often called "bad" cholesterol) present in the blood-stream is most harmful when it becomes oxidized, a process in which the lipid layer surrounding the LDL particle reacts with free radicals and undergoes modification. Once oxidized, LDL particles can cause tissue injury, trigger inflammatory processes, turn white blood cells into atherogenic "foam cells," and cause secretion of sticky adhesion molecules that pull those foam cells into the artery walls. This cascade of effects leads to the formation of arterial plaque and a progressive development of heart disease.

Along with smoking and uncontrolled diabetes, a major contributor to oxidized LDL is a high intake of polyunsaturated fats (PUFAs), especially omega-6 fatty acids. This is due in part to their chemical instability. On a molecular level, the fragile double bonds in PUFAs leave them more prone to free radical attack than saturated or monounsaturated fatty acids, which have more oxidation-resistant structures. When excessive PUFAs are consumed and incorporated into the lipid layers of LDL particles, those particles in turn become vulnerable to oxidation. In contrast to omega-3 PUFAs, which provide enough anti-inflammatory properties to counteract their chemical instability, omega-6 fats are pro-inflammatory and may contribute to cardiovascular diseases through pathways beyond just LDL oxidation.[12]

Here is where a primal diet can provide effortless and automatic correction of a major instigator of heart disease. By avoiding the two most common sources of omega-6 fats for Americans, refined vegetable oils and grains, a primal diet will dramatically lower omega-6 intake and help protect against LDL oxidation and systemic inflammation. The antioxidants supplied by high quality vegetables, fruits, and grass-fed animal products may likewise reduce free radical damage by keeping your LDL particles antioxidant-replete. To date, studies conducted on paleolithic diets confirm they improve cardiovascular risk factors such as blood pressure and lipid profiles, even in the absence of weight loss.[13]

Although some people are more genetically susceptible to heart disease than others, such as those with familial hypercholesterolemia, the reduction of cardiovascular antagonists and increase in protective nutrients will go a long way to reduce your risk and keep you out of the medical labyrinth. What's more, your efforts to ward off cardiovascular disease will help decrease the astronomical costs crippling the nation's health care system.

CANCER

In the span of a lifetime, approximately 1 in 2 men and 1 in 3 women will develop cancer. For the year 2015, a projected 1.6 million Americans will be diagnosed with cancer and nearly 590,000 will die from it.[14] Along with the physical, emotional, and psychological turmoil resulting from diagnosis and treatment, cancer places a significant economic burden upon the country, costing $88.7 billion annually in direct expenses from the disease.[15]

Only 5 to 10 percent of cancer cases are considered genetic in origin, with the other 90 to 95 percent owing to technically "preventable" causes such as tobacco, stress, obesity, physical inactivity, and food.[16] In fact, as many as 35 percent of all cancer cases may be rooted in diet.[17] These astounding figures suggest that our national focus on "race for a cure" fundraising and pharmaceutical treatments may be better spent improving the way we live and eat.

To be clear, we are not promoting a "blame the victim" mentality for those who have been diagnosed with cancer, nor suggesting anyone should feel personally guilty for their condition. You have probably heard anecdotes of health-conscious individuals who "did everything right," avoided smoking, ate pristine diets, exercised daily, and still developed cancer, while others engaged in risky behaviors throughout life and remained free from the disease. Yet for the sake of our discussion on health care, we should embrace the view that cancer has many modifiable contributors and there is much we can do to reduce our risk.

Several elements of the primal lifestyle can lower your exposure to carcinogens as well as boost your body's innate defense system. Getting sufficient sleep, sunlight, and exercise all independently contribute to a reduction in cancer risk.[18,19,20] As with cardiovascular disease, a balanced omega 3/omega 6 ratio, easily obtained by the primal tenets of avoiding vegetable oils and grains, may help suppress cancer progression. In particular, the unique effects of omega-3 fats—which include inhibiting cell growth, halting the transformation of normal tissue into malignant tumors, and counteracting the inflammatory effects of omega-6—may be protective against breast cancer, colon cancer, and potentially prostate cancer.[21]

In animal models, many additives used in processed foods have been shown to cause precancerous DNA damage, and the effects in humans may be similar. Even at low doses, food dyes can damage gastrointestinal organs, while certain fungicides, preservatives, and artificial sweeteners appear to do the same—leading some scientists to call for more targeted research on the safety of such additives for human use.[22] Although reading endless ingredients labels on packaged foods in attempt to avoid known or likely carcinogens would be laborious, simply adhering to primal dietary principles—eating plants and animals as they more or less appear in nature—eliminates these harmful additives by default.

You may have heard fear mongering about red meat raising cancer risk. However, studies that differentiate based on cooking method and meat type suggest it is mainly processed meat and meat cooked at high temperatures that are involved in this link.[23,24] Chemicals called heterocyclic amines (HAs) and polycyclic aromatic hydrocarbons (PAHs) are formed by exposing meat to high temperatures or open flames; these chemicals appear to be mutagenic (causing DNA damage) and could plausibly contribute to cancer risk.[25] Using gentler cooking methods allows you to reap the benefits of high quality animal products without creating dangerous compounds.

Moreover, many plant foods embraced by the primal philosophy have known anti-cancer properties, most notably alliums (including garlic, leeks, scallions, and onions) and cruciferous vegetables (including broccoli, cauliflower, kale, and cabbage). Alliums are believed to owe their effects to organosulfur compounds that modulate enzyme activities, support free radical scavenging, inhibit cancerous mutation, and suppress tumor growth.[26] Likewise, crucifers are rich in glucosinolates, which can block chemical carcinogenesis and reduce susceptibility to environmental carcinogens—particularly after the glucosinolates are converted into isothiocyanates by gut flora.[27] These foods could be thought of as "edible health insurance" due to their powerful impact on immunity and cancer prevention.

Although there is no guaranteed way to cancer-proof yourself or your loved ones, the elements of a primal lifestyle should be considered the first line of defense in preventing this physically and financially devastating disease.

OSTEOPOROSIS

By the year 2025, the cost of osteoporosis-related fractures is estimated to surpass $25 billion—growing rapidly from its current $19 billion as the American population ages.[28] Yet despite its prevalence and high economic burden, osteoporosis remains shrouded in mythology. Conventional wisdom continues to shout at us to "drink your (skim) milk for stronger bones," a message created and propagated by a powerful dairy lobby that offers little help for those actually suffering from the disease. Far from sporting a milk moustache, living primally may be the best defense.

Among the many ways in which primal living benefits bone health, one of the biggest involves vitamin K2, a little-known nutrient critical for protecting against osteoporosis. Studies on vitamin K2 suggest it helps stimulate bone formation, suppress bone resorption (the breakdown of bone tissue), and sustain bone mineral density at critical points in the body.[29] It also works synergistically with vitamins A and D to ensure calcium is deposited into bone tissue instead of arteries, where it may further contribute to heart disease.[30]

Vitamin K2 is found abundantly in liver, butter, high-quality cheeses, egg yolks, and a variety of meats. As a result of national dietary guidelines calling for a reduction in saturated fat and cholesterol, many foods highest in vitamin K2 have been categorically eliminated from the American menu, leaving many people with insufficient intake to support optimal bone health. Fortunately, these nutrient-dense animal foods are wholly embraced by the primal lifestyle, which encourages "nose to tail" eating and reintroduces many products that have been stigmatized by mainstream dietary advice.

Here the primal law of "get adequate sunlight" confers more than just a nice tan. The role of vitamin D in supporting bone health is undisputed, and keeping your levels in the optimal range can help prevent bone loss and subsequent breaks.[31] Additionally, the primal guideline to "lift heavy things," which we will discuss in more depth towards the end of this chapter, is imperative for maintaining bone mass, as well as for developing the balance and strength needed to prevent falls that could lead to fracture.[32]

Although bone density naturally decreases as we get older, osteoporosis need not be an inevitable part of aging. Optimal nutrition and exercise habits, as guided by our ancient roots, can help safeguard against the physical and financial repercussions of thinning bones.

OBESITY

US obesity statistics are nothing short of staggering, with approximately two-thirds of adults considered at least overweight and a full third qualifying as obese.[33] These astronomical rates are reflected in America's health care burden: costs directly related to obesity have surpassed $147 billion annually, encompassing nearly 10 percent of total medical spending.[34] That number is anticipated to reach $344 billion in 2018 if the trends set in motion over previous decades continue into the future.[35] With obesity sitting at the root of many other chronic conditions, curbing the crisis is imperative.

The primal philosophy offers a novel—or perhaps more accurately, ancient—approach to fighting obesity. Rather than attempting to override the body's hunger signals through counting calories, relying on packaged "diet" foods, or embarking on unsustainable quick fixes that rapidly shed water weight, the primal lifestyle tackles obesity from the inside out. The focus on modulating insulin production, becoming a "fat burner" rather than a carb burner, and eating nutritionally dense foods ultimately helps to mobilize fat stores and reduce excess body weight. In contrast to the modern American menu filled with rapidly digesting grain products and sugar, primal eating embraces satiating protein, fat, and slow digesting carbohydrates from whole plant foods. The simple advice to "eat lots of plants and animals" results in a cascade of changes that support a return to a healthier body composition.

Of course, primal eating involves not just the content of the diet, also but the pattern with which it is consumed. Our ability to store and mobilize body fat is rooted in the fact that our ancient ancestors ate sporadically, a stark contrast to the frequent eating and snacking habits of today. This intermittent eating pattern was one of necessity. Because of food scarcity related to seasonal and climatic variation, we evolved the capability to store body fat during times of abundance and to tap into these energy stores during times of scarcity. This adaptation has proven harmful in our modern environment of food novelty and abundance, which has eliminated the "famine" part of the feast-famine cycle that helped sculpt our genome. By eating in a pattern more in line with that of our ancestors, we become capable of skipping meals without hunger and tapping into our fat stores to reduce body weight.

The evidence for primal-style eating as a boon for weight loss extends beyond just theory. In 2007, a short-term trial of paleolithic eating led to spontaneous calorie reduction, as well as improved blood pressure, BMI, and waist circumference.[36] Likewise, a 2010 trial confirmed that on a per-calorie basis, a paleo-style diet is more satiating than a Mediterranean diet, leading to effortless reductions in energy intake.[37]

A primal way of moving can also benefit body weight and composition. This includes the simple but important activity of walking. Anyone who takes up a walking program will experience the positive benefit of fat loss and improved insulin sensitivity, and this may occur not only because of the activity burning off calories, but also because it is sending a familiar signal to our ancient genes that are accustomed to a large amount of low intensity activity. When we engage in frequent low intensity movement, there is a signal that favors leanness, because there is now a diminishing marginal utility to fat storage. Gypsies travel light for a reason: having numerous possessions in storage is of little value if you have to drag it along with you every time you pull up stakes. In a similar vein, even in an environment of food scarcity, the advantage of stored energy in the form of body fat may become less valuable if you have to expend energy hauling it around during frequent daily movement. The signal of repeated low intensity activity reinforces behaviors that optimize body composition. It's not about calories burned versus calories consumed; it's about correct signaling, and this process is key in the fight against obesity.

In 2006, each obese American averaged $1,429 more in medical spending than normal weight individuals.[38] Every effort made to live in accordance with your genes and achieve a healthy weight and body composition will result in less money out of your own pocket as well as that of the nation, not to mention a lifetime of reduced disease risk.

OTHER AILMENTS

As you may quickly discover, following primal tenets can impact conditions you never expected were related to diet or lifestyle, but that together contribute significantly to your health care needs. These include everything from eczema to migraines, asthma, sleep disorders, slow healing and recovery time, pain, and other issues that range from minor nuisances to true disturbances, and which often result in drug prescriptions and time-consuming doctor visits. Upon adopting the ten primal laws, some people see improvements in conditions such as these and find that many of their "minor" health care needs suddenly dissolve. Eye and reproductive health may improve as a result of the higher retinol content of many primal foods—particularly the liver, egg yolks, and full-fat dairy shunned by conventional wisdom but embraced by an ancestral approach to eating. The primal diet's lower glycemic load, a result of excluding rapidly digesting carbohydrates, may potentially benefit acne.[39] The avoidance of inflammatory foods can improve joint health and a spectrum of other issues.

In addition, some people see improvement in mental health as a result of simple changes in diet and lifestyle. In the context of our discussion of health care, this issue deserves extra attention: over 18 percent of American adults suffer from some form of mental illness, and pharmaceutical treatments contribute significantly to annual health care costs.[40] For instance, as of 2011, the CDC reported that 11 percent of Americans above the age of 12 take antidepressant medication, with 254 million prescriptions written annually and national spending nearing $10 billion per year for these drugs alone.[41] Although the causes of mental illness are complex and not always physical or nutritional in nature, there is little doubt that diet and lifestyle can play a role in both the progression and treatment of these disorders. For people with celiac disease, symptoms of anxiety tend to decrease with the avoidance of gluten, a natural consequence of grain-free primal eating.[42] Exercise interventions have long been used as treatment for depression and anxiety, lending credence to the primal laws of "Move Frequently at a Slow Pace," "Sprint Sometimes," and "Lift Heavy Things."[43] The endorphin release triggered by positive social interaction and "play" may also boost mood, as can reduced fructose intake for individuals suffering from fructose malabsorption.[44]

We realize it is unrealistic to expect an entire nation to take upon the diet and lifestyle changes necessary to reduce America's health care burden, just as it is unrealistic to expect sudden change in a health care system that has spent decades in a state of decline. We can only hope to convince you that living in accordance with your genes will greatly reduce your likelihood of needing health care, and may save you from the painful and expensive medical fate that has tragically become accepted as the norm.

A WORD ON EXERCISE

Throughout this chapter, we have mentioned exercise as a powerful way to reduce disease risk and ultimately slash preventable health care costs. Although we are directing you to **www.marksdailyapple.com** for more information on implementing the primal laws, exercise is an area where one of us (Doug McGuff) holds an approach that in some ways diverges from that of Mark Sisson and the primal community in general. Here we will switch off to McGuff's perspective to discuss his approach to exercise as it relates to fitness and disease.

IN DOUG'S WORDS . . .

If I could give only one message to every man and woman that would most impact their health, it would be this: Just Lift Weights. My main area of expertise and interest is in high intensity exercise.

Mark Sisson became aware of me through my work in this area, and we first met at a high intensity exercise seminar. I co-authored a book, *Body by Science*, which discusses in great detail the science behind the benefits of high intensity strength training, as well as the particular protocols that are recommended to reap the maximal benefit from this form of exercise. I would refer any who are interested in the deeper aspects of my work to read the book or visit its website at **www.bodybyscience.net**.

Having shamelessly plugged myself, let me say that I do so also because there are so many benefits to be obtained from this form of exercise, including direct reduction of chronic disease risk and potential protection against some consequences of severe injury or illness. Lifting heavy things aggressively recruits muscle fibers and fatigues them quickly. This recruitment and fatigue produces several downstream benefits, including the rapid use of glycogen, the stored form of glucose. Glycogen is kept in the muscle for on-site emergency use. When needed for high exertion, it is broken down through an enzymatic amplification cascade. One enzyme triggers thousands of secondary enzymes, which in turn trigger thousands of tertiary enzymes, and so forth. This ensures the ready availability of energy for the muscles to use in an emergency.

The result is the ability to quickly use up stored glucose. When this is done, it needs to be replaced. This is accomplished by increasing the number and the sensitivity of insulin receptors on the surface of the muscle cells, which decreases circulating insulin. When circulating insulin (a hormone with many pro-inflammatory effects) is decreased, you will have much less systemic inflammation and reach a state more permissive for fat mobilization, since insulin inhibits hormone sensitive lipase—the enzyme that must be triggered to allow fat mobilization from your fat cells. Other beneficial hormonal cascades, such as HGH and testosterone, are triggered. Increased lean mass raises your basal metabolic rate, protects you from injury, and correlates with organ mass in general.

If for some tragic reason, you wind up in the Intensive Care Unit (ICU) after an illness or injury, your main countdown timer to death is your organ mass at the time you begin. Once this mass is catabolized beyond a certain point, you will die from multi-system organ failure. As your muscles go, so goes every other organ in your body. Increased muscle mass correlates with not only increased organ mass, but also increased bone mass and brain mass.

More organ mass is money in the bank for periods of illness, injury, or prolonged catabolic states. Along with potentially saving your life, this could greatly protect you against the after-effects of illness or injury that would otherwise keep you entangled in the health care system for longer than necessary.

Even more recent evidence shows that skeletal muscle is not just a tissue that produces movement, but rather, is a very active endocrine organ. As we've touched upon in this chapter, exercise—especially that of high intensity—offers protection against type II diabetes and cardiovascular disease, along with multiple cancers and dementia. These effects are mediated by hormone-like substances called "myokines" that are released by contracting skeletal muscle. Myokines have a direct anti-inflammatory effect, as well as inhibitory effects on visceral fat (the fat located in your internal abdominal cavity). Other myokines work locally in the muscle to increase fat oxidation and glucose uptake, as well as counteracting TNF-driven insulin resistance.[45] As the overarching goal of this book is to help you take control of your health amidst the deteriorating health care system, it should now be clear why I am urging you to Lift Heavy Things.

Some proponents of evolutionary based exercise might balk at the recommendation to use machines, pointing out that Grok would never have used a machine, and that it is not "functional." To me this is akin to the recommendation to eat grass-fed meats. The benefit comes from the healthy elements in the meat (omega-3s, CLA, etc.), not in how it was acquired. The argument against machines is like saying that grass-fed meats are only beneficial if we acquire it the same way Grok did, by running it down with a spear. If we chased a buffalo into a ditch and killed it with spear and knife, we would greatly increase our risk of injury or death and not increase the healthful aspect of the meat. Much in the same vein, there is no need to heave and jerk unstable objects, or perform Olympic lifts to exhaustion, or WOD yourself into an unstable delirium. The benefit comes from the aggressive recruitment and fatiguing of skeletal muscle, not by re-enacting the primitive way Grok had to go about it.

In summary, I recommend picking five basics exercises. (I like the Leg Press, Pulldown, Chest Press, Compound Row, and Overhead Press.) Lift and lower the weight in a slow-controlled fashion, trying to keep the muscle under constant tension. Keep doing this until deep fatigue sets in. This will be recognizable by a degree of discomfort that forces you to stop, or an inability to keep the weight moving without cheating. Do only one set. A workout should take between 12 and 30 minutes, depending on how quickly you pace things. Once you get started, you will be almost immediately hooked, because results come quickly. More importantly, you will be living with the knowledge that you are contributing to your own form of "health insurance" for the future.[46]

Apart from some divergence of opinion where weightlifting is concerned, my exercise philosophies align with that of the primal laws. I encourage you to browse **www.marksdailyapple.com** for a fuller discussion on the topics of sprinting, slow movement like walking, and avoidance of "chronic cardio."

At this point, we are going to make a temporary switch in the narration. The material in the rest of Part III derives almost exclusively from the medical training and work experience of the ER doctor, Doug McGuff. Consequently, Chapters 10 to 13 will be written in the first-person singular ("I") to make it easier for McGuff to relate personal observations and anecdotes, as well as to offer educated opinions on medical topics.

Next we will discuss the specific details of how to extract yourself from the health care monstrosity, and how to engage the system for those times when you simply cannot avoid being pulled in. There is much that is great about modern health care. We hope to show you how to get everything good from the health care system as it currently exists, while avoiding as much of the bad as possible. Let's get started!

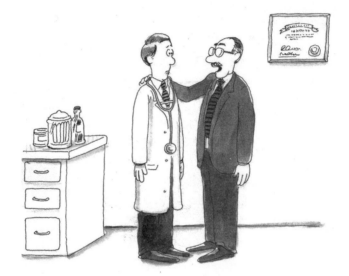

"I'm proud you've become a Doctor, son.
You owe me $200,000 for medical school."

Chapter 10

CHOOSING
YOUR DOCTOR

Picking a doctor is the most crucial step in successfully navigating the health care system. Hopefully, you will never have to get into the belly of the beast, but if you do, you are going to need someone to successfully guide you through the maze. If you have already been pulled into the system, you may need to make some adjustments to get the most benefit and least harm.

The most important step in selecting the right doctor is to have the correct attitude about your potential "health care provider." I put health care provider in quotes because that is a modern term designed to take doctors down a notch. Almost all physicians (MDs and DOs) consider the term a step down from being a physician. Almost all nurse practitioners, physician assistants, chiropractors, nutritionists, psychologists, and so on consider the term a step up. When you search for a health care provider, I want you to choose a physician. You will understand why shortly.

When it comes to physicians, however, I do not want you to have an image in your head of Marcus Welby or House. We are not looking for an authoritarian figure who is going to take charge and tell you how it is. We *do* want the expertise and authority that a physician commands, but we don't want that authority directed at us. Instead, we need that authority directed at the system we may potentially enter.

THINK "SHERPA"

The best model I have for the role of a physician is that of a sherpa. A sherpa is a native guide and servant whom you take on a mountain-climbing expedition. When you have to engage the health care system or enter the hospital, you should view it in that same way: as an expedition. You will be entering a foreign and potentially dangerous environment. You may consider yourself well prepared. You may even work in the health care field and think you know the ropes. But even the most experienced and savvy climbers will use the services of a sherpa on their journey.

A sherpa is a native to the environment through which you will be traveling. He grew up there and retains all the wisdom that his elders passed down to him. He is considered a member of the territory; everyone you will encounter recognizes that your sherpa is "one of them." Your sherpa knows the customs and the rituals. He knows how to introduce you to the natives and help you communicate without unwittingly offending anyone. He knows the environment and how to read it. He knows when to push you and when to hold you back. Most important, he is fully acclimated. When you are limping along in a hypoxic haze, he will be in top form, able to look out for you when you are too tired to be vigilant. Finally, he knows when the expedition should be scrubbed, or at least when you might need a return to base camp.

Despite his superior knowledge, conditioning, and familiarity with the environment, the sherpa knows he is your servant. His authority is always delivered in a subservient fashion, because he knows you are the one paying him. He lets you set the goals and agenda and tries to accomplish them within the constraints of reality. When your goals conflict with the environment, he will tactfully and firmly inform you of the issues. He will present the facts and leave the decisions up to you (or at least make you feel like you are in charge). If your desires pose a danger to yourself or to your sherpa, he will reserve the right to sever the relationship, but will do almost anything to persuade you before he does so. If he is not comfortable with your demands, he will do his best to find a replacement willing to accommodate your wishes.

As you move through your expedition, your sherpa expects to do the heavy lifting and to take the lead facing all the headwinds. However, when you reach the summit, he expects to fade in the background as you stake your flag and pose for pictures. Once the photos have been taken, he will help you pack up and come back down the mountain in the quickest and safest manner possible. The sherpa knows how to get you out of his world and back into yours.

Finding a physician to be your medical sherpa will be difficult. As we discussed in the first section of the book, the political and financial forces in medicine have conspired to make it almost impossible for a doctor to operate this way. First and foremost, you want a doctor who still admits his[1] own patients to the hospital. If you ever have to be admitted to the hospital, you want your hired sherpa directing your journey. Your doctor will have affiliated with what he believes is the top hospital. He knows the system. He knows what floors are best and he has a relationship with the nurses, techs, and ancillary personnel. He knows when the "A-team" is on, when the "B-team" is on, and how to get the most out of both of them.

In addition to selecting the best hospital and guiding your way through it, your doctor will also have developed a referral network with all the different specialists you may need. Your doctor should have a good reputation and a working relationship with the emergency medicine doctors in the ER. Many times, the only entry to the hospital will be through the ER so that stabilizing treatment and expedited testing can be done. If your doctor has the ability to notify the ER of your condition and what workup may be needed, this will accelerate your care and prevent unnecessary testing. Your doctor should also have a relationship with other specialists such as cardiologists, surgeons, and orthopedists. The specialists should be responsive to your doctor because of the prior referrals that represent the "bread and butter" of his practice. If you suddenly rupture your Achilles going for a jump shot on a Saturday morning, it will be great if your doctor can notify the ER and the on-call orthopedist of his choice that you are on your way in.

You can see that having a doctor is something that you must research and establish when you don't need care. This is because a personal doctor is a lot like a tourniquet or a fire extinguisher: you hopefully will never need one, but when you do you, will need it badly and right away. Unfortunately, a doctor of this type is going to be very hard to locate. Combine this with the fact that you will be seeking a doctor with these characteristics who also will be on board with your ancestrally inspired health plan.

In essence, you are looking for a doctor who embraces three characteristics, each of which is rare. To find all three in one doctor is indeed challenging. The three characteristics we are looking for are: 1) a free market orientation, which does not imply particular political beliefs but instead relates to the doctor's views on the provider/client relationship; 2) knowledge and support of a primal, wellness-oriented approach to health care; and 3) someone who still admits his patients to the hospital and has a strong presence within that institution.

A WORD ABOUT "WELLNESS"

In general, the third of our requirements will be the hardest to find. As we discussed in the first part of the book, political forces and price controls have driven doctors from the inpatient side of medicine into the outpatient arena. Many doctors have also become fed up with the "disease management" aspect of medicine, overseeing patients who are unwilling to participate in their own healing. It is therefore quite easy to find primary care doctors who have moved into the outpatient arena and who focus on "wellness." Many of these practices focus on bariatrics (weight loss), hormonal management, and nutraceuticals. However, most of these practices exist for the express purpose of escaping inpatient medicine and thus do not participate in the care of inpatients.

While I obviously support the concept of wellness, and feel these practices offer valid services, I also believe that wellness does not require a physician to achieve. Wellness is your default state that is encoded in your DNA and can be acquired by following the principles of the primal lifestyle and diet. You do not need a doctor to be well. You definitely need a doctor if you become significantly ill or injured. As much as this will rub wellness practitioners the wrong way, medicine exists to treat disease and injury. You simply must choose a doctor who can take care of you when sickness or injury occurs.

Your doctor must also be capable of caring for illness or injury in the office. You should ask your candidate doctor if he is able to sew simple lacerations, or splint non-displaced fractures. Does he have basic lab and x-ray capabilities, or a relationship with a hospital or outpatient lab and medical imaging center? Does the practice hold daily slots open for acute illnesses or injury? You don't want to be told to go to the ER for something that should be handled in an office. If that happens you will incur much more expense, as well as a prolonged wait time because you will be triaged low in the queue.

FREE MARKET ORIENTATION AND "THE GOLDEN RULE"

Finding a free market oriented doctor is challenging and depends on the Golden Rule, to wit: he who holds the gold, makes the rules. The proper relationship between a doctor and patient should be a direct exchange of money for services rendered paid at the point of contact. This makes it crystal clear who the doctor is working for and whose wishes need to be followed.

When the doctor is being paid by a third party to take care of you (as well as thousands of others), the wishes and needs of that third party take priority over the needs of you, the patient. Overall patient demographics and administrative overhead play a major role in determining the type and extent of treatment that you will be offered. In a third-party payment system, the medico-legal risks are collectivized. In order to decrease the overall risk of a malpractice suit, the third-party payer may enforce more extensive workups than you or your doctor might otherwise want. As we will discuss later, more extensive workups have their own set of dangers. When testing is done just for the appearance of thoroughness in order to decrease malpractice risk, you face a greater chance of false positives. These false positives can trigger further testing and treatment that can actually produce harm even though the original intent of the testing was the appearance of safety. Extra radiation and invasive procedures (with risk of injury or infection) are some of the potential harms, but we must also consider the anxiety and worry that go along with unnecessary testing.

A SIMPLE SOLUTION: PAY CASH

The solution to the problems of third-party interference is to seek out a doctor who accepts direct cash payment from his patients and determines the price structure for his practice (as opposed to having a fee schedule that is determined by insurance companies and government payers). This arrangement allows the doctor to bill you directly for services and then provide you with the paperwork to file with your insurance. The physician can then receive payment directly from you without having to go through any intermediary, in turn cutting all of the administrative overhead for the doctor. He doesn't have to file paperwork; he doesn't have to code his medical record and diagnosis in order to apply for reimbursement. There is no prior approval process where he has to figure out if your diagnosis and treatment will even be covered. Also, the payment is received in real time, opposed to the substantial delays with insurance reimbursements. Because of these delays, most doctors have to rely on a billing service to keep track of who has and has not paid and to make sure that payments do not fall through the cracks. In general, the doctor being paid through third party insurance employs a small army of office staff and billing and coding technicians just to try to get reimbursed. These headaches will only increase as the Affordable Care Act's provisions sink in.

The doctor who deals directly with patients can rid himself of all of this overhead expense, and therefore can offer services at a greatly reduced price. Simple office visits can drop as low as $25 to $40 (as of this writing). The requirements for documentation are not as onerous and the treatment you are given (or not given!) can be that which you and your doctor discuss. If you don't want to be on a statin, your doctor can abide by your wishes without risk of third party payment denials for failing to follow "best practices."

Note that you can have traditional employer-based insurance and still participate in this sort of medical practice; you will just have to file for reimbursement through your insurance company. The practice will generally provide you the paperwork and guidance for you to get reimbursed.

More ideally, you can combine this kind of care plan with a "catastrophic" insurance plan. This type of plan generally involves a high deductible ($5,000 is typical) and pays 100 percent of your medical bills and hospitalization after that deductible is met. This makes health care insurance actual insurance again. If you think about your car insurance or your homeowner's insurance, you will see that you are not reimbursed for routine or preventive maintenance such as oil changes or repainting. Instead, insurance is for some catastrophic and unforeseen circumstance that would be financially devastating if you had not paid into a risk pool in exchange for coverage. When you revert to true health insurance, your premiums drop significantly, and when it does kick in, your coverage is complete. As a result, there is less fighting about what is covered. When there is lower risk of premiums being consumed, the payment restrictions are less.[2]

CONCIERGE MEDICINE: THE DOCTOR WILL SEE YOU . . . NOW

Concierge doctors provide care in a manner similar to cash-only plans. The major difference is that they charge an upfront fee instead of charging by the visit. The fee can range anywhere from $500 to $5,000 annually. In exchange for this yearly fee, you get unlimited and unfettered access to your doctor. All visits during the agreed upon contract time (typically a year) are covered under the retainer fee. You will have 24/7 access to your doctor by a cell phone that he carries at all times. The money spent on the retainer may or may not apply towards the deductible of your insurance, and will depend on your policy. The chances are greater for the fee to be deductible if you make these arrangements at the time you are purchasing your insurance policy.

The advantage of a concierge practice is that the higher up-front fee allows the physician to have a much smaller number of patients in his or her practice. Instead of the 3,000 to 5,000 patients that constitute a medical practice, the concierge physician may have only 500 to 2,000 patients. This allows the concierge physician the ability to be available to his patients at all times. Even if you never use the physician during the year, the peace of mind in knowing that your doctor is available to you immediately any time of the day or night may be worth the price of the retainer. Also, many concierge doctors are affiliated with each other and can offer promises of cross-coverage, allowing you similar access to medical care even when you are away from home.

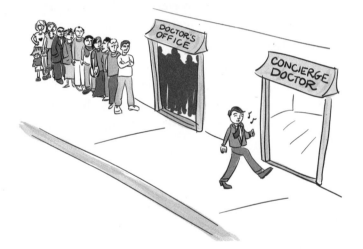

The difference between a concierge practice and a conventional insurance-based practice is about as dramatic as you can get. With the Affordable Care Act going into effect, the pool of patients with insurance coverage will expand greatly. As a result, traditional practices will be seeing much larger numbers of patients at a declining reimbursement rate, which will only make this discrepancy even more extreme.

Although there is a potential conflict in concierge practices—because the patients may adopt a "buffet mentality" while the providers may try to avoid work that is unreimbursed—in practice this does not seem to be a problem. I believe this is because this sort of transaction tends to occur higher in the economic food chain with people who truly understand the value of what they are paying for. This engenders a mutual respect between the physician and the patient, which seems to easily overcome the potential problems we discussed.

WHAT IF YOU ARE OLDER THAN 65 AND ON MEDICARE?

As we have discussed previously in this book, Medicare is the most onerous of the third-party payers and has served as the template for everything bad in commercial insurance. Many, having reached age 65, feel that they have paid into the system all these years and now need to get their money's worth—the "buffet mentality." Also, seniors must consider that the money they have paid in is long gone; the government didn't invest those payroll "contributions" over the years in the S&P500. Any Medicare "benefits" extracted from the system are being paid for by involuntary withdrawals from current workers' paychecks, or (if financed via deficits) by the future tax payments of your grandchildren.

Therefore, I recommend operating outside the system as much as you can. To operate on a cash basis with your doctor, you must either rely on your doctor for services not paid by Medicare (routine preventive care or cosmetic procedures), or you must sign a private contract agreeing to give up Medicare payment for services rendered by your doctor and instead pay the fee set privately by your doctor. This is at best a general discussion on how to get care outside of Medicare and you may want to contact HCFA (Health Care Financing Administration) directly for further detail. Many physicians who provide cash services have opted out of Medicare entirely, and because of CMS regulations and how hospitals are funded, many are disallowed from inpatient care. The solution for many independent physicians who have opted out of Medicare is to simply not bill for inpatient services provided to the patients in their care. Others may rely on a hospitalist service that they stay in close communication with, should you be hospitalized. I prefer the former arrangement, but if the hospitalist route is necessary it should not be a deal breaker, especially because most traditional insurance-based practices rely on hospitalists as well.

WHAT IF YOU ARE ON MEDICAID?

You need to acknowledge that Medicaid is not insurance; it is welfare. As such, you are not participating in a market exchange and thus have no real right to input regarding your care. You are stuck taking what you are given. You are utterly at the mercy of the government and health care bureaucracy, and that's why—for both your financial and medical wellbeing—you need to exit this situation as quickly as possible.

Having said that, the most important thing you can do is take any job or jobs that become available and begin to purchase your health care through a cash-only approach. In fact, many Medicaid beneficiaries cannot get care because so few physicians are accepting Medicaid patients. (The reimbursement is so low that a practice cannot see Medicaid patients and expect to keep their doors open.) Many patients that attend charity clinics are actually on Medicaid but end up there because of the lack of Medicaid-accepting doctors. Likewise, many cash-only practices have a significant number of Medicaid patients because the care is so affordable. The only good advice I can give about Medicaid is to use it for what it was intended to be: a temporary situation to give you a "hand up," so that you can become productive and self-sustaining again.

WHAT KIND OF DOCTOR?

When I say what kind of doctor, I mean what specialty. I must preface my recommendations by informing you that what follows is not based on the scientific literature, but instead is my opinion based on a quarter century in the trenches interacting with generalists and specialists from all different fields.

When selecting a personal physician, you want someone whose training has given some direct experience in all the different specialty fields. This makes the physician able to deal with problems from almost any specialty. If you have a mild to moderate problem, your doctor can usually handle things as well as a specialist. If the problem is severe—such as a perforated ulcer—then your general physician won't be doing your surgery, but he or she will have done several months of surgery rotation in residency and know what to expect, whom to call, and how to expedite your transition to specialist care. In short, I am talking about someone trained in family medicine.

Family medicine or family practice-trained doctors rotate through all the specialties of medicine, but with a special emphasis on office practice. They are trained to be "team leaders" and to coordinate the care of specialists. Not all family practitioners take on the role of team leader: many will "punt" you to a specialist and defer entirely to the specialist's opinion. However, their training at least grants them direct experience in other specialties, the ability to coordinate care between multiple specialists, and the competence to accept or reject their consultants' opinions based on a patient's overall needs. Having been in this position in the past, family physicians will have developed a network of specialist consultants who they feel are the best among those available to them. Further, since these specialists depend on family physicians for referrals, they are very responsive to their requests for consultation. This all serves to benefit you, the patient.

Another advantage of family medicine specialists is that their practice is not constrained by age, gender, or body system. This may make them a "jack of all trades/master of none," but it also gives them a broad and integrative overview of medicine. This means that one doctor can oversee your entire family from infancy to adulthood and old age. Some still provide excellent obstetrics services as well. Doctors using a cash practice are very rare, so if you find one that can provide care for your entire family you can save yourself from a potentially time-consuming search.

If you are an older adult, an internal medicine specialist may be a good choice as well. Their training is not as broad as a family medicine specialist, but their experience with the diagnosis and treatment of medical conditions is very extensive. Since most adult illnesses are medical in nature, internists can be a very strong choice. General internists tend to function well as referring doctors for surgical or non-medical issues just based on necessity and experience in community practice.

Pediatricians are excellent choices for your children, but once your kids reach their mid to late teens, you may need to transition to an adult physician (family or internal medicine).

I generally discourage women from using their OB/GYN doctors for their primary care. I do not think their breadth of training is sufficient for general medical care. It works fairly well until you get sick outside the realm of gynecologic issues. (I strongly think OB/GYN doctors should be used for pregnancy care and gynecologic conditions.)

Once again this is a personal opinion, but I definitely recommend relying on an obstetrician or family physician for prenatal care and delivery of your baby. Nurse midwives and doulas are fine as long as their care is provided in (or affiliated with) a hospital and with some form of physician backup.

I realize that many people—including those in the primal community—hold a negative view of hospital-based deliveries. Even so, I advise against home or out-of-hospital deliveries even when performed by physicians (but especially when practiced by non-physicians). When a baby comes out blue, breach, or in respiratory failure, 911 gets called and the crisis is dumped in my lap in the ER.

MID-LEVEL PROVIDERS

Your doctor may employ mid-level providers such as physician assistants or nurse practitioners. I think this is fine. These people are well trained and can offer excellent care, often even better than their physician counterparts.

Their training, however, is directed toward the less serious conditions. As such, I think they are great for your routine office care and even rounding on you in the hospital. Yet I recommend that each of your visits to the office at least involve a brief encounter with the supervising doctor and some indication that he or she is overseeing your care. If you become more seriously ill, you will need the physician's direct care, and that care will benefit from having prior familiarity with you as a patient and as a person.

ALTERNATIVE PROVIDERS

There are alternative providers of health care such as chiropractors, naturopaths, homeopaths, nutritionists, and numerous other therapists. They certainly may have a place in your health care and wellness plan. However, they should not serve as a substitute for a physician who will care for you when you are sick. Despite the move towards "wellness," medicine is still about caring for the sick or injured. If you face a serious health crisis (especially if you require hospitalization), you will need a doctor. You will be best served if you have established a proper relationship with a great doctor who is on your payroll, and you establish the relationship long before you actually need it. Do everything you can to be well, but be prepared for when things don't go as planned.

Finally, an acid test to apply when selecting a physician is his willingness to avoid prescribing medications, or to help you wean yourself off prescription medications if you are already taking them. This is such an important issue that we devote the next chapter to it.

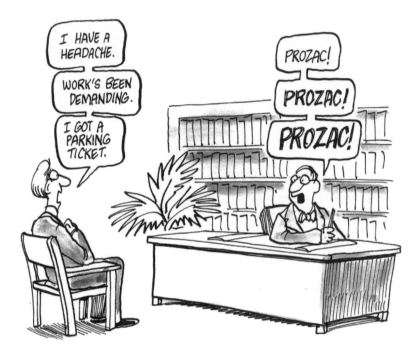

Chapter 11

GETTING
OFF YOUR MEDS

One of the main criteria you should use in selecting (or de-selecting) your doctor is a willingness to seek non-pharmacologic solutions to your health-related problems. Whenever a disease state exists, the emphasis should be on addressing and correcting an underlying cause, not on immediately prescribing a drug to treat the symptoms or to "manage" the disease. Being healthy and drug-free should be our expected default state, but our drug-oriented culture takes it for granted that being on prescription medications is just a part of life. The orientation away from prescription medications is a simple heuristic that you can apply when selecting your doctor.

The logical extension of this heuristic is that if you are currently on a list of medications, your doctor's first order of business should be to look at your list with an eye toward what can be eliminated. This is something your doctor is almost never asked to do, but should be incredibly excited to attempt. Physicians are much more accustomed to patients who leave an office visit angry if they don't have a prescription in hand. *Trouble sleeping? Here's some Ambien. Trouble staying awake? Here's some Provigil. Trouble concentrating? Here's some Adderall. Life stressing you out? Here's some Xanax. Eyelashes not long enough? Ask your doctor if Latisse is right for you.*

Even in my practice of emergency medicine, I get daily visits from patients requesting prescriptions for things that are not medical emergencies. Heck, they aren't even medical events. Instead, people show up in the ER daily requesting prescriptions for *life* events. In the mind of the modern American, these life events are emergencies to them. For example, a typical case is a male in his early 20s who signs into the ER at 3 a.m. with a complaint of insomnia. He is requesting Ambien for sleep, but can also commonly be seen sipping a Mountain Dew or Red Bull while staring at the screen of his laptop. Another common situation is a request for Xanax for anxiety. This commonly occurs after family deaths or funerals during a grief spike. I have to explain to the patient and family that their emotions and symptoms are appropriate to their level of loss, and that suppressing that response with drugs will only complicate and drag out the grieving process. Many times, however, Xanax and other anxiolytics are requested simply for the stressors of daily life. I am left explaining why prescribing a highly addictive medication that can produce a deadly withdrawal syndrome is not appropriate.

Even though most people can endorse the goal of a medication-free routine in the abstract, it can be difficult for people to climb out of the prescription drug pit once they've fallen in. The rest of this chapter provides guidance for escaping.

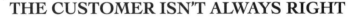

THE CUSTOMER ISN'T ALWAYS RIGHT

Although in this book we have called for a return to a market-based relationship between doctor and patient, this doesn't mean that the proper treatment is always the one demanded by the customer, especially when so many Americans now believe that pills are the solution to all of life's woes. In this context, the shift toward "patient satisfaction surveys" as an important element in doctor performance and reimbursement is ominous:

"[B]y 2017, Obamacare's "pay for performance" program mandates that hospitals will lose 2 percent of their Medicare payments if they perform poorly on quality measures—some 30 percent of which will be based on patient satisfaction scores. Hospitals are

investing in capital upgrades like escalators to improve the "cus-
tomer" experience.   Meanwhile, doctors are under even more
pressure to "please the customers"—even if it means unnecessarily
scoping them, irradiating them, or plying them with toxic and ad-
dictive pills."[1]

GETTING A LAY OF THE LAND

The first step in the process of reducing your medications is to get an aerial view of what is going on. You should schedule a 30- to 60-minute appointment with your doctor for the purpose of reviewing your medications. The longer the appointment, the better, as this can actually get quite complicated. The complication arises from the fact that medications are often given without consideration for the potential interactions with other medicines or supplements you already take. A further complication is that your prescribed medications may be coming from multiple doctors who may not be aware of all of your medications or why other doctors originally prescribed them. You are likely to uncover some scary potential interactions and have some tough decisions to make, so setting aside more time with your doctor will be to your benefit.

Making efficient use of this appointment is up to you, however. You can have a more productive experience by preparing well ahead of time. This process involves you collecting *all* of your (1) prescribed medications, (2) over-the-counter medications, and (3) supplements, and putting every pill bottle or container into one of three bags according to these categories.

Next you need to make a spreadsheet for each category that will list each drug by number, and as well as columns or headings for each drug to include the following descriptors:

1. <u>Generic name and trade name</u>. For whatever reason, most doctors will be familiar with a drug's generic name or its trade name, but seldom both. For example, most doctors will immediately identify with

Lasix but hesitate when they see *furosemide*. Operating in the most familiar terms will make applying our new heuristic easier.

2. <u>Prescribed by or recommended by whom</u>. Knowing who prescribed or recommended a drug offers important information. Something prescribed by your primary provider whom you have seen over the years may hold more weight than something written by a specialist whom you saw one time for an acute problem. Many medications, once started, get refilled and are very hard to make go away. Also, your doctor knows the reputation of many local prescribers. Their extent of medical knowledge, general orientation, and whether they are a "quick draw" with a prescription pad will be relevant knowledge when going over your list.

3. <u>When the medication was started</u>. Assembling a timeline for all of your medicines can be quite revealing. It may expose what are legitimately chronic conditions versus acute conditions. It may give some weight to those medicines that are truly important versus medications that have fallen through the cracks of scrutiny and have simply been refilled as a matter of course. Medications that you have been on for short periods of time could be for acute conditions that are now gone, or may be plays towards the medicinal flavor of the week as new drugs come out. A timeline could uncover something that was supposed to replace a prior medicine, but instead was added without stopping the old prescription. This is commonly exposed by overlaying your oldest and your newest medications. Needless to say, a lot can be revealed with a medication timeline.

4. <u>The indication for the medicine</u>. In other words, why were you put on the medicine, and what condition or symptoms was it meant to treat? This provides incredibly useful information. You can see if the medicine is to treat a specific disease or if it is used to treat the symptoms of a disease. You can see if a medicine is aimed at symptoms generated by life itself or life progression. Such a medication should be relatively higher on your list for elimination. Even more important, if

you do not know why the medicine was started, then say so by writing "unknown" in this category. Do not look up the drug's usual purposes and assert this. You can never assume that you were started on a medicine for its usual indications, because there can be multiple indications for a drug and there are many "off label" uses of drugs (both legitimate and not). A drug in this category is also high on the list for elimination. Finally, make sure to note whether a particular drug's indication is to treat the side effects of another medication, as this creates an opportunity for a Primal Rx two-fer! If you are prescribed one med for a lifestyle issue and another to treat the side effects of the lifestyle medicine, these are high on the list to *both* be eliminated.

5. <u>Is the medication working for its intended purpose</u>? This question is particularly germane if the medicine in question is for treating life events as opposed to true disease or illnesses. Are your eyelashes really longer? If not, get off that med. Still moody before your period? Maybe you should try a non-pharmacologic solution. If the med in question is for a bona-fide medical condition (such as hypertension), then the dose may be inadequate. However, before that conclusion is reached, we need to look at the other medications on your list. It is possible that one of the other drugs has an equal but opposite effect or side effect. It is also possible that one of your other drugs is up-regulating the metabolism of the drug or blocking its binding site. One thing is for certain: if a drug is not doing what it was intended to do, we need to find out why and make appropriate adjustments.

6. <u>How is the medication metabolized</u>? This step is somewhat related to step 5 and is a major reason for drugs becoming either ineffective or toxic. This may sound like something that only your doctor can do, but with a little help from your Internet search engine or Wikipedia, you may be able to give your doctor a head start; it is incredibly hard to remember how the myriad of drugs out there are metabolized. Simply enter the term "metabolism of" along with the name of the medication in question. You do not even have to understand the terms; just scribble the answer in the appropriate box. You

may find a term such as "hepatic cytochrome P450 pathway" or "renal secretion at the distal tubule" or "Hoffman degradation" or "serum protein binding with renal elimination." This will become important as your doctor sees the aerial view of your list. Some metabolic pathways get stronger with use (like lifting weights), and if you have one drug eliminated by such a pathway and you add another eliminated by the same pathway, the serum concentration of your first drug may drop because it is metabolized more rapidly. This can happen in cytochrome P450 metabolism, for instance. However, after a certain number of drugs are added, the system can become overwhelmed (similar to overtraining with weights), causing metabolism to drop off and create toxicity issues. This is why some alcoholics can go into liver failure from a therapeutic dose of Tylenol. The normal effect of one drug can accelerate the elimination of another, such as a diuretic increasing the excretion of a drug eliminated through the kidneys. Also, many pathways that involve excreting active metabolites into the gut rely heavily on intestinal bacteria to assist with a drug's metabolism. Going on a round of antibiotics for a bladder infection or pneumonia can wipe out your intestinal flora and affect the metabolism of some of your medications. Knowing this ahead of time will allow you to prepare by concurrently taking probiotics and prebiotics. One thing is certain: seeing the metabolism of all of your medications on one page can be very informative, and may create an opportunity to eliminate or at least optimize your drug regimen.

7. <u>Drug-drug interactions</u>. While you are looking up a drug's metabolism, just scan down the page and you will probably find a listing of drug-drug interactions. Most likely, this section will scare the crap out of you (and it should). The scariest part is how long the list can be. You do not have to write down every single drug that a particular drug interacts with; just write down the first three to five. You may be shocked to find that some drugs listed in the top three are also in your own medication list. If so, you will have some choices to make because you definitely want a list where no medications have any high-risk interactions with each other. (Ideally, you want to work for *no* list.)

8. <u>Eliminate? Yes/no. Wean? Yes/no</u>. After you have gone through steps 1 through 7 with each of your medications, it's decision time. Should it stay or should it go? If you decide a medication should be eliminated, keep in mind that some medications should not be discontinued abruptly. Stopping certain blood pressure medicines cold turkey can cause rebound hypertension. Certain anxiety medicines have to be weaned very slowly in order to avoid a potentially life-threatening withdrawal syndrome. Narcotic medicines also need to be weaned very slowly to avoid an extremely unpleasant withdrawal syndrome. In some cases, weaning will need to be done with the help of an addiction specialist in order to avoid dangerous or challenging withdrawal effects. Needless to say, the discontinuation of any of your medications should only be done with the knowledge and help of your doctor. This section of your worksheet will help orient your doctor toward decision-making and serve as a reminder to consider whether weaning is appropriate.

9. <u>Replace with? Supplement or lifestyle change or nothing</u>. Some medications don't need to be replaced with anything because they were never needed in the first place. They may have been intended for conditions that were purely aesthetic (eyelash length) or for conditions that were physical manifestations of psychic conflicts. Other medicines may have been for conditions that commonly resolve with the application of a primal diet and lifestyle. These include acne, irritable bowel, eczema, psoriasis, arthritis, type II diabetes, elevated triglycerides, and a host of other conditions that often disappear or improve to the point that medication is no longer needed. Other conditions may be addressed by a supplement instead of a prescription medication. Instead of Ambien for sleep, how about magnesium citrate and melatonin washed down with some chamomile tea? How about dropping your statin in favor of discontinuing grains and taking a fish oil supplement? Instead of Viagra, how about zinc, selenium, Brazil nuts, and egg yolks? As you remove some of your medications, you may find that what remains was actually treating the side effects of the medication you just stopped and that the others are now unnecessary. The same vicious cycle that got you on so many medications can be turned on its head and work to

your favor. You may not be able to get off all of your medicines. There are true disease states that legitimately require prescription drugs. However, it is not uncommon for those following a primal lifestyle to healthfully eliminate their medications.

With the spreadsheet in front of you and your doctor, it should be fairly easy to decide what medications can be eliminated by following the guidelines we've provided. If in doubt, cut it out. Think about what primal lifestyle, dietary, and supplemental adjustments you might make instead of using a given medication. You may be able to get off all medications or, more realistically, you will be left with one, two, or perhaps three that treat legitimate conditions such as hypertension or type II diabetes.

WHAT TO EXPECT: PSYCHOLOGICAL IMPLICATIONS

Expect to be scared when you first go off some of your medications. You may feel overwhelmed, worrying that everything might spin out of control if the delicate balance of your medicine routine is disrupted. This is sort of a medical version of Stockholm syndrome, where you become dependent upon and thus sympathetic to your captors and tormentors. Over time, you may have come to feel that your life depends upon your medications and that your body will not function properly without them. You did, after all, take them diligently twice a day with food. You had a special pill container and an alarm set on your iPhone to remind you to take them. Certainly all this attention to detail signals some importance to your wellbeing, if not your very existence! When you suddenly stop, you really fear that your physiology might go haywire. As a result, you will be on high alert and likely to interpret every bodily sensation as an impending disaster.

Rest assured this is almost never the case. You may have some symptoms, as even medication that does not produce physical dependence and withdrawal will still produce *psychological* dependence and withdrawal. Communicate these potential fears with your doctor in advance. A little reassurance will go a long way in terms of heading off these feelings. If you can get through this initial phase of anxiety and realize that everything will be OK, after a week or two your physiology will settle out and you will be reaping the benefits of a less drug-dependent lifestyle. At this point, the major issue left to deal with is the anger arising when you think back on all of the time you spent meticulously taking your medications and fearing you would fall apart if you missed even a single dose. Indeed, this anger will also likely happen. All I can recommend is to just let it go. You as a patient could never have been expected to figure this out on your own. Just be glad that you and your doctor are taking steps toward discovering the healthy you that is encoded in your ancient DNA.

WHAT TO EXPECT: PHYSICAL MANIFESTATIONS

Psychological issues are not the only obstacles you will encounter when you attempt to discontinue a long-standing medication; there can be real *physical* consequences as well. This does not mean you shouldn't try stopping a certain medication, or that the attempt should be abandoned if there are immediate signs of minor worsening of the disease state. If the medicine is withdrawn gradually, and if you give your body a chance to recalibrate, you may be able to successfully go off a given medicine. Let me explain why.

Medications often work by blocking receptors that bind hormones or other physiologically active chemicals in your body. Hormones, neurotransmitters, and certain proteins work by binding to specific receptors in a lock-and-key type fashion. In this case, the active chemical is the key and the receptor is the lock. Many medications work by blocking a receptor, or in our example, by covering up the keyhole on the lock. Under normal conditions when key and lock can come together, the lock becomes active and either directly or through another chemical released from the lock (called a second messenger) triggers a physiologic reaction. With a second messenger system, there may be release of a much larger number of active chemical messengers, or a series of similar lock-and-key reactions that result in an amplification of the

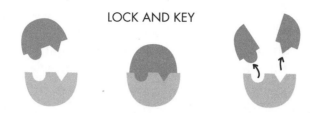

LOCK AND KEY

effect of binding the original receptor. In this way, binding a single receptor produces a bigger bang for the buck in terms of the desired physiologic reaction. Conversely, this means that blocking just a small percentage of a given receptor produces an amplified therapeutic effect.

This creates two advantages for a medicine that works by this mechanism. First, you don't have to bind all, or even many, of the receptors to produce a desired therapeutic effect. Second, the fact that just a small percentage of receptors needs to be bound to produce the effect means that you have the opportunity to fine-tune the results by increasing or decreasing the dose of the medicine. The term that defines this second advantage is "dose-dependent."

However, there is a downside to medications that work by this dose-dependent receptor mechanism, and that downside is termed "tachyphylaxis." Tachyphylaxis means that your body builds a resistance to medication over time, requiring a gradual increase in dose to achieve the same level of therapeutic effect. This effect is highly variable in drugs that work by a receptor-blocking mechanism, and may be somewhat related to the magnitude of the amplification of the second-messenger system. The way this resistance to receptor-blocking drugs occurs is as follows. When receptors (locks) get blocked, you will have a situation where you have more keys circulating around than there are locks for them to bind with. The way your body *can* respond to this (I italicized "can" because it does not always happen) is by synthesizing more new receptors or locks to engage the surplus of keys floating around. Your body may also respond by synthesizing more keys to overcome the blockade or to match the increase in locks. When your body mounts such a reaction, the medication may lose its therapeutic effect and require an increase in dose. Commonly, the dose is not changed, and the patient continues to take a medication that is no longer generating the desired therapeutic effect.

The important point to recognize is that this response of generating more receptors and/or making more keys has implications for the discontinuation of such medications. No biologic system works on an all-or-nothing basis, but instead operates across a variable spectrum. In our lock-and-key analogy, there will always be circulating keys and there will always be both bound and unbound locks, even when we intervene by using a medicine that blocks the locks' keyholes. In a situation where you are on such a medicine and you body has responded by manufacturing more locks and/or synthesizing more keys, there are consequences when you abruptly stop the medication and uncover all of the available locks. You may suddenly have a situation where there are more locks, more keys, or a combination of both. In this instance, the physiologic response that the medicine was originally started for may return; in some cases it may return with a vengeance. The trick to discontinuing a medication that works by this mechanism is a gradual weaning of the dose. In so doing, you allow the response of making more locks and/or keys to slowly ratchet back until things return to a natural baseline and the dose can go from tiny to nothing without untoward consequences. This is why any discontinuation of a medicine needs to be done under the supervision of your doctor and usually should be done gradually. When done properly, you won't have to worry that the rebound response represents continued existence of a disease state rather than an adaptive response to the medication.

The sort of withdrawal syndrome we've described here occurs to varying degrees with different medications. Typically, the withdrawal will simply be a return of the disease symptom that the medicine was designed to treat, and this likely represents the adaptation to the medicine (tachyphylaxis) and not persistence of the disease state (naturally, this is assuming that you have had a long period of living and eating in a way that's compatible with your primal genes). Most of the time, this reaction will be a minor worry or produce symptoms that are merely a nuisance. In other cases, the withdrawal syndrome can produce symptoms that are nothing short of agonizing, sometimes reaching life-threatening levels. I will discuss some examples for illustrative purposes. This is not intended to put you, the patient, in the position of identifying specific instances where such dangers exist, but rather to reinforce that withdrawing medication should only be done under the supervision of your physician.

One of the more common, highly uncomfortable withdrawal syndromes involves narcotic pain relievers. This class of medication results in profound tachyphylaxis by increasing the number of narcotic receptors. These receptors don't just involve pain transmission, but involve other bodily functions such as gut motility, tear production, attention and sedation, and many others.

When a narcotic medication is discontinued abruptly or weaned too quickly, a very unpleasant withdrawal syndrome occurs. It includes an intense craving for the drug as a result of a plethora of unoccupied brain receptors. The predominant withdrawal symptom is, naturally, a higher level of pain throughout the body. This is the result of excess pain receptors all over the body, including in the brain. The pain receptors in the peripheral nervous system send more pain signals to the brain, and the receptors in the brain amplify the effect of the signals sent from all regions of the body. The end result is agonizing diffuse body pain. Other symptoms also arise from the presence of narcotic receptors throughout the body. Abdominal cramping, nausea and vomiting, and diarrhea occur secondary to narcotic receptors in the gastrointestinal tract. Gooseflesh, sweating, and excess tear production occur as a result of skin and mucous membrane receptors. None of these withdrawal symptoms are in and of themselves life threatening, but they are so profoundly unpleasant that almost no one can make it through going "cold turkey"; most will require a supervised detox program to come off of this class of medications.

Most life-threatening withdrawal syndromes occur in medications that act upon the sympathetic ("fight or flight") arm of the nervous system. The chemically active components of this system are usually adrenaline, or adrenaline-like excitatory neurotransmitters. After using a medicine that blocks receptors for these kinds of excitatory chemicals and facing an increase in receptors (locks) or keys as a result, abrupt cessation can cause a massive binding of adrenaline-like chemicals to their receptors. The result is a major sympathetic outflow that drastically raises blood pressure and heart rate. At the brain level, threshold for neural transmission lowers due to the excess binding of epinephrine, norepinephrine, and serotonin, in turn leading to excitability, agitation, hallucinations, and seizures. A full-blown withdrawal from abruptly stopping such medication can result in a heart attack, hemorrhagic stroke, kidney failure, sudden congestive heart failure (causing you to drown in your own fluids), brain swelling from the aggressive rise in blood pressure, and intractable seizure activity.

Medications that fall in this category include the benzodiazepine class of anti-anxiety medicines, such as Valium, Ativan, and Xanax. Alcohol withdrawal is almost identical to benzodiazepine withdrawal, to such an extent that starting high-dose benzodiazepines and then slowly weaning them is the treatment for alcohol withdrawal. Sudden discontinuation of Clonidine, a centrally (meaning brain level) acting blocker of adrenaline-like activity can result in severe and life-threatening rebound hypertension. Other blood pressure medicines that block alpha or beta receptors (called alpha- or beta-blockers) can produce a milder withdrawal effect. There are several other examples as well; the important point is that you should only withdraw medications under the direction of your doctor. I offer this explanation so that you might remind your doctor to be extra cautious when withdrawing medications that act on the sympathetic ("fight or flight") system.

I hope this discussion has impressed upon you the idea that stopping your medications can have real physical effects. Most of these effects are mild and not life threatening, and should not thwart your attempt to go off a drug as long as you have been adherent to primal lifestyle and dietary principles for several months. Some medications can produce dangerous, unpleasant, or life-threatening withdrawal syndromes that definitely require the help of your doctor or even inpatient detoxification.

In most cases, attempts to come off medications occur because you and your doctor made an active decision to give it a try. In other cases, your improving health will force the need to stop a medication upon you. To understand how this might occur we will need to revisit the concept of number needed to treat.

WHAT TO EXPECT: NUMBER NEEDED TO TREAT (NNT) REVISITED

As people undertake primal dietary, exercise, and lifestyle changes, it is not uncommon for them to begin to exhibit side effects from their long-standing medications that had previously not given them any problems. To understand why, let us return to the concept of the number needed to treat (NNT), which we introduced back in Chapter 2 in our discussion of the FDA. NNT basically refers to the number of patients that need to take a given medication in order to achieve a therapeutic benefit or harmful side effect. The number needed to treat to benefit (NNT-B) and the number needed to treat to harm (NNT-H) depend partly on how powerful the medication in question is, but they mostly depend on the severity of the disease state for which the medicine is being used.

We must remember that drugs are not just chemicals that produce a single disease-oriented effect. The body is very complex and has numerous interconnecting feedback loops. As such, any drug has a wide constellation of physiologic effects. If there is a significant disease state that one of the drug's effects addresses, this action will be called the drug's *therapeutic effect*. All the other effects of the drug will become the drug's *side effects*. As we discussed previously, if the disease state is relatively severe, the drug's therapeutic effect will overshadow its side effects and the NNT-B will be smaller than the NNT-H, thus making the medicine worthwhile to take. If a disease state becomes less severe, there is some point at which the drug's therapeutic effect diminishes and the NNT-B becomes greater than the NNT-H. For the individual, this will mean that the drug's side effects will become more pronounced than its therapeutic effect. If a disease state completely resolves, then all of the drug's effects will revert to side effects, including the former therapeutic effect—which will then, typically, become the new predominant side effect. For instance, if you were taking a blood pressure medication and your hypertension resolves, then the major side effect will become light-headedness and fainting as a result of unhealthfully low blood pressure.

This discussion shows why people undertaking Primal Blueprint changes to their lifestyle will often face the *need* to stop medications.

Two of the most common conditions where this occurs are hypertension and type II (adult onset) diabetes.

In hypertension, primal dietary changes involve dropping many components of the modern Western diet that cause vascular inflammation. Eliminating grains and gluten plays a big part here. In addition, avoiding massive doses of fructose from processed foods and sweeteners results in decreased uric acid production. Uric acid has a side effect of inhibiting nitric oxide synthetase, an enzyme that produces nitric oxide. Nitric oxide's main action is to relax and dilate blood vessels. The decrease in nitric oxide is a major driver in the development of hypertension. Beyond that, changes induced by high intensity exercise, sprints, large amounts of low intensity activity, and other elements of a primal lifestyle also act to decrease blood pressure. These kinds of activities result in muscle growth and a process called neovascularization. Neovascularization is a fancy term for the growth of new blood vessels. This occurs at the level of the smaller blood vessels, including venules, arterioles, and capillaries. The end result is greater vascular surface area and blood vessel volume. The increase in vascular capacity at a given level of blood volume results in a lower blood pressure, due to a fixed volume of fluid now being held inside a larger container. Also, the act of exercising improves the pumping efficiency of the heart and the elasticity in the walls of the blood vessels. All of these things contribute to a natural reduction in blood pressure. For a hypertensive patient adopting primal diet and lifestyle practices, this means the severity of his or her disease is decreasing. As that severity decreases, the therapeutic effect of lowering blood pressure starts to become an unhelpful side effect, as the dose that was once proper becomes excessive for the degree of disease. The NNT-H begins to exceed the NNT-B and the patient will face the side effects of hypotension. With a blood pressure that is now too low, our budding Grok or Grokette will begin to experience lightheadedness. To avoid this, a hypertensive patient will need to work with his or her doctor to decrease or discontinue blood pressure medication.

In the case of type II diabetes, patients undergoing a primal lifestyle overhaul will also experience a decrease (or resolution) in the severity of their disease. The primal dietary changes largely eliminate foods that produce elevations in blood sugar and the consequent overproduction of insulin. When insulin is no longer over-produced, the pancreas gets a chance to rest and recover, and the insulin receptors get an opportunity to become unoccupied and rejuvenate their effectiveness. Further, primal exercise induces a significant emptying of glycogen stores from the muscle. This raises the muscle's number of insulin receptors, which need to engage with the existing circulating insulin to replenish the sugar stores (glycogen) inside the muscle. The result is greater sensitivity to insulin and a consequent lowering of blood glucose. If an oral hypoglycemic (which works by flogging the pancreas to produce more insulin) is still being taken in this scenario, the excess insulin will be bound and produce hypoglycemia. I have seen numerous cases of clients at *Ultimate Exercise* (my personal training facility) begin to experience spells of hypoglycemia and require a dose reduction (and many times a discontinuation) of their oral hypoglycemic medication. Those with type II diabetes who undertake primal lifestyle changes need to be aware of—and vigilant towards—this phenomenon. You should notify your doctor of your lifestyle changes, so that together you can closely monitor your blood sugar and make adjustments before you become symptomatic. It is much better to make dose adjustments ahead of time than it is to experience your first episode of hypoglycemia when you are driving home from the gym. The good news is that for many type II diabetics, there is the possibility that you may cure your disease and be able to completely go off your diabetic medications.

WORST CASE SCENARIO: IT'S NOT SO BAD

We have spent the bulk of this chapter discussing the desirability of eliminating as much medication as possible. I do not want to construe this discussion to mean that I think medication is bad or evil. In my work as an emergency physician, I am heavily reliant on pharmaceutical agents and would have so much less to offer patients if I were cut off from this technology. Pharmaceutical agents have enormous power to help patients, but remember what Uncle Ben said to Peter Parker (aka Spider-Man): "With great power comes great responsibility."

So, just as we should not come to think of being on medications as a normal part of life and trust that there is a pill for every problem, we should not think of being on medication as a sign of weakness. There will be many readers of this book who have very real disease states that will require ongoing medication. These disease states are usually not brought on by the action or choices of the patient, but are commonly due to a genetic predisposition that is activated by some environmental trigger. Primal principles can go a long way toward eliminating or mitigating these environmental triggers, but some are simply part of our world and cannot be eliminated (or have not yet been discovered). As such, a given person may have a disease state that must be managed with pharmaceutical agents.

Many health and fitness enthusiasts—including some of those who consider themselves part of the primal community—think nothing of taking biologically active supplements that have as powerful a therapeutic effect as many prescription medications. Some will consume creatine, branched-chain amino acids, thermogenic agents, and hormonally active substances without a second thought. These same people, however, might consider it a personal failure to need a medication. If you have to be on a medication, whether it is an antibiotic for an infection or a blood pressure medicine for hypertension, it should not make you feel any worse than taking a biologically active agent that you bought over the counter. Ultimately, all of the rules that apply to prescription medications also apply to biologically active substances, so you need to be cautious with both. We would love to see you go off all prescription medications as you advance along your primal journey, but you definitely should not beat yourself up if you ultimately have to stay on some (or even all) of your medicines. No matter how things turn out, you will only stand to benefit by incorporating primal principles into your life.

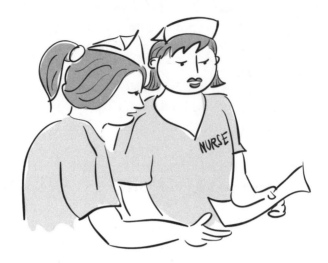

"Make sure Room 350 gets 500cc every hour."

"Right, 500 for 350."

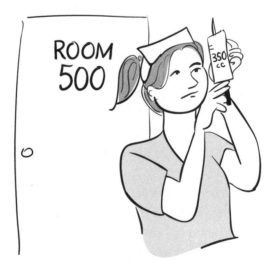

(WHOOPS)

Chapter 12

SURVIVING THE HOSPITAL

Being hospitalized is a truly scary experience, even beyond the obvious fear from the issue causing the hospitalization itself. As you are admitted, you realize that the people taking care of you are not actually superheroes; instead, they are normal people doing a work-a-day job just like you. You realize that errors made on the lowest level of the medical food chain may be the ones that get you killed. A registration clerk can accidentally miss a keystroke that changes your middle initial, leading to the wrong blood type being administered to you or the wrong patient's medication being delivered to your room. You begin to think about how your own motivation and job performance wanes after fighting with your spouse or yelling at the kids before dropping them off at school. With everyone you encounter, from the registration clerk to the lab tech, your assigned nurse, and the doctors in charge of your care, you hope against all odds that they are all having a good day.

As you worry about these things, you are simultaneously reluctant to verbalize your fears to those caring for you: you don't want to piss off the lady who is about to draw your labs or the young man about to start your IV. Instead, you vow to be very vigilant and watch them all like a hawk. However, you realize two things. First, this is a very foreign environment, and you have no idea what is being done to you or the nuances of the technology involved in doing it. Second, you are sick or injured! You may feel too poorly or be in too much pain to focus on the details of your care. You may be forced to concede your vulnerability and simply hope and trust that everyone cares enough to do his or her best job.

THE PERSPECTIVE OF THE PROVIDER

Your hospitalization represents one of the biggest events of your life. Yet to those who are caring for you, you may be the 40th patient of the day. Your surgery may be the third that morning after two emergency cases that kept your surgeon awake all night. To you, it is frightening to think that your crisis may be mundane to your health care team. At the same time, you want them to be experienced enough so that treating you *is* mundane, from their perspective.

Members of your health care team have to walk an emotional tight-rope where they are able to demonstrate care and compassion, yet not experience so much empathy that they develop "compassion fatigue." Compassion fatigue is a real risk for doctors and nurses who empathize too deeply with patients. They eventually become unable to absorb one more tragic story or handhold one more patient through a personal crisis. Even if a provider does not over-empathize, an excess volume of work or expectations can overwhelm the capability to care. I remember secretly confessing to my fellow medical students and residents that I had at times wished a patient would die so I could just get some sleep. I was shocked to find that all of the people I confided in admitted to having similar thoughts at some point in their training or careers. Even now, almost daily, an ambulance will get called out for a cardiac arrest, and when the paramedics arrive and call back a "signal 9" (indicating a patient dead too long to resuscitate), the entire ER work station will erupt in a cheer.

I realize these statements may alarm some readers, but they are the truth, and I want you to trust that *I am telling the full story*. We are dropping a lot of "cold hard reality" on you in this book, telling you many things you probably don't want to hear, but at the very least I hope we are conveying the sincerity of our claims. While my anec-dotes about medical school and life in the ER surely seem incredibly calloused to someone outside the field, it is in fact a normal defense mechanism for those who work in a "pressure cooker," where the stakes are life-and-death and the acceptable error rate is nothing short of zero.

This stress and pressure is exacerbated in situations where the demand for services greatly exceeds the ability to supply them. For reasons we discussed in the earlier parts of this book, there are many flawed policies that led to exactly this situation. As if the stress of taking care of critically sick and injured people were not enough, modern health care workers are now burdened with a truckload of government mandates, many of them contradictory. They are required to use a cumbersome system of electronic medical records (EMRs) for all order entries and documentation. Of all the things I hear patients comment negatively on, the most common is the fact that their nurses, technicians, and doctors seem to spend most of their time at a computer screen and very little time at the bedside. Ironically, the "patient safety movement" has created so many redundant mandates that patient care is actually being compromised.

A NEW WAY TO THINK ABOUT HOSPITAL SAFETY

Despite all of these downsides, hospitals perform incredibly well and are very vigilant. Nowhere else do you find such good outcomes where the odds are so stacked against those engaged in a challenging endeavor. We must remember that the majority of people in this country die in the hospital—60 to 70 percent, depending on the source. It is very common for patients who are in hospice to end up in the ER near the moment of death because families are not familiar or comfortable with the death process. At least a couple of times per month I am placed in the position of shepherding the family of a hospice patient through the dying process. This is now such a prevalent part of emergency medicine that it is becoming a subspecialty interest for some emergency physicians.

I bring up these realities to point out that hospitals are filled with sick and dying patients. Most of the patients there have multiple medical illnesses and have been in decline for a long time. As we discussed in Chapter 2 with the concept of NNT, drugs never have just a single effect. When you have a patient with multiple illnesses, it is very likely that you will worsen one disease process through the act of treating another. As a patient becomes sicker and sicker, the attempt to treat one problem may disproportionately worsen another, producing the appearance of medical error. Ultimately, in hospitals across the country, patients will die and they will do so in proximity to some sort of medical intervention. When these sorts of things happen it is very easy to interpret them as medical errors that caused injury or even death. This is somewhat akin to storming the beaches at Normandy expecting that no one will be injured or killed. Just because people are dying in hospitals does not mean that hospitals are killing people.

I don't mean to belittle the dangers of medical errors or suggest that a hospital is a safe place to be, as there *are* real dangers. However, becoming overly freaked out, or overstating a danger, actually makes it harder for patients and their health care providers to be vigilant against dangerous mistakes. The patient safety movement, while well intentioned and important, has created new dangers.

THE ALARMS THAT CRIED WOLF

"The constant beeping of medical devices in hospitals is causing "alarm fatigue" and putting patients' lives at risk.

Hospital workers have become desensitized to the noise, which sometimes causes them to ignore the alarms, and has resulted in at least two dozen deaths each year, according to a new report by the Joint Commission, the national organization that accredits hospitals."[1]

To understand how to rationally address your risks while in the hospital, we need to understand how we became so concerned about risk that we have impeded our ability to mitigate it. To understand this phenomenon we have to go to the source: the Institute of Medicine.

TO ERR IS HUMAN: HOW TO PROPERLY PROMOTE PATIENT SAFETY

In 1999, the Institute of Medicine published a report on the scope and nature of medical errors, along with suggestions for decreasing their risk.[2] One of the laudable aspects of the report was the focus on systems errors rather than blaming individual actions.

Even so, the report's preamble contained the shocking statement that "at least 44,000 people, and perhaps as many as 98,000 people, die in hospitals that could have been prevented. . . . [P]reventable medical errors in hospitals exceed attributable deaths to such feared threats as motor-vehicle wrecks, breast cancer and AIDS." You can probably guess that the media focused on *this* part of the report, rather than the nuanced treatment of systems errors versus individual mistakes. It is this statistic that has been used repeatedly by journalists and others to represent patients being killed as the equivalent of a jumbo jet loaded with passengers crashing every day for a year.

The result of this report over the past 15 years has been a bonanza of patient safety initiatives and activity. An entire cottage industry has sprung up around this report, and now hospitals have entire floors of wall-to-wall cubicles of ex-nurses, social workers, and administrative types entirely devoted to patient safety initiatives.

Let me give two examples of the well-intentioned but ultimately counterproductive outgrowths of this report. First, there was a national movement to label all liquids on a procedure tray. This was in response to a single case report of a surgeon who accidentally injected epinephrine instead of saline from cups placed on the surgical tray. As a result, I now have to label betadine (a brown cleaning solution) that is in a cup and lidocaine (a clear liquid) that is in a syringe on every suturing procedure I perform. Failing to do so is a firing offense, even though it is impossible to mix up the intended purposes of a brown liquid in a cup and a clear liquid in a syringe. It is also extremely difficult to accomplish under sterile conditions. The solution has been the production of kits with pre-made labels at enormous expense when calculated on a nation-wide basis.

The other example I'll give of an inappropriate application of rules that do not truly promote safety is the expansion of the "time out" procedure. This was born from the experience of wrong site or wrong patient surgeries. The "time out" has been a ritual amongst the best surgeons for a very long time; this was not something that was recently invented. The way it works is that you identify the patient appropriately, and if there is to be a surgery on any paired limb or body part, you write "yes" on the limb or part that has the procedure and "no" on the incorrect side. Before you begin the procedure, you take a "time out" to confirm the patient identity and surgical site. However, since the IOM report came out in 1999, the "time out" ritual has been applied to every single procedure imaginable, even those cases where common sense dictates it is not necessary. For instance, time outs for laceration repair in a non-paired body site are patently ridiculous. Even when the body site is paired, it is pretty easy to see which side needs the laceration repair. Nonetheless, the ritual must be performed—and most important, documented—to satisfy an arbitrary rule that does not serve the original intent.

Do not misunderstand me: I can fully appreciate the public's horror at the idea of waking up and realizing your surgeon amputated the wrong leg! It is entirely appropriate that hospitals adopt procedures to make sure this type of outrage is exceedingly rare. (Many readers would have wanted me to say "impossible" rather than "exceedingly rare," but that would only be true if we stopped amputations, period. Is that the right solution?) What I am saying is that we have to use our heads when devising the safety protocols. It makes perfect sense to insist on a "time out" when it comes to leg amputations, but it does *not* make sense to do so for stitching up a gash in the neck. The sad effect of over-applying a great idea to inappropriate situations is a gradual desensitization to the process in general. It is the same phenomenon we discussed in Chapter 2 regarding the FDA's rules on advertising. When it comes to things that can significantly affect your health, you want the safety rules to be as crisp and sensible as possible; ironically, this is the *worst* area to cast too wide of a net.

Let me be clear: I do want to emphasize that medical error is a real problem, and that those convened to address the problem are in fact well-meaning people doing important work. Further, actual improvements have occurred since the advent of the IOM report. It is important to create a culture where error analysis can be done openly. Different lines of work carry different risks when an employee has a bad day: a birthday cake may have a misspelled name, a steak may be undercooked, or an investor may lose money. A bad day at the hospital means someone's child can die.

However, there is a downside with anything you do, and as we have learned, those downsides are magnified when you implement change in a top-down fashion. One of the biggest problems with this campaign is that things are not as bad as the 1999 report made them out to be. A hospital is a place where critically ill and dying patients are cared for. A medication or procedural error can occur with a critically ill or dying patient. If you retrospectively go back and discover such an error in a patient who has died, it is very easy to attribute the death to the error. This is especially true if you have been commissioned to write a report on the problem of medical errors. In some cases, off-protocol treatments given as a last-ditch effort in a dying patient may have been scored as an error.

Overstating dangers can also create *real* dangers. Being too quick to sound the alarm—crying wolf—makes us not respond to the alarm any more. There are so many safety procedures and precautions in hospitals nowadays that it actually impedes patient care and exhausts the ability to be truly vigilant. When safety measures are feared or resented, they will not make you safer. When the ER doctor and nurse have to go through an arduous "time out" ritual and documentation to relocate your obviously dislocated right index finger, then safety has actually suffered.

To make sure I'm not losing any readers, let's make a quick detour into the "real world" that you all know: flying on a plane. How many readers carefully listen to the stewardess before the plane takes off, as she explains *how to operate the seat belt?* This is exactly the kind of thing I am talking about in this section. The government—in this case, the FAA—mandates absolutely absurd "safety protocols" that the airlines must obey, or else they go out of business. Flying passengers can sense that these drills are patently absurd, and so tune them out. Now, does this mean flying carries no risks? Of course not; the whole plane can crash into the Pacific Ocean—that's pretty dangerous! My point is that slapping on a bunch of nonsense regulations so that we feel we're "doing something about safety" is not only silly, but it actually crowds out possibly meaningful information that the flight attendants *could* give during those announcements.

The patient safety movement has spawned numerous private agencies that rate hospitals on their safety. In principle this sounds great, but in practice it too produces unintended consequences. For example, every region has smaller community hospitals that boast on their billboards some safety award from one of these agencies, while regional referral centers are lambasted in the papers for their safety record. But consider that when patients are too sick or unstable for the community hospital, they end up being transferred to the referral center. When you take sicker patients, who have been hospitalized multiple times and who have had multiple rounds of antibiotics at the community hospital, then your infection rates are going to be higher than other centers, and you may have to administer treatments that do not fall into "best practices" parameters.

As our new safety culture unfolds, we are seeing truly excellent surgeons who have unfavorable safety statistics because they are willing to take on the sicker and more challenging cases. People of lower socioeconomic status are more likely to be such sicker patients. How many specialists are dropping off ER call to avoid uncompensated care of patients who might damage their safety profile? How long can a referral center withstand the bad press that is their only reward for serving as backup for a community hospital? The biggest danger emerging from the patient safety movement that the sicker you are, the less anyone in the medical profession will want to associate with you.

THE DANGERS NO ONE IS TALKING ABOUT

In contrast to the often-exaggerated dangers, in this section I want to focus on the *real* things you should worry about if you must be hospitalized:

- Your doctor does not work for you. Your doctor is not paid by you. His treatment of you is based on protocols and "best practices" that are required by the government, third-party payers, and hospital administrators. These protocols may contradict the type and extent of treatment that you desire or that you and your doctor think are best. If your doctor deviates from protocol—even when it is per your desires—he may not be paid, could be financially punished, or could even face firing or loss of privileges. Your doctor may be faced with a tough choice between your wishes and practice standards. This is even truer of the hospital. There are ever-tightening criteria for what constitutes a "legitimate" hospitalization and what will be paid for. Even when you are hospitalized, the hospital will only be reimbursed for a certain number of days or a fixed amount. This creates immense pressure to treat and discharge you within the allotted time frame. An army of case managers is continually looking over the shoulders of inpatient doctors in attempt to discharge patients "in a timely manner."

- The patients are sicker than ever. Most of the patients will (hopefully) be sicker than you. The sickest patients have chronic diseases of civilization and have been dying slowly for decades. This creates an environment that expects patients to just be tuned up until their next hospitalization. The idea of treating and curing an acutely ill person is becoming more and more foreign. Because the staff is used to dealing with people with much poorer protoplasm, you face the risk of over-treatment, and because the staff is used to sending patients home who are still experiencing signs of illness, you face the risk of premature discharge. As patients have gotten sicker and resources more scarce, the acceptable criteria for admission have become more stringent (you have to be sicker) and the criteria for discharge have become more lax (you can be sent home less well). The presence of these sicker patients means that they may distract care from patients who do not come from a background of chronic illness and may appear to be lower risk. Finally, patients who are in and out of the hospital become colonized with multi-drug resistant organisms—organisms that you will be exposed to during your hospitalization.

• The system is overburdened with patients. Overcrowding combined with reduced funding results in understaffing relative to the demands. Your caretakers will be pushed to the limits of their attention and coping ability at all times. They are constantly just one small surge in volume away from tipping into disaster mode. Fatigue combined with frenzy puts you in real jeopardy.

• The system is overburdened with rules and regulations. As if mountains of chronically ill patients are not enough, there are also endless regulations and requirements to be met in the process of caring for this tsunami of sickness. Irrelevant documentation requirements have been set in place to try to deny payment to hospitals, meaning the hospitals must insist on following the requirements if they want to get compensated for their work. This leads staff to ask a patient who is having a heart attack about ringing in the ears, or a history of domestic abuse; or asking a person with a laceration about smokers in the family, seatbelt usage, or presence of guns in the house. The time staff spends doing these sorts of things translates to attention diverted away from your real problem.

• EMRs (electronic medical records) have crippled efficiency. As we discussed previously, the government has pushed EMRs down the throats of providers without any evidence of improved efficacy. The result has been cumbersome systems that have all but ground clinical care to a halt. If you are ever hospitalized, take note of how much time your doctors and nurses spend tapping a screen. These inefficient systems and government mandates have turned these professionals into the highest paid data entry clerks in the world. EMRs also increase the risk of improper data or simple data entry errors being populated forward with each new encounter. Worst of all, the system is fragile. One power outage, computer outage, or sunspot event could bring an entire hospital to its knees. All of which poses a danger to you.

• Doctors and patients have both been made fungible. The third-party payment system has subverted any true price system where value is objectively calculated. A top-notch orthopedic surgeon who has done thousands of hip replacements gets reimbursed the same amount as an orthopedist just out of residency who has to read the product insert of the prosthesis and be guided by the product rep. Payment for your illness as a patient will be based on your diagnosis, regardless of how complex your case may have been. The fact that both you and your doctor have been made into interchangeable cogs means that you have little means of detecting the best health care providers, and you run the risk of being the square peg that gets rammed through a round hole.

• You have been made the enemy. As is inevitable with price controls, there is resentment between the provider and the consumer. To the provider of inpatient care, you essentially represent an overwhelming risk of financial loss. You also represent medico-legal risk, as well as potential fraud allegations from a government that does not want to pay out what it has promised—and that has created a web of impossible-to-follow laws that reclaim paid-out funds and levy fines so that the system can limp along.

STEPS YOU CAN TAKE TO PROTECT YOURSELF

Finally, after laying all of this groundwork to dispel some of the hysteria surrounding the IOM report, as well as making you aware of the dangers no one has previously informed you of, we can now discuss some specific measures you can take to protect yourself in the unfortunate event that you, or a loved one, are hospitalized.

HAVE A PERSONAL PHYSICIAN

This is first and foremost. If you are hospitalized, you want someone who is familiar with your health, personality, and wishes at the helm. Ideally, this will be a doctor who still admits his or her own patients to the hospital. When your own doctor is writing admission orders and doing daily rounds, you will have a greater chance of influencing care. Hopefully, this will be predicated on having selected your physician by the criteria we discussed in Chapter 10. When this is the case, your prior discussions and meetings will be in your doctor's consciousness, and will make their way into your treatment plan. It is quite uncommon for primary care doctors to admit their own patients for reasons we have covered previously. Even if your doctor does not do his own admissions, the fact that you have a doctor will positively influence those providing your inpatient care. Your doctor's practice style and philosophy will be known and this will influence your care in a positive way. Your doctor provides referrals to the specialists who may be called in on your case, and these specialists will be more responsive and will operate in a way that keeps your doctor happy.

The ideal circumstance is that you have a primary care doctor who participates in a cash-only plan or concierge practice, has opted out of Medicare and Medicaid, and does not file directly with insurance. This means you will have to pay your doctor out of pocket and get reimbursed by your insurance. In some cases, these doctors avoid all the hassle by having an agreement with their patients that they will not bill for inpatient services. In this case, you will have someone at the helm of your care that can be more resistant to government-mandated treatment protocols and length-of-stay requirements.

DO NOT BE HOSPITALIZED UNLESS ABSOLUTELY NECESSARY

The best way to avoid the dangers of hospitalization is to avoid being admitted in the first place. For instance, if the reason for admission is the need for IV antibiotics, then try to accomplish this on an outpatient basis at an infusion center. If you have a blood clot in your calf or thigh and need anticoagulation, see if you can be self-taught how to administer your Lovenox (blood thinner) injection at home. If you have a respiratory illness that requires breathing treatments and oxygen by nasal cannula, see if this can be set up through a home health agency. Many times hospitalization occurs only because of technical issues with treatment. If there is no difference between treatment in the hospital versus similar treatment administered at home or at an outpatient facility, then you should not be hospitalized. Before agreeing to hospitalization, make sure there is something that is going to be done to you in the hospital that cannot be done elsewhere.

DIRECT ADMISSION OR ER ADMISSION?

Which is the better route? The answer is: it depends. If your admission is elective or for the performance of an inpatient procedure, and you are stable, then direct admission is the way to go. You can be seen at your admitting doctor's office and your doctor can make arrangements for you to go directly to an inpatient room with his admission orders in hand (or transmitted electronically). If, however, you are acutely ill, unexpectedly ill or injured, or unstable in any way, then it is best to be admitted through the ER. In some cases, you may have to go directly to the ER and your doctor will become aware of your illness after the fact. In other cases, your doctor may send you to the ER for stabilizing treatment and workup. In such situations, the ER can carry out treatments quickly that cannot be accomplished on the floors. Lab tests, x-rays, and other tests can be acquired in a much more expedited fashion, and their interpretation by the emergency physician can guide your treatment and determine the setting to which you should be admitted. Advance notice from your doctor before your arrival at the ER can help represent the acuity of your situation, so that you are triaged appropriately and your evaluation is expedited. ERs around the country are bursting at the seams, but if you are unstable or acutely ill, it is where you need to be.

HAVE AN ADVOCATE

This is where developing the strong social connections implicit in a primal lifestyle will come in handy. You need to have established the sort of close personal relationships that ensure a support system will rally around you when you are hospitalized. You really want to have a close friend or family member with you throughout your hospitalization. Not merely for the moral support, but also to help look out for your best interests. If the person(s) staying with you have a medical background, all the better. Your advocate needs to be very defensive of you, and unafraid to ask questions on your behalf. Your advocate can be a watchdog who makes certain that the people who care for you have washed their hands and properly identified you before administering treatment. Your advocate can be on point when you are too tired or ill to concentrate fully. Your advocate can help communicate your wishes when you feel too vulnerable to assert yourself. Just the mere presence of someone who looks intelligent and interested will be enough to make the people involved in your care bring their "A" game. Ideally, your advocate(s) will be with you at all times, even if this means friends and family are working in shifts. If this cannot be achieved, then try to have your advocate present for the medical team's morning and afternoon rounds, where scarce time should be applied. If you are hospitalized away from home, or are otherwise unable to have such a support system, ask the nurse in charge of your care if the hospital is able to assign a patient advocate to you.

BRING YOUR STUFF

Make sure you bring (or have been brought by someone else) your cell phone, tablet, and/or laptop, along with their respective chargers.

These are your connections to the outside world. If you have selected the right doctor, he will also be your connection to the person in charge of your care. He will likewise be a source of entertainment during the long boring stretches. You can look up issues related to your treatment on the Internet, investigate any potential drug-drug interactions, or check out websites like thennt.com. Also, do not forget other "stuff" like your toiletries, a change of clothes for when you are discharged, and your favorite pillow and comforter.

BRING A FACT SHEET

I highly suggest preparing ahead of time a "fact sheet" to bring with you to your hospital admission. This is a sheet that you can hand to anyone filling in information on your chart. All of this information is required for documentation in the medical record. Some of it is incredibly important, while some is utterly ridiculous. All of it is mind-numbingly tedious for whoever is stuck entering this data. The fact that it is such an agonizing part of your admission makes it error prone, and like an early mistake on a trigonometry test, its impact will be passed forward throughout this—and possibly any future—hospitalizations. Your admitting nurse or doctor will be incredibly pleased if you hand over a document with the following information:

- Full name
- Birthdate/current age
- Social Security number
- Race (it can actually be relevant)
- Gender
- Religion (if any)
- Your primary language
- Marital status
- Occupation
- Allergies (medication, food, or anything else); include the nature of the reaction (extremely relevant)
- Prior exposure to general anesthesia and if there were any problems

- Your current weight in kilograms (your weight in pounds divided by 2.2)
- Your current height in inches and centimeters (multiply inches by 2.54)
- If you use tobacco or alcohol. Specify type and amount (can be relevant). Include exposure to second hand smoke
- If you have been subject to domestic violence in the past two years (only if you wish to disclose)
- If you have firearms in the household (only if you wish to disclose)
- Your last tetanus booster
- If you have had this season's flu or pneumonia vaccine
- Your preferred emergency contact and medical power of attorney if you become incapacitated
- If you have a living will or advanced directive
- Your preferences for resuscitation status (full code, CPR, ventilator, do not resuscitate)
- Organ donation status/preferences
- Your insurance and policy number
- Your family doctor and his office phone number

If you can hand a sheet like this to the person doing your intake documentation, he or she may fall down and kiss your feet.

BRING YOUR MEDICATION LIST

Be sure to bring the worksheet you composed if and when you were trying to come off medications. This should include all of your medications with both trade and generic names. Include the dose, how taken (oral, transdermal, etc.), and the dosing interval. Also include all supplements that you take, even those you fear might make you look odd. For example, fish oil may postpone an invasive procedure because of its blood thinning properties. Vitamin K may be relevant if you are going to receive prophylactic therapy for deep vein thrombosis, and olive leaf extract has calcium channel blocking properties. The possible interactions are extensive, so list all of your supplements. Any medications that will be continued in the hospital, along with the medications that are ordered during your admission, will be combined on a "medication reconciliation form." Make certain that a hard copy of this is kept in your paper chart. Also request a hard copy you can keep on your person. If the hospital's computer portal or EMR crashes, a hard copy of this form can be a real life saver. At the time of discharge, you should receive another medication reconciliation form that includes your prior medications and any new medicines you will be sent home with, along with how long you will be on these new medications. Make sure you have such a form to take home at discharge. Use it to update your medication worksheet.

NAME, RANK, AND SERIAL NUMBER

Whenever someone enters your room to do anything for you or to you, demand that they confirm your full name and birthdate. Do not let this slide, even if your nurse has seen you 20 times that day. Remember he or she is overburdened and likely does not remember your name. Every so often, give them a fake birthdate or wrong middle name and make sure they catch it. If they do, just give them an "I was just testing you" tease and then provide the proper information. If they let it slip by, let them know they screwed up and that you don't want it to happen again. If you are blown off, request the charge nurse or hospital administrator.

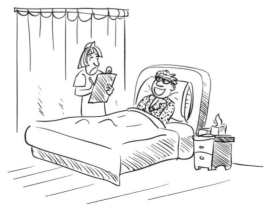

"My full name is Denzel Washington."

BE "THAT GUY" (OR LADY)

Some readers may not be the "pushy" type, and may think the suggestion to quiz every nurse and doctor on your name and birth-date is just too awkward. But consider this: the mere fact that you *ask this type of thing* will keep everyone on his or her toes when dealing with you. That is **exactly** what you want. If the nurses all chuckle and roll their eyes behind your back, it means *they are thinking about your case even after they've left the room*. The following statement is critical to understand: if something bad (and preventable) happens to you in the hospital, it's *not* going to be due to a malicious intent to hurt you. Rather, it will be caused by an honest mistake due to fatigue or overwork. The best way to prevent that from happening to *you* is to make yourself stand out from the moment you show up. This is one of the rare situations where yes indeed, you want to be "that guy" (or lady).

WALK, COUGH, AND DEEP BREATHS

If your condition permits it, make certain to get out of bed and walk around the ward or hospital at least two times per day. Every two hours that you are awake, practice coughing and deep breathing. The walking helps to prevent venous blood from pooling in your legs where it could form a blood clot or deep venous thrombosis. The walking, along with the coughing and deep breathing, prevents a condition called atelectasis. When you lie in bed for a prolonged time and do not breath deeply enough, the lower segments of your lungs do not ventilate fully. As a result, the tiny air sacs do not expand and will fill with fluid. When this happens, you can develop a fever that can create confusion about your condition. Even worse, the fluid can colonize with bacteria from the hospital environment and actually develop into pneumonia. Hospital-acquired pneumonias tend to be more virulent and difficult to treat than community-acquired pneumonias and represent one of the greatest dangers of hospitalization.

BRING YOUR HAND GEL

On the wall of your room, right by the door, should be a dispenser of an alcohol-based instant hand sanitizer. Anyone who enters your room should hit that dispenser before touching you or anything in your room. If they fail to do so, immediately offer them a hit of your hand gel before they touch you, the bed rail, or the computer keyboard. The last thing you want is some MRSA or multi-drug resistant bacteria from your neighbor down the hall deposited on you or on any surface in your room.

BE PREPARED FOR ROUNDS

You may only be able to communicate with your doctor or team of doctors once or twice per day. This is the time where discussion about tests, procedures, and treatments will occur. It is your sole opportunity to be prepared for what is going to happen, and to bring your preferences into the equation. As such, make sure you discuss with your doctor when to expect rounds to occur. Let your nurse know this information as well, and make sure that it is confirmed by his or her experience. Let your nurse know that you want to have a heads-up about rounds, and under no circumstances should you be allowed to sleep through rounds or be off the floor when they occur.

When the team comes to your room, you need to have all of your questions and concerns prepared. Rounds are performed in a rapid-fire fashion and can be over before you know it. Make sure you get the opportunity to have all of your questions answered and for the next stage of your hospitalization to be clearly laid out. Ask if you can use your smart phone to record the discussion so you will have it for future reference. Also, make sure your advocate(s) are present for rounds. The presence of articulate and well-dressed friends and family will put everyone on notice that all involved need to be on their toes.

FOOD

Hospital food is almost universally horrible. It is generally straight out of the ADA guidelines, minus any hope for palatability. Ask your doctor if you can have your own food brought in for you. Your advocate(s) can keep you on an optimal primal diet that will help speed your healing and recovery. If you must eat hospital food, specify a gluten-free diet and then pick around with primal principles in mind.

DISCHARGE PLANNING

As important as the admission process is, the discharge process can be even more important. Unfortunately, many patients' experience of discharge planning is having a nurse walk into the room to announce "congratulations, you are being discharged." The next thing you know, you are in a wheelchair on the way to the front entrance of the hospital while you frantically dial your cell phone for a ride home.

One of the reasons for this is the extreme push to get patients out of the hospital as quickly as possible: the inpatient payment formulas only allow payment for a certain number of days for a given diagnosis. Therefore, make certain that you are truly ready for discharge. You may simply still feel ill, or you may not have been able to make the appropriate social arrangements at home. When you check in for admission, you will sign a form acknowledging your right to block any discharge that you feel inappropriate—which is based on Medicare law, but is often given to all patients. If you state that you do not feel ready, and yet you are still pushed to leave, then tell your nurse, doctor, and discharge planner that you wish to exert your right to appeal the discharge. This will usually buy you more time. If this fails, bring the issue to the hospital administrator.

In general, though, you should be happy to be discharged at the soonest possible time. Even so, you need to leave with a clean and well-planned transition. Your discharge medications and home instructions for self care, as well as exact dates, places, and times for follow-up, should all be provided in an easy to read (legible) format. A specific discharge time, arrangements to gather all of your belongings, and a way home should all be in place the day before (or the morning of) your discharge. Again, make sure all of your questions and concerns are addressed before leaving. Once everything is in order, grab your bag of belongings along with your get-well balloons and climb into the wheelchair for your ride to the front awning.

Congratulations! You survived.

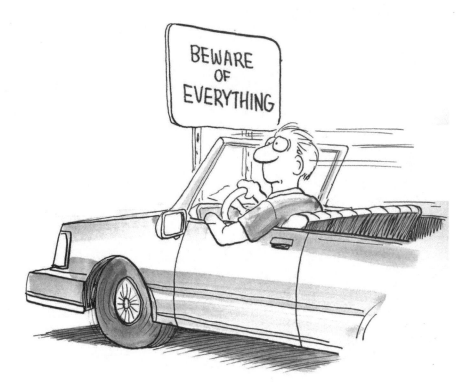

Chapter 13

MEDICAL SCREENING
& ELECTIVE PROCEDURES:
WORTH THE RISK?

O ne of my professors in medical school once quipped that the major difference between doctors and the rest of humanity was doctors' ability to order tests. In a classic case of "supply creates demand," the number of tests that medicine is able to offer has increased exponentially in the past few decades. Not surprisingly, the public's demand for medical testing has kept pace accordingly, and in many cases has even overtaken the current capabilities of medical technology. The result is an extreme push to develop new diagnostic and screening technologies. As these new technologies become available, doctors and hospitals begin using them even before data is accumulated to determine the risk-to-benefit ratio of the test in question.

Our overuse of medical screening and testing stems partly from massive public health and media campaigns. The notion that early detection saves lives has been promoted heavily by medical societies, public health officials, and celebrities. Millions of people get a warm and fuzzy feeling participating in walk-a-thons, earning money that will be spent on the promotion of medical screening. All of the publicity emphasizes the benefits of medical screening, but completely ignores the potential risks.

The result has been a mindset amongst the general public and health professionals alike that a given test will just give an answer, and that answer will be correct and make a difference in our lives. In this popular view, things are either yes or no, positive or negative. The public dutifully marches in to get their mammographies, Pap smears, PSAs, and colonoscopies. If the test comes out negative, we are reassured and vindicated. If the test comes out positive, we believe we have averted disaster by "nipping it in the bud."

The reality can be quite different. In Chapter 4, we briefly walked through the statistics on Pap smears from an economic cost/benefit perspective, but in this chapter let me give some real-world examples on a more personal level.

COLONOSCOPY: A SUCCESSFUL CAMPAIGN

In 1998, Jay Monahan, the husband of popular NBC Today Show host Katie Couric, died tragically as a result of colon cancer. Mr. Monahan was only 42 years old. Having suffered through the arduous treatment protocol and premature death of her husband, Ms. Couric, understandably, sought to give meaning to her husband's death by doing everything she could to make sure that others might avoid a similar fate.

Ms. Couric became a tireless worker and promoter of colorectal cancer awareness and screening. She co-founded the National Colorectal Cancer Research Alliance, a part of The Entertainment Industry Foundation. She also helped to establish The Jay Monahan Center for Gastrointestinal Health at New York City's Cornell Medical Center. Ms. Couric's biggest influence in the battle against the disease that took her husband is most likely to be her advocacy of screening colonoscopies. In March of 2000, she underwent an on-air colonoscopy on The Today Show in an effort to promote the importance of this screening test.

Three years later, authors from the University of Michigan School of Medicine published an article in the July 14, 2003 issue of *The Archives of Internal Medicine* confirming the effectiveness of Ms. Couric's promotional efforts.[1] They showed a 20 percent increase in colonoscopies after the March 2000 show and from Ms. Couric's ongoing efforts. The effect was strongest amongst women. The authors coined the term "The Couric Effect," and concluded that a celebrity spokesperson can have a substantial impact on public participation in preventive programs. (Note that the study made no comment on whether the increased screening was positive on net.)

When we consider increased participation in medical screening, we need to assess whether it actually reduces morbidity or mortality. We also need to consider the risks and side effects of testing. In doing so, we should keep in mind that the concept of number needed to treat (NNT) applies to testing in the same way that it applies to taking medication. The likelihood of a disease being present greatly affects the NNT. As we convince more people to undergo screening, we are more likely to include people who are at lower risk for disease. When this happens, the NNT to harm may actually become smaller than the NNT to benefit. Increased participation in screening may not always be a good thing. Stated differently, if more people who are less likely to have the disease participate, the benefits of screening will decrease, but the side effects (or complications) of the test go up. This is because the rate of side effects remains constant regardless of risk of disease, and with more people participating, the absolute number goes up.

Understand that I am *not* making a blanket statement that one should never undergo screening colonoscopy or that the guidelines for colonoscopy are incorrect. I *am* saying that we need to be careful when we push for broader and broader applications of a test. Too often, the public discussions of such matters make the assumption that medical screening has all benefits and no costs.

Currently, the guidelines for colonoscopy recommend that screening begin at age 50. This is probably reasonable, since about 90 percent of colon cancer occurs after the fifth decade of life. Simply being 50 or older is likely enough of a pre-test probability to swing the NNT numbers towards benefit over harm. This may be little consolation for Katie Couric whose husband died at 42, and it is understandable that she would feel those younger than 50 should get screened. (In fact, she was only 43 at the time of her on-air colonoscopy and had no other symptoms or risk factors that would put her at increased risk.)

AN ER DOCTOR REPORTS FROM THE
FRONT LINES . . .

"As an emergency physician, I am in the unique position of actually being pulled into the loop when complications do occur with medical screening procedures. In the past 20 years, I have responded to four cardiac arrests in the colonoscopy suite (all four were successfully resuscitated). In the past year I have seen about four post-endoscopy GI bleeds. This typically occurs several days after polyp removal, when the eschar at the biopsy site sloughs and allows an underlying vessel to bleed. This results in significant blood loss that can potentially require ICU admission, blood transfusion, and emergent endoscopy to cauterize the bleeding site. Over the years I have also seen four bowel perforations, two splenic lacerations, and one liver laceration resulting from elective screening. These complications are indeed rare, and my observations are courtesy of the selection bias of being in the ER, but they are nonetheless real. When such complications occur in low-risk patients encouraged to undergo testing by public health campaigns, it highlights the dark side of the push to increase participation in low-risk populations."

—Co-author Doug McGuff

Another thing to consider with regard to screening is whether early detection actually decreases the mortality from disease. Some polyps have pre-cancerous or cancerous cells in them, and the presumption is that removal is curative and prevents a colon cancer that would have gone undetected. Polyps that are left alone can undergo adenomatous change where they form cancerous cells, and cancerous polyps can grow into full-blown colon cancer. It would only seem logical to seek these out and remove them. However, the March 5, 2008 issue of CA-A Cancer Journal for Clinicians (the Journal of the American Cancer Society) notes that "[t]here are no prospective randomized controlled trials of screening colonoscopy for the reduction or incidence of colorectal cancer." Gina Kolata, science writer for The New York Times, noted in a 2006 article: "The patients in all studies had at least one adenoma detected on colonoscopy but did not have cancer. They developed cancer in the next few years, however, at the same rate as would be expected in the general population without screening."[2]

Another troubling fact is that the American Cancer Society in 2007 noted that the annual incidence of colorectal cancer has risen by 30,000 cases annually, a 22 percent increase since 1999.[3] On the face of it, this suggests the possibility that the Couric Effect might be *negative*: the incidence of colorectal cancer has increased precisely during the period when screening increased. We must remember that when we discuss the incidence of a disease, that is a figure that should be constant and unchanged by testing; the benefits of screening are supposed to allow us to catch an existing disease early and improve mortality, *not* to change our assessment of what fraction of the population has the disease. The increase in cancer rates amidst increased screening suggests one of two things: first, that increased testing is overcalling the diagnosis or discovering lesions that were previously clinically insignificant and did not progress to disease. (For instance, if doctors started giving pregnancy tests to millions of men annually, it's possible we would measure a slight uptick in the rate of pregnancy nationwide—due to false positives.) The second possibility is that the screening procedure itself may be doing something to increase the incidence of the disease.[4] The first possibility is the much more likely one, namely, that the public campaigns urging people to be screened for colorectal cancer have resulted in a higher *proportion* of false positives among test recipients, since people in lower-risk populations are receiving the screening than would have occurred in the absence of the public campaigns.

I personally believe that the removal of a polyp is likely indicated and is most likely beneficial when it is found to have cancerous or pre-cancerous cells. But I also believe that screening should be done only in those with an elevated pre-test probability of disease (age greater than 50, strong family history, history of rectal bleeding, positive fecal occult blood screening, or another positive screening test). When you cast too wide of a net, the real and theoretical risks of screening are more likely to manifest.

Thus when we consider undergoing screening colonoscopy, we must not only consider the potential benefits (real and imagined); we must also consider the real and imagined downsides. The real downsides include the possibility of bowel perforation, acute bleeding after polyp removal, delayed bleeding after polyp removal, infection, sepsis, or complications related to the bowel prep. A recent study investigated the frequency of these complications and reported the following:

> Of the 16,318 eligible colonoscopies (96% performed by board-certified gastroenterologists), the incidence of serious complications was 5/1000 procedures. The 82 cases of serious complications that occurred involved 15 perforations, 6 cases of postpolypectomy syndrome, 53 cases of bleeding requiring hospitalization (15 requiring surgery or transfusion), 38 cases of bleeding requiring inpatient observation, 6 cases of diverticulitis, and 2 unusual complications (1 snare caught in a large polyp requiring surgery and 1 case of diabetic ketoacidosis associated with the colon preparation). There were 10 deaths within 30 days of the procedure, but only 1 of these was directly related to colonoscopy (a patient with congestive heart failure and sepsis after a transfusion for postpolypectomy-related bleeding).[5]

Finally, although it is not likely a major contributor, we have to consider at least the theoretical possibility that the sharp rise in detected cases coinciding with more widespread screening is due to a perverse effect of the "safety first" approach itself: specifically, that polypectomy may directly *cause* disease. There are many types of cancer capable of spreading by a mechanism called "seeding." Cancers can erode through local tissue barriers or into blood vessels, resulting in metastasis (spread to other body sites). Recent research seems to indicate that tumors can also undergo "self-seeding," where a tumor grows or spreads by a process of local chemical signaling that causes tumor cells to re-infiltrate primary tumors or surrounding local tissue. A recent journal article noted that breast cancer, colon cancer, and melanoma have this self-seeding capability.[6] Melanoma lesions are commonly excised with a wide margin to prevent seeding. If colon cancer has similar capabilities, I worry about the possibility that "nipping colon cancer in the bud" may actually result in scattering cancer cells to the four winds.

As we can see from this review, there are genuine risks of colonoscopy, meaning that the decision to be screened is more complicated than the public awareness campaigns would have you believe. This is especially true for someone who has successfully incorporated healthy primal laws. One of the major factors raising your risk for colorectal cancer is your lifestyle. If you are a smoker, drink alcohol to excess, are obese, have a poor diet that includes lots of inflammatory mediators, and are deficient in nutrients and antioxidants, then your risk goes up. If you eliminate these risks factors over a period of time and eat a primal diet that is anti-inflammatory and full of antioxidants, then your risk of disease diminishes. That means you are becoming part of a category that should be more *reluctant* to undergo testing, because the benefits of the screening (i.e., early detection of existing disease leading to early treatment and better outcome) go down, while the costs are the same.

What we can now understand is that is a widespread general recommendation should actually be a complex decision involving risk-benefit analysis. This is not a decision that you should be expected to make on your own. Hence why we spent an entire chapter on physician selection. A personal physician who knows you well and has a sense of your own risk/benefit orientation can help you determine when you might personally have enough of a pre-test probability to indicate a need for screening colonoscopy. You and your doctor might consider other testing, such as fecal occult blood testing or fecal DNA testing, as a threshold that must be crossed to trigger colonoscopy. Only by considering all the risks, the benefits, your pre-test probability of disease, and your own personality and preferences can you make the best decision about colonoscopy.

MAMMOGRAPHY: HOW TO SCARE THE HELL OUT OF YOURSELF

Every once in a while, I will have a distraught woman check into the ER after having completed a mammogram. When a woman is told that she has a positive mammogram, she naturally assumes she has a very high likelihood of having breast cancer. Typically her first action will be to call her husband or significant other in tears. Visions of mastectomy, loss of her femininity, and baldness from chemotherapy rush through her mind. Then she considers that even after all the disfiguring treatment, within a few years she may still be dead, leaving her husband a widower and her children motherless. As these thoughts race through her and her loved one's heads, there arises the small hope that it is just a false positive. Perhaps it is all just a scare and life can return to normal. Typically, the patient will then call the office of the family doctor, OB/GYN, or surgeon that ordered the test. If she is lucky enough to get hold of the doctor, the results will not have been sent to them yet and they will not know what to say. Typically, an appointment will be set for days or weeks away to review the results and decide the next step. These will be among the longest days of a woman's life, filled with ruminations of suffering and death. Sleep will be near impossible, and when it occurs, it is haunted with fitful dreams. Some women cannot face this prospect and will come to the ER in hopes of expediting the process. Sometimes we are able to help; sometimes we are ineffective. Most of what I have to offer is a discussion of the actual possibility that her positive mammogram indicates cancer. We will go over that later.

AN ER DOCTOR REPORTS FROM THE FRONT LINES . . .

"One of the best surgeons I have ever known had a policy of only ordering mammograms on a specific day of the week and holding a batch of open appointments at his office on that day. The purpose of this was so that he could be able to see any woman who

had a positive mammogram immediately. If there were a positive mammogram, he would set a same-day appointment for the patient and perform an immediate needle aspiration (or biopsy) so the woman would not be left hanging. Most times, the needle aspiration reveals fluid that is typical of a benign cyst and the woman can be immediately reassured. If things are less clear, the results of fine needle aspirate can also return fairly quickly and are most often negative. If things are inconclusive, the surgeon can perform an excision biopsy or lumpectomy, which is also negative the majority of times. This surgeon recognized that the biggest risk associated with a positive mammogram is the morbidity of worry and dread. If you have selected your doctor appropriately, and you decide to undergo screening mammography, I highly recommend that you make similar arrangements with your doctor. Many hospitals now have Breast Centers that are set up to function in exactly this way."

—Co-author Doug McGuff

The reason that a positive mammogram instills such fear is that the general public and even many physicians misinterpret the statistics of screening mammography. Our natural misinterpretation of statistics has been amplified by the politicization of breast cancer, as well as by the numerous pink ribbon walk-a-thons and awareness campaigns. Even NFL players spend an entire month of their season playing in pink shoes. Certainly if something is so important and commands such attention, then the screening that is being pushed by these "awareness" campaigns must be reliable—right? In truth, it depends on context and a proper understanding of statistics.

I remember my favorite surgeon telling me that if you perform mammography on a woman with known breast cancer, the mammogram will detect the cancerous lesion about 95 percent of the time. This statistic is what launched mammography as a potentially reliable screening test in the first place, because the rate of false negatives is low. Most people, including many physicians, assume that if this statistic is true, then its converse is also true—but no, this is not really the case. In other words:

if a woman with known breast cancer undergoes mammography, her tumor will be visualized some 95 percent of the time; but that does *not* mean that a woman with a positive mammogram will have a 95 percent chance of having cancer. *The actual figure is closer to 9 percent.*[7] Thus we see that a mammogram is not very likely to miss it if you actually have breast cancer, but at the same time *a mammogram very often reports false positives, warning of cancer even when you are fine.* I should also point out that even though the 9 percent figure is a much more reassuring number, it still does not quell the anxiety for a woman receiving a positive mammogram, because there is still the very real possibility that she has cancer. After all, if an individual is part of the 9 percent, it is 100 percent for her.

A 2013 article in the *Annals of Family Medicine* quantified the negative impact of "false positive" results, as well as its duration long after the women had been notified that the initial "positive" result had been a mistake.[8] Specifically, the researchers recruited 454 women who had received a "positive" result (both true and false) on a mammogram during the course of a year, and for each such woman recruited an additional two others from the same clinic who had been screened the same day but who initially received a "negative" result on the mammogram. Because some of the women who had initially received a "positive" result were later given the good news with a follow-up "negative" result, the researchers could use surveys administered to the three different groups to assess the psychosocial impact on a woman of believing (incorrectly) that she might have breast cancer. The researchers followed the three groups of women for a full three years after the final diagnosis. They concluded:

> False-positive screening mammography causes long-term psychosocial harm. In a period of 3 years after being declared free of cancer suspicion, women with false positives consistently reported greater negative psychosocial consequences compared with women with normal findings. The first half-year after final diagnosis, women with false positives reported changes just as great in existential values and inner calmness as women with breast cancer.

In other words, these researchers found that not only were women objectively harmed (psychologically) by the experience of receiving a "false positive" result on a mammogram, but that this harm was empirically detectable a full three years after the erroneous diagnosis had been corrected. Furthermore, on two of the indicators examined, the women who had received the false positive were just as rattled as women who really had breast cancer, for a full six months *after* the two groups of women received their final diagnoses. Acco rding to this study, then, frequent administering of mammograms carries quite serious and lasting costs; the harm of a "false positive" result is not mere angst until a follow-up exam reverses the initial (and erroneous) finding.

With such a negative impact of false positives, there must be a very positive impact of early detection if we are to justify the practice of frequent mammograms. We would hope that the harm of false positives is offset by the lives saved through the early detection of true positives. The best place to answer such questions is to search the database of The Cochrane Collaboration. This is highly regarded as a good source of unbiased information on many medical and scientific topics. They have produced over 5,000 Cochrane Reviews, which involve scouring the literature for the best studies to answer a given question. They are meticulous about addressing potential areas of bias and confounding data.

Their summary on mammography (along with many other summaries) can be found at their website (www.cochrane.dk). Their original summary published in 2008 reads:

> It may be reasonable to attend for breast cancer screening with mammography, but it may also be reasonable not to attend, as screening has both benefits and harms.

> If 2000 women are screened regularly for 10 years, one will benefit from the screening as she will avoid dying from breast cancer.

> At the same time, 10 healthy women will, as a consequence, become cancer patients and will be treated unnecessarily. These

women will have either a part of their breast or the whole breast removed, and they will often receive radiotherapy, and sometimes chemotherapy.

Furthermore, about 200 healthy women will experience a false alarm. The psychological strain until one knows whether or not it was cancer, and even afterwards, can be severe.[9]

Not exactly a strong endorsement of the value of mammography screening, is it? This goes completely against the grain of public sentiment, which has largely been framed by advocacy groups, the government, and the media. The message women have had pounded into their heads is that it's their responsibility to get frequent mammogram screenings, and that there are no downsides to this except the hassle involved. But as we have explained, this popular message is simply wrong. There are quite real harms from mammogram screening, which must be balanced against the potential benefits.

Recently, the evidence against mammography as a screening intervention has gotten even stronger. In 2013 the Cochrane group updated their summary with the following:

> **We believe that the time has come to re-assess whether universal mammography screening should be recommended for any age group.** Declining rates of breast cancer mortality are mainly due to improved treatments and breast cancer awareness, and therefore we are uncertain as to the benefits of screening today. Overdiagnosis has human costs and increases mastectomies and deaths. **The chance that a woman will benefit from attending screening is small at best, and— if based on the randomised trials—ten times smaller than the risk that she may experience serious harm in terms of overdiagnosis.** Women, clinicians and policy makers should consider the trade-offs carefully when they decide whether or not to attend or support screening programmes.[10]

It seems clear that default screening mammography for all women is not the way to go, but what is an individual woman to do? Two things will help you decide on the correct answer for yourself. The first is to go through the process of selecting a good physician who understands your personality and health history. The second is to return to our notion of NNT. In order for the NNT to benefit to predominate over the chance for harm, there must be significant risk factors for the disease for which you are testing. Clearly, mammography applied as a general screening test across the general population does not meet this standard. However, a given individual may have enough risk factors to tip the scales in favor of screening. Such risk factors include prior confirmed breast cancer or a history of breast cancer or ovarian cancer in primary family members (a mother or sister), especially if the cancer occurred at a young age. Such a history might trigger genetic screening that can uncover the presence of the BRCA1 or BRCA2 mutations, which increase risk for this disease.[11]

Even then, we must consider that, with the improved treatment protocols, there may not be a demonstrable benefit to earlier diagnosis. In other words, if you don't have mammography and the cancer is not discovered until it is larger and obvious, the cure rate may be no different.[12] In this case the only benefit of mammography may be additional years of anxiety and worry.

One of the mainstays of a primal mindset is not to follow general recommendations intended for the population at large. You must always consider any screening or treatment in light of the number needed to treat and your own risk for disease. Sometimes you can reach these conclusions on your own; at other times, you may need to consult with your physician. What you should never do, however, is jump on a bandwagon because of media or celebrity endorsement.

ONE FOR THE MEN: PSA TESTING

Women are not the only ones who have the opportunity to scare themselves with false positive screening tests; men get their chance as well. Prostate cancer screening via the PSA (prostate specific antigen) has also been promoted as an early detection tool. Like our other screening tests, it falls down when we cast too wide of a net. What was hoped to be a means of early detection to help avoid progression and spread of prostate cancer actually had no influence on long-term survival. Further, false positives and the diagnosis of what would most likely be small and/or slow-growing tumors resulted in many men being treated unnecessarily. We found out only after the fact that many men suffered the risk of radiation and or chemotherapy, as well as incontinence and impotence, for no corresponding benefit.

To cut right to the chase, the Cochrane summary for prostate cancer screening (including digital rectal exam and prostatic ultrasonography) was as follows:

> Prostate cancer screening did not significantly decrease prostate cancer-specific mortality in a combined meta-analysis of five RCTs. Only one study (ERSPC) reported a 21% significant reduction of prostate cancer-specific mortality in a pre-specified subgroup of men aged 55 to 69 years. Pooled data currently demonstrates no significant reduction in prostate cancer-specific and overall mortality. Harms associated with PSA-based screening and subsequent diagnostic evaluations are frequent, and moderate in severity. Overdiagnosis and overtreatment are common and are associated with treatment-related harms. Men should be informed of this and the demonstrated adverse effects when they are deciding whether or not to undertake screening for prostate cancer. Any reduction in prostate cancer-specific mortality may take up to 10 years to accrue; therefore, men who have a life expectancy less than 10 to 15 years should be informed that screening for prostate cancer is unlikely to be beneficial. No studies examined the independent role of screening by DRE.[13]

Even the American Urological Association has backed off from routine screening, but still recommends that men from ages 55 to 69 consider screening, noting that the risks and benefits require shared decision making. They stated in a 2013 guideline:

For men ages 55 to 69 years, the decision to undergo PSA screening involves weighing the benefits of preventing prostate cancer in 1 man for every 1,000 men screened over a decade against the known potential harms associated with screening and treatment.[14]

My own addendum would also include the loss of the downstream revenue generated by these harms caused by screening and treatment.

One of the best sources for getting to the bottom of most questions of efficacy in the medical field is the website www.thennt.com. They review the strongest literature and boil it down to a summary that shows the benefits in percentages and the harms in percentages. Reviewing their evaluations of many of the treatments I use on a daily basis makes me wonder what the hell I am even doing in medicine, as much of what is considered standard of care is not supported by the evidence. I strongly suggest visiting this site when you are considering any medical treatment.

With regard to PSA testing, www.thennt.com details the benefits as follows: 100 percent saw no benefit; 0 percent were helped by preventing death from any cause; 0 percent were helped by preventing death from prostate cancer. With regard to harms, 20 percent were harmed by undergoing a prostate biopsy for a false-positive test.

IF YOU GET TOO CLOSE TO THE PROM QUEEN YOU WILL SEE HER WARTS

I can draw on my experience in emergency medicine to give a perfect example of the problems with indiscriminate screening: the widespread use of CT scanning in trauma. In the past, we always screened for pneumothorax—an air collection in the chest cavity from a punctured lung—with a plain chest x-ray. When a pneumothorax was seen, we evacuated it by placing a plastic chest tube about the size of your index finger or thumb between the ribs, into the space between the lung and chest wall. With the advent of CT scans, we started to identify very small pneumothoracies that were previously not visible on chest x-ray.

As a result of the increased sensitivity of this test, we started to turn up a lot more tiny pneumothoracies that we didn't know what to do with. Knowing that they were there, it was hard to do nothing, especially with the medico-legal consequences should anything go bad. This was especially true for any patient entering the OR who was going to be on a ventilator with positive pressure ventilation, as this could theoretically expand a small pneumothorax into a large tension pneumothorax that might cause cardiac arrest. The consequence was that for almost a decade, large numbers of trauma patients needlessly underwent a painful invasive procedure with a high complication rate.

As we accumulated more cases of pneumothoracies diagnosed on CT that were not visible on plain chest x-ray, we did start to wonder, "Where were all the bad outcomes before the advent of CT scanning?" Eventually, through both retrospective and randomized trials, we came to realize that such tiny pneumothoracies could be watched expectantly and required no intervention.

The conceptual common denominator to keep in mind when considering screening is the idea of prior probability. The more sensitive you make a test for a disease, the more important it is *not* to apply it as a population-wide screening test. The "better" a test is, the more important it is only to apply to people who have an elevated risk of the disease in question.

GENETIC TESTING: A SCREENING TEST FOR A SCREENING TEST?

Our discussion of prior probability begs the question, "Is there anything that can be done to determine my prior probability other than the presence of symptoms or a strong family history?" There exists technology to screen for genetic mutations or variations that increase risk for certain diseases. Some of these are diseases for which screening tools exist, like the examples discussed in this chapter.

Currently, the biggest supplier of genetic testing technology is the company *23andMe*. The name refers to the 23 gene pairs that we all possess. Your genes are analyzed using a saliva or cheek swab sample.

Your DNA goes through a process where it is broken up into pieces and mixed with known DNA base pairs that bind to known gene variations. These are labeled with a fluorescent tag that identifies "SNiPs," known as single nucleotide peptides, which are basically segments of DNA that correspond to certain gene variants.

Much of what is identified is just information that is cute or interesting. Things such as your ability to make asparagus pee, or your capacity to taste bitter, or the geographic region from which your ancestors came. However, more ominous things are also reported. These include your risk for Alzheimer's disease, type II diabetes, and colon cancer, and especially the presence of the BRCA1 and BRCA2 genes that define a markedly increased risk for breast and ovarian cancer. The presence of this gene variant (along with a strong family history) is what led Angelina Jolie to undergo a prophylactic mastectomy.

The following are my general thoughts on how you should go about forming your own decision when it comes to genetic testing:

→ If you are trying to collect information to get around the issue of low prior probability, you still need to remember that you are gathering this information through . . . a process of screening. So unless you have symptoms or a family history that makes you want to go looking, then all the problems of false positives still exist. Further, genes do not just operate on a yes/no basis. Environmental conditions probably contribute 70 to 80 percent towards whether a gene will express disease or not. Thus, the detection of a disease-prone genotype does not necessarily help you quantify a family history that you already know you have.

→ Before you dive in and take the test, you really need to consider how you might react to results that you do not want or like. You might fancy yourself as the type of person who doesn't care or who can shrug off ominous findings. But perhaps things will be different when you see unexpected results. The psychic toll of such knowledge is legitimate, and can cause your mind to generate real physical symptoms that can ultimately put you on the road to increased medical testing. False signals of greater prior probability raise the odds of false positives or incidental findings that, again, set into motion psychosomatic symptoms that can only be quelled by testing that comes back negative. In the process, there is risk for iatrogenic injury, more false positives, infection, and radiation exposure that greatly outweigh the risk for any real disease.

➔ Will the results of a genetic test alter your behavior? For example, suppose you undergo genetic screening and find yourself at risk for type II diabetes and Alzheimer's dementia. What should you do? It turns out the answer is to follow primal principles that ensure proper dietary, exercise, and environmental signaling. If you are already diligently following the primal lifestyle, then your new knowledge will not change what you are doing whatsoever. So, if testing does not change what you should be doing, why do it in the first place?

WEIGHING THE PROS AND CONS OF ELECTIVE PROCEDURES

We have established that how you behave during hospitalization is of critical importance. Your mindset and demeanor can have a profound influence on the degree of risk that you will encounter while in the hospital. When you undergo (or consider undergoing) an elective procedure, your mindset and demeanor are even more critical.

When you are in the hospital, you are more likely to be at greater risk because you are sick or injured, and most likely did not arrive there by your own volition. While it is generally true that you will have to be in better condition to undergo an elective procedure, the more critical issue is that you don't necessarily have to be there. You are there of your own choosing. The risks may or may not be as great as a hospitalization, but the decision to take the risks is entirely one of free will. Thus, if any of those risks come to fruition, then the damage that occurs will seem much more bitter, because they will then seem totally unnecessary. For this reason, your orientation and approach to elective procedures is of extreme importance.

In this section we will provide general guidelines for deciding whether to undergo an elective procedure or not. You will be taught how to gather information on the risks and benefits of a given elective procedure, as well as how to seek out alternative treatments. Should you decide to undergo treatment, we will discuss how to locate the most qualified professional to perform the procedure and how to find the best price.

There are two general categories of elective procedures. First, there are those procedures that are elective in terms of their timing and location, but are otherwise mandatory. Elective in the medical world means "not emergent." In other words, the surgery or procedure does not have to be done immediately, but instead, can be put off until a later date. The second category consists of those procedures that fit the lay definition of "elective." Not only is their timing optional, but whether to do them at all is also an option. (If we apply the strictest of definitions, nearly all procedures fall into this second category.)

Some examples of procedures that are of the first category (optional timing but must be done) are the elective repair of a torn ACL knee ligament in a professional athlete or laborer who depends on knee stability in high force situations. Another example might be a professional baseball pitcher who has a torn labrum in his shoulder. Or perhaps an anesthesiologist with a compressed C7 nerve who has lost pinch strength and can no longer perform an intubation procedure.

The exact same procedures listed here may fall into the second category under different context. If the ACL injury or torn labrum is in an office worker, or even in an athlete who does not place severe stresses on the joints in question, it is truly optional to undergo corrective surgery. I once trained a professional BMX racer who competed several seasons with bilateral torn ACLs.

In most cases, almost all elective medical procedures are in this second category. Even conditions that produce a lot of pain or impairment will heal themselves if given enough time. This includes conditions that many doctors will tell you will not self-correct. For example, I know of an ER doctor who suffered an L5 disc herniation that produced such severe nerve compression that he developed atrophy of the muscles, foot drop, and partial paralysis. He refused to undergo surgery or even take a Tylenol. He suffered through the pain and drug his leg around on ER shifts over 18 months, when suddenly one day all of his symptoms resolved. Within a few weeks his muscle mass and function returned to normal and he has been symptom-free since. What seems like a matter of necessity is really a matter of our unwillingness to endure the pain and suffering for the period of time it takes Mother Nature to heal the injury.

SHOULD YOU HAVE THE PROCEDURE AT ALL?

The most important question to first answer is: should you have the elective procedure in the first place? In the setting of this book, it is not practical for me to discuss every possible procedure that one might face. Instead, let us lay out some general guidelines for deciding whether to undergo a procedure or to let nature take its course.

REVISIT THE NNT

One of the first places I suggest you start is to visit the website www.thennt.com. The concept of number needed to treat (NNT) has come up repeatedly throughout this book; this website looks at the scientific literature, dissects the raw data on clinical issues, and then expresses the results in a NNT format. When you visit the website, don't just look for the clinical issue or procedure that concerns you. Instead, peruse the entire website (especially the blog) to get a flavor of how uncertain and often completely backwards the standard practices are for medicine in general. Another pattern to notice is that the conclusions of many medical studies—even in renowned journals—are actually inconsistent with the raw data within the study. The vast majority of medical practitioners and institutions accept these conclusions at face value, and this is generally what will be recommended to you when you speak to physicians. Yet the raw data in even the most definitive studies may actually point in the opposite direction. I suggest that you use this website to investigate the procedure or therapy that you are considering, along with similar therapies. Each analysis is summarized and represented by a traffic signal type system. A green light means benefits exceed harm, a yellow light means benefit is uncertain, a red light means there is no benefit, and the black triangle/exclamation point means that harms exceed benefits.

Many times, a visit to this website, along with reading some of the literature itself, will be enough to make the decision for you. If the issue is still uncertain, you can proceed to the next step and consult with a physician.

ASK AN EXPERT

If your question is not answered by visiting www.thennt.com or searching the literature, then it is time to pose the question to an expert. You cannot, however, just schedule an appointment with a local specialist, especially if this is the same person that may be doing your procedure. Most doctors are very objective and honest, but the bias that occurs when you ask a barber if you need a haircut is very hard to overcome. This is especially true because such bias is usually of a subconscious nature. Even if the physician is a close personal friend, this bias cannot be escaped.

I generally recommend asking your local specialist, "Who are the most renowned practitioners in the field?" Another route is to ask who is the chairman of the department or the director of the residency where they trained. Once you find these names, perform some Internet searches, or look at a listing of their publications on PubMed. Soon this will lead to discussion articles that will help reveal who the thought leaders are in the field that pertains to the procedure you are considering.

Once you have decided on a leading authority, attempt to schedule an appointment at their clinic for consultation. If you have decent health care coverage, you will find these appointments easier to acquire than you think. Even better, pay out of pocket, and offer to pay the full cost of the appointment ahead of time. Offer to give your credit card information over the phone to schedule the appointment. You will be surprised how much this can expedite your appointment or move you up in the queue. As to the content of the consultation, just let them know your clinical situation and that you are seeking counsel on whether or not an elective procedure would be recommended. Offer to send all of your pertinent medical records and studies ahead of time. At the very least, assure them that you will bring all of these records with you. The best option is to do both.

Here is the catch that you do not want to discuss until the day of your appointment. You are there just to get their expert opinion on whether or not to undergo a procedure. If the procedure in question is recommended, you will not be having it done at their institution. Most academic physicians are salaried and thus do not have a financial interest in the decision to have the procedure or not. However, they are usually at the helm of a residency or fellowship and are always actively seeking cases for their residents and fellows. By stating your intention to have the procedure done elsewhere, you diminish the risk of any bias, conscious or unconscious. Also, your consulting physician will also feel great relief knowing that he will not have to wrestle with the conflict associated with trying to draw in new cases.

There is one major precaution to this approach, and that is the overwhelming desire you may develop for this world expert to be the one to perform your procedure. If and when such a desire develops, I generally advise not to succumb to it. There are a couple of reasons for this. First, becoming a department chairman, director, or otherwise famous physician requires much more in the way of charisma and political cunning than any sort of clinical or technical excellence. Second, someone who has risen to this level is usually not very clinically active, and in any event the bulk of your actual procedure may be done by a fellow or residents in training.

Another tip for your meeting with your renowned expert is to try to speak with his or her colleagues, and especially the residents. Commonly, an upper level resident will be present during your evaluation and discussion. Watch the demeanor and expressions of the consultant. Sometimes, a department chair will have gained so much power and influence that they may have "gone off the reservation" without any real resistance. Such is the dark side of tenure. If this is the case, it will be evident in the body language of the resident. You may even get a tell-tale head shaking directed at you or an eye rolling. Often, you may be left alone in the room with the attending resident. Take the opportunity to ask if they are in agreement, or if this is an unorthodox view. The resident may self-deprecate and try to bow out, but you should insist on their input. In most cases, if something is amiss, they will be dying to tip you off. If everything lines up, you can feel confident that the advice you have received is good. If it does not, you can most likely rely on the opposite advice, but can seek confirmation elsewhere if you feel the need. In either case, the information obtained will be very worthwhile and the trip will have been worth the time and effort.

BRING IT HOME

Once you have had your meeting with the most renowned expert you could find, bring the information and records back home with you. Your next step is to contact your family doctor (the one you have picked by the criteria previously discussed). You can either set an appointment or request a phone conversation. Simply request a referral to your doctor's preferred specialist for the procedure you are considering. This referral is especially important if your expert has recommended in favor of performing the procedure.

Ideally, your family doctor will have a strong referral relationship with the specialist, which should result in an expedited appointment. When you have this appointment, tell the specialist that you want his or her opinion on the situation. Let the specialist know you have visited a renowned expert in the field, but do not name that expert or what was recommended to you. Also, inform the specialist that you intend to pay in full for the appointment, but will not commit to having the procedure done by him or her. Ideally, and most commonly, the specialist will reach a conclusion that is the same or very similar to your renowned expert. Gather up all of the recommendations, pay for the appointment by cash or credit card, and state that you will be in touch.

DISCUSS WITH YOUR LOVED ONES

Assuming that the recommendations seem in agreement and solid, the next step is to discuss it with the other stakeholders in your life: your loved ones. Ideally, they will have already been along for the ride. Even so, a good heart to heart can help solidify your decision. If you are at odds about the decision to undergo a procedure, I strongly advise not to proceed until the conflict has been fully resolved. If you are married or otherwise in a committed relationship, and your spouse or partner strongly opposes, then I would yield. Most times this person is seeing something that you are refusing to see or are incapable of seeing. If you do not wish to yield, then keep working on the debate until it is amicably settled. Once settled, spend a few days or weeks letting it sink into your consciousness. Sleep on it. Let your gut and the content of your dreams deliver any data that is still needed. Once everything falls into alignment, then and only then make your final decision.

PICKING YOUR SPECIALIST

The remainder of this discussion is predicated on the assumption that you have decided to go ahead with your elective procedure. There are many considerations with regard to selecting a specialist and an institution for your procedure. The reputation and experience of the specialist and the institution where the procedure will take place, insurance and preferred provider status, comfort and ease of travel, cost, and post-procedural care are but a few of the considerations that need to be made.

EXPERIENCE AND REPUTATION

The importance of experience can vary somewhat based on the elective procedure in question. Procedures that are "bread and butter" for a given specialty or that involve automated technology are less dependent on the absolute number of cases involved, and because they are routine, almost any specialist will have exceeded the minimum number of cases to be proficient. Cholecystectomy (gallbladder removal), appendectomy, Lasik, and cataract surgery fall into this category.

Procedures that are less commonly performed, are technically complex, and are at the mercy of the specialist's technique are more dependent on experience. Also, procedures that are new or cutting edge make it more challenging to accrue enough cases to be truly facile and experienced. Total hip replacements are a good example of the former. New endovascular procedures or keyhole surgeries are examples of the latter.

For the more bread-and-butter procedures, you would like to see the high double digits performed per year (ideally, in the hundreds) and thousands of the procedure done to date. For the newer or more unusual procedures, you would like to see at least a dozen a year with total procedures in the hundreds. Also, you would like to know that the training for the procedure in question exceeded a weekend course. Instead, ideal is some evidence of supervised advanced training (even if obtained outside official or credentialed channels), or perhaps a mini-fellowship. You should not be shy about asking for this sort of information.

With regard to reputation, a simple Google search of the physician's name will turn up a variety of consumer rating organizations. Don't expect anything like Angie's List where you get detailed descriptions from satisfied customers. Instead, be on the lookout for any bad reports or evidence of bad outcomes or losing privileges. The best source for reputation is any friend that you might have in the medical field, or who works at the hospital where you may be getting your procedure. If you can find out who certain physicians or nurses are going to for the procedure in question, that is worth its weight in gold. Even if your connection is not "high in the food chain," they can still provide useful reconnaissance. Hospitals are like small towns: everyone knows what's what. The janitorial staff could very likely tell you who is best and who to stay away from.

Keep in mind that as you collect this data, you may not be looking just for a particular person who is best. Sometimes you will be looking for who does a particular *procedure* the best. The best overall surgeon may not be the one who does the best gallbladder removal. One surgeon may be best for gallbladders, and another may be preferred for lumpectomies. In the vast majority of cases, there will not be an issue of having to root out a bad player. Usually, the issue is just finding who is best for your particular procedure.

INFECTION RATES

While you are deciding on a physician, check into the infection rates of the facility in which your physician will be operating. The national average for surgical infection rates is around 2 to 2.5 percent. Ideally, you want to be cared for in a facility that has an infection rate of 1 percent or less. This is not based on any scientific studies or data; rather, it is only my personal opinion. I just do not think any elective procedure is worth more than a 1 in 100 chance of post-operative infection. A higher infection rate does not necessarily reflect poorly on the institution. In fact, quite the opposite may be true, since taking on a higher volume of tougher cases will naturally drive the infection rate higher. The tricky part is to find a physician with a caseload that supports the right amount of experience, practicing in an institution with a lower infection rate. Many times this can be achieved by engaging that physician in an outpatient surgery center. While it may not be the fault of the institution with a higher infection rate, it is not your fault either. Also, the higher infection rate is an indirect indicator that the infections are more likely to be from multi-drug resistant organisms. In an elective procedure, such a complication would be truly tragic.

PRICING

If you are still in an employer-sponsored, third-party payment insurance program, then pricing will be less of a concern for you. You will just need to be aware of any deductibles and co-pays you may have. You will also need to get "prior approval" for your procedure. Make sure that you obtain your prior approval from your insurance company in writing. *Do not* rely on the doctor's office staff to secure this for you and *do not* proceed simply on their say-so that your procedure has been approved by the insurance company. You do not want to be stuck with the full bill—which will run into the tens of thousands, commonly—when you find out that your procedure did not receive proper authorization. *This is why you should obtain prior authorization from the insurance company in writing.*

If you have taken my earlier advice and purchased true insurance with a high deductible, or if your insurance company would not approve to pay for your elective procedure, the price of your procedure will become very important to you. If insurance is not picking up the bill after a deductible, you will probably find it very difficult to fund your elective procedure.

In order for pricing to work, third-party payment needs to be removed from the equation. Fortunately, there are surgery centers that accept only cash payment. This removes the entire overhead of government and third-party payment systems and allows prices to come down to true market levels. The flagship example of this model is the Surgery Center of Oklahoma (www.surgerycenterok.com) located in Oklahoma City. They have devised an all-inclusive pricing system that gives a single price for all components of your procedure (surgery, anesthesia, facility fees, and any others). There are a handful of similar facilities scattered throughout the country. If insurance and pricing are a problem, traveling to a facility like this is probably the ideal solution. In general, I have found that it is the very best doctors who resent the current system the most. As a result, centers like the Surgery Center of Oklahoma tend to attract some of the best practitioners available. However, as we will discuss later, there are downsides to traveling away from home for an elective procedure.

You may not have to leave home in order to benefit from the Surgery Center of Oklahoma's price structure. The incredible thing about competition is that its effects can be felt far and wide. At their website, the Surgery Center of Oklahoma lists its price structure. Patients are already having success printing off their price list and bringing it to their local surgery center or hospital. Present the quoted price for the procedure you wish to have and let them know that you would love to have your procedure done at their facility, but will travel to Oklahoma if they cannot match their price. Allow them a little extra in their pricing to account for the expense that would be incurred traveling to Oklahoma. Let them know that you want a single price and that you will pay in full at the time of the procedure. Even though the entity you are dealing with may still take Medicare, Medicaid, and commercial insurance, they will likely jump at the chance for immediate cash without all of the expense and hassle of filing with a third-party payer. They will quickly realize that their net profit is likely to be higher than what they obtain through the current system. If you cannot strike such a deal, I highly recommend that you plan a trip to Oklahoma.

Speaking of travel, another option for free market medical procedures is *international* medical tourism. This is not something with which I have personal experience, but I refer interested readers to start with Timothy Ferriss' book *The Four Hour Body*, which has a chapter on medical tourism entitled, "How To Pay For A Beach Vacation With One Hospital Visit."

POST-OPERATIVE COMPLICATIONS

One thing to always remember is that things may not go as planned. You may develop an infection, your wound may open up, or you may develop pneumonia or a deep vein thrombosis. You need to discuss ahead of time with your physician what will happen in the event that you have a complication and how that will be paid for. This is especially true if you are going the cash route. Most cash practices will eat the cost for complications. Third-party insured patients will rack up a bill, with substantial co-pays potentially heading your way.

If you are having your procedure done locally, find out from your doctor how you will be handled if you develop an after-hours complication. You should have a written agreement if your doctor will meet you at his office or ER if you have problems. If your doctor has arrangements with an on-call partner or uses the ER for post-operative complications, this needs to be discussed ahead of time. This is perfectly acceptable, provided the coverage is pre-arranged. No one expects a surgeon or doctor to work 24/7/365, but he does need to have appropriate arrangements during after hours. If your doctor utilizes the emergency department to help manage his post-operative care, this is also acceptable. You may, however, want to contact the emergency department director to make certain that it is common practice for them to evaluate your doctor's post-operative complications. Usually, there is a collegial and cooperative process in place. Not uncommonly, however, some doctors just instruct their patients with post-operative complications to go to the ER without any prior agreement or communication with the ER physician. They abuse EMTALA to have their after-hours patients cared for, and then if they need to be admitted, the problem gets passed to the on-call surgeon (who they may not have a prior agreement with), or worse yet, the hospitalist service. You do not want to be the "hot potato" in one of these dumping scenarios, so make certain you have this ironed out ahead of time.

If you are traveling to have your procedure done, the issue of post-operative complications is even more critical. As an emergency physician I can tell you that one of my most hated scenarios is the patient who had surgery done at the Mayo Clinic or Duke or another mecca and who shows up with a post-operative complication. I perform my workup and contact the surgeon at the mecca, only to be told to admit them to the local surgeon. This is totally unacceptable, and no surgeon wants to be stuck with another surgeon's post-op complication. Usually, I arrange an aeromedical transport back to the surgeon of record. You do not want to go through this.

One option, although very hard to arrange, is for the physician performing your procedure to contact one of your local specialists to establish an agreement to see you for any complications. The compensation would have to be arranged between all three parties ahead of time to make this work. Many times, professional courtesy alone will allow this plan to be successful.

More ideally, you should arrange to stay in the area after your procedure for a period of time that equals or exceeds the time period where complications would be expected to occur. That way, if anything untoward happens, you can be seen by the physician responsible for your care. It may be a little less convenient, and cost a little more, but the peace of mind will be well worth it.

I will offer one final precaution about traveling to have a medical procedure. That involves the risk of travel itself, especially as it relates to your procedure. Undergoing surgery or an invasive procedure is an inflammatory process that activates many inflammatory mediators affecting healing and blood clotting. As such, you are at greater risk for developing blood clots. Post-operative deep vein thrombosis (clots in the deep veins of the legs) is not uncommon, and the risk is greatly amplified by prolonged sitting or immobilization. The type of sitting that occurs in air travel and car travel in particular increases the risk of deep vein thrombosis, so much so that the term "coach class syndrome" has been used to describe DVTs obtained during airline travel. These blood clots can break free and become lodged in the lung, known as a pulmonary embolism or PE. A PE can trigger severe respiratory distress, low blood oxygen, and even cardiac arrest. Changes in cabin pressure and oxygen levels can prove dangerous for patients who have undergone any vascular procedure or who have any history of lung disease or a pulmonary procedure. If you have abdominal surgery, it may take time for your intestines to become fully mobile. Any gas trapped may expand at low cabin pressure, causing severe discomfort or even obstruction or perforation. Remember, even if traveling by auto, you need to consider risks. If you had blepharoplasty (eyelid surgery), consider the consequences of a face full of air bag. With a healing incision, or a leg full of pins and wires, consider the effects of even a minor traffic accident. Travel is probably one of the greatest risks associated with having a procedure done away from home. Be sure to discuss with your physician these risks and any provisions that should be made to mitigate them.

FINAL WORDS ON ELECTIVE PROCEDURES

The decision to undergo an elective procedure is one of the most important decisions you will ever make. The likelihood of anything going wrong is truly small, but the consequences are significant, and will be amplified after the fact by the knowledge that you chose to do this thing. So the first step in considering an elective procedure is to really think about whether you want to have it done. Consider that the problem may self-correct given enough time, and your urge to do something may be born out of impatience. If the issue is cosmetic, consider that it may be a much bigger issue for you than it is for anyone looking at you from the outside. What you deem undesirable may actually be an attractive, defining feature for you.

Do your research. Find out the chances of your problem self-correcting. If the decision is not clear, seek out the best consultant in the field and solicit his or her opinion in a circumstance where the consultant does not stand to materially or financially benefit. Once you have that opinion, confirm it with the expert's colleagues and trainees, as well as with your local expert.

If everything lines up and you decide to go ahead with the procedure, investigate where you wish to have it done and with whom. Check out the statistics and reputation of the physician and the facilities available. Finally, negotiate the price. Consider private pay centers or medical tourism. Even if you do not end up traveling, you may be able to use their price structure to negotiate a better deal at home. Finally, make certain that you have made appropriate arrangements for any post-procedural complications. Elective procedures are just that: elective. Ensure that you have them on your own terms.

PART IV

FREEDOM IS THE ANSWER

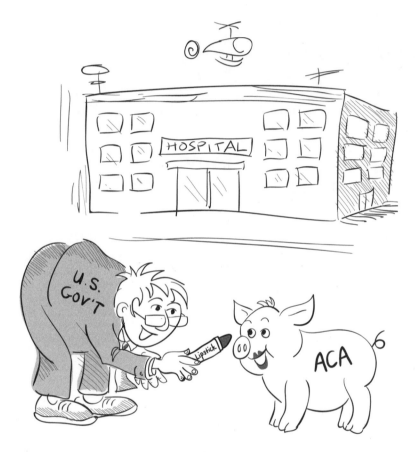

"There, that'll take care of everything!"

Chapter 14

ROLLING BACK
BIG GOVERNMENT AND
BIG PHARMA

I n this chapter, we will list and briefly explain several policies that the federal and state governments could take that would immediately and significantly improve the delivery of health care, simultaneously boosting quality and slashing prices.

We are deliberately keeping this chapter relatively short, because the purpose of this book is to educate and empower *you, the individual reader*. We actually think it is counterproductive for people to engage in excessive "evangelism," even on a topic of this importance.

Nonetheless, we recognize that some readers will want this type of list for completeness. Furthermore, there are always critics ready with the zinger: "If you don't have a solution, quit complaining!" Without further ado, here is our list of policy proposals that would dramatically improve our health care and insurance markets:

1. Repeal the Affordable Care Act. This legislation cannot be tweaked. It needs to be repealed, period.

2. Abolish the FDA and its associated powers. We showed in Chapter 2 that the FDA is quite literally responsible for the deaths of many thousands of lives, through both its acts of commission and omission. Consumers should have the freedom to try whatever drugs, devices, or procedures they wish, without getting permission from Washington. On the other hand, private sector groups would do a much better job of warning the public about genuine safety hazards—especially once the spell of the authoritative FDA disappeared and the public realized it needed new sources of information. This is not speculation on our part; we already see private-sector ratings outperforming the FDA in this crucial role.

Abolition of the FDA would cut drug development costs by more than half, virtually overnight, and without a sacrifice of safety. In practice, the current system involves a revolving door and cozy relationship between large pharmaceutical companies and their government overseers. Getting rid of the FDA would not only make popular drugs cheaper, it would allow for the development of "niche" drugs that cater to rare conditions and are currently not profitable for pharmaceutical companies to pursue.

3. Eliminate the Department of Agriculture's influence on the American diet. Perhaps the only thing more horrifying than federal bureaucrats telling you what pills are safe is having them tell schools the ideal daily allowance of carbohydrates. To understand exactly *why* the supposed experts in DC keep getting things so wrong when it comes to nutrition would require a full study of the government's long-standing tradition of subsidizing farmers. Don't worry; people would still grow food and sell it for money even without oversight and encouragement from Washington. Whatever genuinely useful nutritional functions the USDA currently serves could be filled (at lower cost) by private-sector analogs in a competitive field. There is nothing magical about being employed by the federal government; experts would have the same skills working for private inspection agencies, insurance companies, and consumer watchdog groups.

4. Abolish all government medical licensing and certification. If two adults of sound mind want to engage in a voluntary transaction involving health care, this should not land one of them in a cage just because he doesn't have the government's seal of approval. In a free market in medicine, *private, voluntary* certification organizations would thrive. Major hospitals and clinics would no doubt insist that their staff have the appropriate educational background and residency experience, and insurance companies would do the same before offering malpractice coverage.

With this simple change, the floodgates of medical supply would open, driving down prices with a surprisingly small drop (if any) in *average* quality. People who wanted to hire the best surgeons could still do so; those highly trained experts wouldn't suddenly forget how to use a scalpel just because the government no longer issued medical licenses. The difference is that patients would now have the *option* of hiring lesser-qualified medical personnel at a fraction of the previous price.

Furthermore, in combination with abolition of the FDA and Department of Agriculture, this step would remove most of the power that many cynics currently associate with "Big Pharma." As we stressed back in Chapter 2, we wholeheartedly acknowledge that there are devious characters inside *and* outside the halls of government; the private sector is not composed of angels, especially in the health care field. But the crucial fact remains that without the government's club to stamp out "unsafe" products (like raw milk) and "unqualified" practitioners (like homeopaths), companies like Monsanto would not be the menace that so many currently fear. [1]

5. Remove legal restrictions on organ sales. Yes, we realize this particular proposal may strike some readers as absurdly radical. But the current arrangement is nonsensical and deadly. If someone needs a kidney and finds a compatible donor, it is perfectly legal to pay the donor for his travel expenses and hospital bills. But it is illegal to throw in a "little something for the effort" (as Bill Murray might say). Studies suggest that some 9,000 Americans die *annually* because of an organ shortage.[2]

It's no mystery how to cure a shortage: the government just has to get out of the way. Currently there is an effective price ceiling of $0 set on the compensation (above genuine expense reimbursement) for the sale of a spare kidney. If Jim Smith is going to die without a transplant and would gladly pay (with the help of his insurance) up to $100,000 for a kidney, while Bill Martin has two perfectly healthy kidneys and would be willing to sell one of them for anything above $60,000 as this would allow him to move his family to a nicer neighborhood, then there is a great scope for these two men to strike a deal, where they both walk away feeling like big winners. It would take a serious busybody to step in between and insist that Jim dies and Bill stays stuck in his crime-ridden building.

6. End legal restrictions on health insurance portability. Although part of the problem comes from the health insurance companies themselves (which are, in fairness, merely responding to the incentives they face), certain legal barriers prevent people from buying truly portable health insurance policies that follow them even after losing a job. In this suggestion we also have in mind the legal prohibitions on "selling health insurance across state lines," as the issue has been discussed in political campaigns.

7. Give citizens the option to permanently (and irrevocably) "opt out" of Medicare, at a large "gain" to the taxpayer. The Medicare Ponzi scheme will eventually come crashing down; it is only a question of *when*. Current workers are keenly aware that they are not going to receive the full benefits they have been promised. The government could let them relinquish their claims on those future benefits in exchange for being exempt from payroll taxes for the rest of their careers. Not only would this move improve the (properly calculated) government's financial position, but it would spur faster economic growth as the lower marginal income tax rate made the worker in question more eager to sell his labor. Naturally, there would be complications about very young workers who are just starting to pay in and thus who (after the accounting footwork of the ACA) might cost the government money, even in a "present discounted value" accounting sense, if they opted out. Our purpose here is not to issue a white paper policy proposal, but just to spur creative thought on solutions.

8. Reform the tax code to minimize the advantage of employer-provided health insurance. As we've explained, the tax code is one of the primary reasons health insurance is tied to employment. A popular suggestion among policy wonks is to level the playing field by giving individuals the right to pay for health insurance with pre-tax dollars. The problem here is that there will always be exceptions to the exceptions, and the government will end up further micromanaging the whole system with its tailoring of the "loopholes." In any event, a general *cut in the marginal tax rates* would help all around. The reason people jump at the chance to have their employer pay for health coverage—rather than receive those dollars in salary—is to avoid the high marginal income tax rate. If the top rate were, say, 10 percent, then far more individuals would prefer cash wages.

9. Allow physicians and health care facilities to deduct all charity care from their tax liabilities at market rates, perhaps using Medicare formulas as the initial baseline. We certainly hope our analysis in this book didn't appear as a denial that there are genuinely needy people who require help from others in order to receive decent medical attention. We simply feel that the best solution involves *private* charity, rather than government sources.

10. Repeal EMTALA. This would immediately solve the financial crisis of today's hospitals. However, in conjunction with the other steps suggested, the poor would still receive adequate care. Prices would be far, far lower for comparable quality of care, and the tax code changes would motivate health care workers to offer pro bono services.

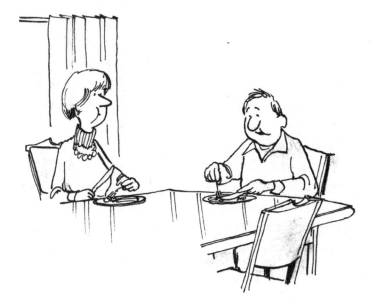

"Ooo, I just felt the good cholesterol
kick the bad cholesterol."

Chapter 15

LIVING HEALTHY AND FREE

We have covered a lot of territory in this book, and now at the end we can summarize some of the major themes. First, we hope you noticed the parallel between government intervention in the health care and insurance sectors and medical intervention in the human body. Although it's not always wise to draw analogies between different fields, in this case we think the comparison is a good one. As our historical survey demonstrated, each successive wave of federal "solutions" only spawned more problems—side effects, if you will. The public didn't realize that the festering problems with US health care and insurance would largely resolve themselves if the natural forces of the market economy would only be allowed to function.

The public's relative ignorance on such matters is entirely understandable, however, because legions of "experts" in academia and prestigious agencies assured them repeatedly that their tinkering would make things better. Over the decades, the US markets in health care and insurance had grown so hamstrung with mandates, penalties, regulations, and taxes that many Americans felt utterly dependent on their benefactors in Washington.

This pattern is exactly what happens at the level of personal well-being—viewing the human body as its own complex system, with its natural ability to self-regulate when operating in the proper framework. Here too, minor problems fester into major crises with successive waves of intervention from the medical industry. As we have documented in this book, it is tragically commonplace for a person to suffer from various medical conditions that are largely due to the "remedies" themselves. Here again, such people are not merely victims of their own foolishness; they have been led down this path by countless (and often well-meaning) scholars and professionals who don't realize that their recommendations are only exacerbating the problem. Over the years, some people become enmeshed in so many layers of treatments that they feel helpless with their own bodies and become utterly dependent on outside benefactors—such as medical professionals and pills.

The second theme of the book is that a true solution must start with you, the individual. Only you have the knowledge of personal circumstances and the interest to ensure that a proper decision is made regarding your well-being. However, there is still an obvious need for you to seek out trustworthy information and to obtain needed health care services from qualified professionals. That is why we have equipped you in this book with the analytical framework and information sources to make such decisions.

We encourage you to widen the focus beyond nutrition and exercise, or even health care broadly conceived. The message of this book isn't just about staying fit and out of the hospital; it's about reducing stress and embracing independence as a way of life. Benefits will spill over into other areas of life, including your career and personal relationships.

Now that you have seen firsthand how to pierce through the jargon of government reports on the Affordable Care Act, and how to evaluate the pros and cons of medical screening, we hope you can generalize this approach to other areas. Yes, there are always going to be true experts in every walk of life who know more than you, but you must develop the ability and confidence to identify sincerity and reject charlatans. With the explosion of information available on the Internet, you have what you need to make an informed decision—but you need to know how to find and *recognize* the right information when you see it.

As a final takeaway message, let us caution you about the dangers of "evangelism." Although it may be tempting for you to spread our message to your relatives, friends, and co-workers, there is a downside here as well. (Isn't there always?) Knowledge can be both a blessing and a curse, and sometimes people who have had their myths shattered—as we hope we've done for you in this book—are eager to warn as many others as they can. The problem here is that you may burn yourself out agitating for political action, or arguing on the Internet, and thus forfeiting some of the reduced stress that our message *should* have produced for you. Moreover, depending on how you approach various issues, your confident jabs at the "conventional wisdom" might serve only to reinforce the prejudices of those you are trying to help.

As much as we'd appreciate more book sales, we think the best testimony you can give to others is the transformation our suggestions have effected in your own life. Whether in markets, human health, or interpersonal relationships, the great news is that we don't have to choose between idealism and pragmatism. Freedom and independence are appealing aesthetically, but they also *work*.

NOTES

Chapter 1

1. John F. Fulton, "History of Medical Education," *British Medical Journal*, August 29, 1953, pp. 457-461, available at: http://www.ncbi.nlm.nih.gov/pmc/articles/PMC2029428/.

2. Milton Friedman, *Capitalism and Freedom*, 1962, Chapter 9, available at: http://books.cat-v.org/economics/capitalism-and-freedom/chapter_09.

3. Milton Friedman, *Capitalism and Freedom*, 1962, Chapter 9, available at: http://books.cat-v.org/economics/capitalism-and-freedom/chapter_09.

4. The history of government policies on physician/population ratios is contained in Kevin Grumbach, "Fighting Hand to Hand Over Physician Workforce Policy," *Health Affairs*, 21, no. 5, 2002, pp. 13-27, available at: http://content.healthaffairs.org/content/21/5/13.full.pdf.

5. The history of government policies on physician/population ratios is contained in Kevin Grumbach, "Fighting Hand to Hand Over Physician Workforce Policy," *Health Affairs*, 21, no. 5, 2002, pp. 13-27, available at: http://content.healthaffairs.org/content/21/5/13.full.pdf.

6. Key dates obtained from Ross (2002) and EBRI (Employee Benefit Research Institute)' 2002 "History of Health Insurance Benefits," available at: http://www.ebri.org/publications/facts/index.cfm?fa=0302fact.

7. Melissa Thomasson, "Health Insurance in the United States," edited by Robert Whaples (EH.Net Encyclopedia), April 18, 2003, available at: http://eh.net/encyclopedia/article/thomasson.insurance.health.us

8. John C. Goodman, "Health Insurance," The Concise Encyclopedia of Economics, 2008, available at: http://www.econlib.org/library/Enc/HealthInsurance.html.

9. John Goodman, *Priceless*, pp. 125-126.

10. John Goodman, *Priceless*, pp. 125-126.

11. For details of the Christopher Sercye case, see Mickey Ciokajlo, "Ignoring bleeding teen costs hospital," Chicago Tribune, May 2, 2003, available at: http://articles.chicagotribune.com/2003-05-02/news/0305020332_1_ravenswood-hospital-medical-center-christopher-sercye-trauma-center; and American Urbex, "Ravenswood Hospital," available at: http://americanurbex.com/wordpress/?p=1676.

12. For text of the act see: https://www.govtrack.us/congress/bills/105/hr3937/text.

13. See the January 31, 2012 issue of the Center for Public Integrity's *Weekly Watchdog*.

14. See: http://www.hhs.gov/news/press/2012pres/09/20120917a.html.

15. See: http://www.hhs.gov/news/press/2014pres/05/20140507b.html.

Chapter 2

1. Opening chapter quotations from Robert Higgs, *Hazardous to Our Health? FDA Regulation of Health Care Products* (Oakland, CA: Independent Institute), 1995, p. 1.

2. Health expenditure data taken from Centers for Medicare and Medicaid Services historical tables, available at: http://www.cms.gov/Research-Statistics-Data-and-Systems/Statistics-Trends-and-Reports/NationalHealthExpendData/Downloads/tables.pdf. Accessed June 20, 2014.

3. The FDA's origins are described at: http://www.fda.gov/aboutfda/whatwedo/history/default.htm. Accessed June 20, 2014.

4. 4. FDA mission statement taken from: http://www.fda.gov/AboutFDA/Transparency/Basics/ucm192695.htm. Accessed June 20, 2014.

5. Joseph A. DiMasie, Christopher-Paul Milne, and Alex Tabarrok, "An FDA Report Card: Wide Variance in Performance Found Among Agency's Drug Review Divisions," Manhattan Institute, Project FDA Report No. 7, April 2014, p. 4.

6. The history of the thalidomide tragedy, and the role played by the FDA, is taken from Linda Bren, "Frances Oldham Kelsey: FDA Medical Reviewer Leaves Her Mark on History," FDA Consumer Magazine, March-April 2001, available at: http://permanent.access.gpo.gov/lps1609/www.fda.gov/fdac/features/2001/201_kelsey.html. Accessed June 21, 2014.

7. Linda Bren, "Frances Oldham Kelsey: FDA Medical Reviewer Leaves Her Mark on History," FDA Consumer Magazine, March-April 2001, available at: http://permanent.access.gpo.gov/lps1609/www.fda.gov/fdac/features/2001/201_kelsey.html.

8. Milton Friedman, *Free to Choose* (New York: Harcourt Brace Jovanovich, 1980), p. 206.

9. Quotation and earlier statistics about New Drug Application (NDA) from Joseph A. DiMasie, Christopher-Paul Milne, and Alex Tabarrok, "An FDA Report Card: Wide Variance in Performance Found Among Agency's Drug Review Divisions," Manhattan Institute, Project FDA Report No. 7, April 2014, pp. 3-4.

10. "FDA Issues Public Health Advisory on Vioxx as its Manufacturer Voluntarily Withdraws the Product," FDA News Release, September 30, 2004, available at: http://www.fda.gov/NewsEvents/Newsroom/PressAnnouncements/2004/ucm108361.htm. Accessed June 21, 2014.

11. DiMasie et al., p. 4.

12. The FDA's online glossary defines a NME as "an active ingredient that has never before been marketed in the United States in any form" and a therapeutic biological product as "a protein derived from living material (such as cells or tissues) used to treat or cure disease." See: http://www.fda.gov/Drugs/InformationOnDrugs/ucm079436.htm.

13. Some of this difference in average approval rates is no doubt due to the initial backlog of applications that were reviewed early in the PDUFA era, but even correcting for this, the Vioxx scandal seems to have had a demonstrable effect.

14. See: http://www.fda.gov/AboutFDA/CommissionersPage/ucm113239.htm.
15. The Procter & Gamble raid is described in James Bovard, "Double-Crossing to Safety," The American Spectator, January 1995, available at: http://www.jimbovard.com/Bovard_American_Spectator_1995_FDA_Double_Crossing_to_Safety.htm.
16. Paul H. Rubin, "FDA Advertising Restrictions: Ignorance Is Death," in Robert Higgs, *Hazardous to Our Health?*, pp. 29-53.
17. Rubin, pp. 32-33.
18. Rubin, p. 47.
19. Quoted in Dale Steinrich, "Playing God at the FDA," Mises Institute Daily Article, May 2, 2005, available at: http://mises.org/library/playing-god-fda.
20. Graham quoted from a 2005 interview in, "The FDA Exposed: An Interview With Dr. David Graham, the Vioxx® Whistleblower," Life Extension Magazine, October 2012, available at: http://www.lef.org/Magazine/2012/10/The-FDA-Exposed-An-Interview-With-Dr-David-Graham/Page-01. The text of Graham's 2004 Senate testimony is available at: http://www.finance.senate.gov/imo/media/doc/111804dgtest.pdf.
21. See: http://www.fda.gov/drugs/developmentapprovalprocess/default.htm.
22. See: http://www.worstpills.org/includes/page.cfm?op_id=552#table1.
23. For just two examples, see: Sarris, J. et al. (2014) "S-adenosyl methionine (SAMe) versus escitalopram and placebo in major depression RCT," *J Affect Disord*, Aug; 164:76-81, and GISSI-HF investigators (2008), "Effect of n-3 polyunsaturated fatty acids in patients with chronic heart failure (the GISSI-HF trial): a randomised, double-blind, placebo-controlled trial," *Lancet* August 2008, DOI: http://dx.doi.org/10.1016/S0140-6736(08)61239-8.

Chapter 3

1. See: http://www.sec.gov/answers/ponzi.htm.
2. See Diana B. Enriques, "Madoff Is Sentenced to 150 Years for Ponzi Scheme," *New York Times*, June 30, 2009, available at: http://www.nytimes.com/2009/06/30/business/30madoff.html.
3. Krugman referred to Social Security's "Ponzi game aspect" in a 1997 column, and later in 2011 tried to walk back the comment when conservative critics began circulating the quotation. For the original quote, Krugman's explanation, and Krugman's reference to Paul Samuelson saying the same thing, see Paul Krugman, "The Ponzi Thing," NYT blog post, September 14, 2009, available at: http://krugman.blogs.nytimes.com/2011/09/14/the-ponzi-thing/.
4. The CBO projections in this section all come from the June 2009 Congressional Budget Office "Long-Term Budget Outlook," available at: http://www.cbo.gov/sites/default/files/cbofiles/ftpdocs/102xx/doc10297/06-25-ltbo.pdf.
5. From page 202 of "2009 Annual Report of the Boards of Trustees of the Federal Hospital Insurance and Federal Supplementary Medical Insurance Trust Funds," available at: http://www.cms.gov/Research-Statistics-Data-and-Systems/Statistics-Trends-and-Reports/ReportsTrustFunds/Downloads/TR2009.pdf.

Chapter 4

1. Covering office visits and other "preventive" care measures is in a sense understandable because a health plan may cover so many *other*, non-catastrophic events, but it is still worth pointing out the discrepancy with traditional insurance.
2. John Goodman, *Priceless*, p. 61.
3. Goodman, *Priceless*, p. 65.
4. The analogy with life insurance is also due to Goodman, p. 124.
5. Sources of health insurance coverage data obtained from Kaiser Family Foundation website: http://kff.org/other/state-indicator/total-population/. Accessed September 5, 2014. The total does not equal 100 percent because of rounding.
6. Data on drug shortages from John Goodman, *Priceless*, pp. 78-79.
7. John Goodman, *Priceless*, p. 63.
8. Goodman, *Priceless*, p. 24.
9. End-of-life statistics obtained from Helen Adamopoulos, "The Cost and Quality Conundrum of American End-of-Life Care," Medicare News Group, June 3, 2013, available at: http://www.medicarenewsgroup.com/context/understanding-medicare-blog/understanding-medicare-blog/2013/06/03/the-cost-and-quality-conundrum-of-american-end-of-life-care.
10. Avik Roy, "How the FDA Stifles New Cures, Part I: The Rising Cost of Clinical Trials." Forbes, April 24, 2012, available at: http://www.forbes.com/sites/aroy/2012/04/24/how-the-fda-stifles-new-cures-part-i-the-rising-cost-of-clinical-trials/.

Chapter 5

1. Mitt Romney, "Health Care for Everyone? We Found a Way." *Wall Street Journal*, April 11, 2006, available at: http://online.wsj.com/news/articles/SB114472206077422547.
2. Specifically, the "medical care" component of the CPI went from 250.0 in June 1999 to 375.177 in June 2009, for an annualized increase of 4.1 percent. In contrast, the CPI for "all items" went from 166.00 in June 1999 to 214.79 in June 2009, an annualized increase of only 2.6 percent. Data accessed from the St. Louis Federal Reserve (as originally released by the Bureau of Labor Statistics) at http://research.stlouisfed.org/fred2/data/CPIMEDSL.txt and http://research.stlouisfed.org/fred2/data/CPIAUCSL.txt on September 2, 2014.
3. Health expenditure data taken from Centers for Medicare and Medicaid Services historical tables, available at: http://www.cms.gov/Research-Statistics-Data-and-Systems/Statistics-Trends-and-Reports/NationalHealthExpendData/Downloads/tables.pdf. Accessed June 20, 2014.
4. C. Schoen, A.-K. Fryer, S. R. Collins, and D. C. Radley, "State Trends in Premiums and Deductibles, 2003–2010: The Need for Action to Address Rising Costs," The Commonwealth Fund, November 2011. Available at: http://www.commonwealthfund.org/Publications/Issue-Briefs/2011/Nov/State-Trends-in-Premiums.aspx.

5. For a discussion of the various figures cited on the size of the Affordable Care Act legislation itself, see Tom Giffey, "Is 'Obamacare' really that long?" Leader-Telegram, July 17, 2012, available at: http://www.leadertelegram.com/blogs/tom_giffey/article_c9f1fa54-d041-11e1-9d01-0019bb2963f4.html. For a discussion of the pages of regulations pertaining to the ACA, see Glenn Kessler, "How many pages of regulations for 'Obamacare'?" Washington Post Fact-Checker, May 14, 2013, available at: http://www.washingtonpost.com/blogs/fact-checker/post/how-many-pages-of-regulations-for-obamacare/2013/05/14/61eec914-bcf9-11e2-9b09-1638acc3942e_blog.html.
6. Quotations taken from: http://www.hhs.gov/healthcare/facts/timeline/timeline-text.html. Accessed September 4, 2014.
7. The interaction of the limits on age and smoking "discrimination" led to a funny if depressing outcome: apparently there was (yet another) programming glitch in the Healthcare.gov website, such that a 64-year-old smoker could not be charged a premium more than three times that of a 19-year-old nonsmoker, even though the intention of the rules was to allow an insurance company to charge a hypothetical 64-year-old smoker 4.5 (= 3 x 1.5) times as much. This "smoker's glitch" possibly made smokers' premiums lower (and nonsmokers' higher) in 2014 than would otherwise have been the case, and smokers may see more significant changes as HHS fixes the programming glitch. See Avik Roy, "Smokers Rejoice! Latest Obamacare Glitch Forces Non-Smokers To Subsidize Your Health Coverage," Forbes online article, July 13, 2013, available at: http://www.forbes.com/sites/theapothecary/2013/07/13/smokers-rejoice-latest-obamacare-glitch-forces-non-smokers-to-subsidize-your-health-coverage/.
8. Quotation concerning the individual mandate fee schedule taken from: https://www.healthcare.gov/what-if-i-dont-have-health-coverage/. Accessed September 4, 2014.
9. See: http://obamacarefacts.com/obamacare-taxes.php. Accessed September 4, 2014.
10. In the appendix to this chapter, we will reproduce a key chart from the CBO's headline-grabbing analysis and pinpoint this enormous gross/net distinction.
11. A note for purists: strictly speaking, in the event of large losses, the actual compensation payment from the government involves a flat 2.5 percent payment of the target amount, in addition to the 80 percent coverage of remaining losses. But the simpler treatment in the text above, along with the diagram in Figure 5-2, explain the reason for using the term "risk corridor" to describe the program.
12. Joseph Salerno, "What You Were Never Told About Obamacare," Mises Economics Blog post, January 14, 2014, available at: http://bastiat.mises.org/2014/01/what-you-were-never-told-about-obamacare/. Note that the "official" information from the government concerning the federal risk corridor program and the state-administered risk sharing programs is available at: http://www.cms.gov/cciio/resources/files/downloads/3rs-final-rule.pdf.
13. Specifically, the Treasury allocates $2 billion in 2014, $2 billion in 2015, and $1 billion in 2016. See: http://www.cms.gov/cciio/resources/files/downloads/3rs-final-rule.pdf.

14. The actual details of the employer mandate are quite complicated, such that law firms were issuing qualified guidance as the legislation's teeth began to kick in. See for example Sacks Tierney Attorneys, "Prepare Now for the Obamacare Employer Mandate," March 2013, available at: http://www.sackstierney.com/articles/obamacare1.htm.

15. For example, in 2013 the CBO responded to an inquiry from House Republican Paul Ryan, telling him that repeal of the ACA would increase the deficit. The media and political reaction to that exchange reinforced the idea that the ACA "paid for itself" through frugality. See Elise Viebeck, "CBO: Repealing Obama healthcare law will increase budget deficit," The Hill, May 15, 2013, available at: http://thehill.com/blogs/floor-action/healthcare/299895-cbo-obamacare-repeal-will-increase-the-deficit.

16. As we will explain thoroughly in chapter 6, the inflow of money to the Treasury resulting from the tax on so-called Cadillac plans comes primarily from *workers*, not the employers on whom the tax is directly levied.

17. Specifically, the CBO predicts that the ACA on net will cause fewer workers to receive health insurance from their employers. When things settle down, this will mean that workers tend to get more of their compensation in the form of taxable wages or salary, rather than non-taxable health insurance packages. This factor will cause the Treasury to receive more tax payments than it otherwise would have. We will return to this alarming feature of the ACA in the next chapter.

18. Our classification here—when disregarding the "insurance coverage provisions" dimension—comports exactly with the CBO's own summary, as relayed in its 2012 cover letter to John Boehner. (Available at: http://www.cbo.gov/sites/default/files/cbofiles/attachments/43471-hr6079.pdf.) As a note for purists, we mention that the $890 billion in "direct spending" seems to include the subsidies to the state insurance exchanges, which take the form of refundable tax credits. To classify a refundable tax credit as government "spending" might seem illegitimate to some readers, because (in principle) a refundable tax credit consists of a mix of a tax reduction and a government spending increase.

Chapter 6

1. Frédéric Bastiat, "The State," in *Selected Essays on Political Economy*, available at: http://www.econlib.org/library/Bastiat/basEss5.html. Accessed September 7, 2014.

2. See the "final rule" relevant to premium pricing issued on February 27, 2013 summarized at: https://www.cms.gov/CCIIO/Resources/Files/Downloads/market-rules-technical-summary-2-27-2013.pdf.

3. Linda J. Blumberg and Matthew Buettgens, "Implications of Limited Age Rating Bands Under the Affordable Care Act," Robert Wood Johnson Foundation / Urban Institute, March 2013. Available at: http://www.rwjf.org/content/dam/farm/reports/issue_briefs/2013/rwjf404637/subassets/rwjf404637_1. We note that this analysis is drawn from a publication that *supports* the ACA's 3-to-1 restriction.

4. Angie Drabnic Holan, "Lie of the Year: 'If you like your health care plan, you can keep it,'" PolitiFact, December 12, 2013, available at: http://www.politi-fact.com/truth-o-meter/article/2013/dec/12/lie-year-if-you-like-your-health-care-plan-keep-it/.

5. To reiterate what was explained in the earlier block quotation: strictly speaking the ACA allowed catastrophic plans issued before the passage of the ACA to be grandfathered in, but any modification to the plan (including raising the premium, as typically happens year to year) would cause it to no longer be "the original plan." This nuance is part of the explanation behind the very misleading statement, "You can keep your plan…"

6. See: https://www.healthcare.gov/glossary/essential-health-benefits/. Accessed September 18, 2014.

7. Jess Bravin and Louise Radnofsky, "Court Backs Obama on Health Law," WSJ, June 29, 2012, available at: http://online.wsj.com/news/articles/SB100014240 52702304898704577480371370927862.

8. For purists, we note the distinction between the number of people lacking health insurance *because of whom* a tax penalty is assessed versus the number of people *upon whom* that tax penalty is assessed. For example, a single mother with a high income and three children under the age of 18, all of whom lack health insurance, will see a higher tax penalty than a similar woman with no children. The CBO estimates in Table 6-1 refer to the total number of unin-sured people triggering the penalty, even if another person (such as a parent) is responsible for paying the penalty.

9. CBO, "The Budget and Economic Outlook: 2014 to 2024," February 2014, p. 117, available at: http://www.cbo.gov/sites/default/files/cbofiles/attach-ments/45010-Outlook2014_Feb.pdf.

10. A "full-time equivalent" job means that multiple workers could collectively cut back their hours the equivalent of one worker losing a full-time job.

11. Paul Krugman, "Labor Supply and the Meaning of Life," NYT blog post, Feb-ruary 6, 2014, available at: http://krugman.blogs.nytimes.com/2014/02/06/labor-supply-and-the-meaning-of-life/.

12. David R. Henderson, "Obamacare's 'Disincentive' Scheme," Hoover Institu-tion *Defining Ideas*, February 18, 2014, available at: http://www.hoover.org/research/obamacares-disincentive-scheme.

13. Joseph Rago, "The Economist Who Exposed ObamaCare," *Wall Street Journal*, February 7, 2014, available at: http://online.wsj.com/news/articles/SB1000142 40527023046809045793671438805322248.

14. Paul Krugman, "Beyond the Lies," New York Times blog post, August 19, 2014, available at: http://krugman.blogs.nytimes.com/2014/08/19/beyond-the-lies/.

15. Statistics of Income (SOI) SOI Tax Stats - Individual Income Tax Returns Publication 1304 (Complete Report), IRS, available at: http://www.irs.gov/uac/SOI-Tax-Stats-Individual-Income-Tax-Returns-Publication-1304-(Com-plete-Report)#_pt1. Accessed September 18, 2014. Note that the figure in the

text of 5.2 million overstates the precise number of tax returns that will be hit with the ACA tax hikes on upper income earners, because the IRS data didn't break out the returns for $250,000 and above, only for $200,000 and above. (Married couples filing jointly are only hit with the new taxes if they earn above $250,000.)

16. As we explained in regard to Table 6-1, these estimates include uninsured children who are triggering a higher tax bill for those responsible for them.

17. CBO, "Updated Estimates of the Effects of the Insurance Coverage Provisions of the Affordable Care Act, April 2014," p. 13.

18. CBO, "Updated Estimates of the Effects of the Insurance Coverage Provisions of the Affordable Care Act, April 2014," p. 7.

19. CBO, "Updated Estimates of the Effects of the Insurance Coverage Provisions of the Affordable Care Act, April 2014," p. 13.

20. The actual details of the employer mandate are quite complicated, such that law firms were issuing qualified guidance as the legislation's teeth began to kick in. See for example Sacks Tierney Attorneys, "Prepare Now for the Obamacare Employer Mandate," March 2013, available at: http://www.sackstierney.com/articles/obamacare1.htm.

21. Note that as of this writing, the employer mandate in 2015 is only partially phased in, because employers with 50 to 99 full-time equivalent employees are exempt from the penalty so long as they certify that they did not strategically adjust their employee counts because of the ACA. See CBO, "Updated Estimates of the Effects of the Insurance Coverage Provisions of the Affordable Care Act, April 2014," p. 13.

22. Lisa Myers and Carroll Ann Mears, "Businesses claim Obamacare has forced them to cut employee hours," NBC News, August 14, 2013, available at: http://www.cnbc.com/id/100962203.

Chapter 7

1. For example, in October 2013 the Heritage Foundation released a study that used published premiums for state exchanges to estimate that the average premium in 2014 for 27-year-olds in 11 states would *more than double*, while it would fall at least 28 percent in three states (Colorado, New York, and Rhode Island) that already had tight regulation of insurance premiums but did not (before the ACA) impose an individual mandate. (See Drew Gonshorowski, "How Will You Fare in the Obamacare Exchanges?", Heritage Foundation, Issue Brief on Health Care, October 16, 2013, available at: http://www.heritage.org/research/reports/2013/10/enrollment-in-obamacare-exchanges-how-will-your-health-insurance-fare.) In contrast, in September 2014 Ezra Klein trumpeted a new study from the Kaiser Family Foundation (which projected 2015 premiums would be slightly lower than those in 2014) and announced, "But less than 10 months after major media outlets were hosting debates with headlines like 'Is the Affordable Care Act Beyond Repair?', Obama's signature accomplishment is succeeding beyond all reasonable expectation." See Ezra

Klein, "The Obamacare train keeps not wrecking," Vox, September 20, 2014, available at: http://www.vox.com/2014/9/5/6108493/obamacare-premiums-lower-2015.

2. US Department of Health and Human Services, "Health Insurance Marketplace Premiums for 2014," ASPE Issue Brief, September 18, 2013, available at: http://aspe.hhs.gov/health/reports/2013/MarketplacePremiums/ib_marketplace_premiums.cfm.

3. The summary of the Manhattan Institute analysis of the HHS data, as well as the quotation from Douglas Holtz-Eakin, come from Avik Roy, "Double Down: Obamacare Will Increase Avg. Individual-Market Insurance Premiums By 99% For Men, 62% For Women," Forbes.com, September 25, 2013, available at: http://www.forbes.com/sites/theapothecary/2013/09/25/double-down-obamacare-will-increase-avg-individual-market-insurance-premiums-by-99-for-men-62-for-women/.

4. Amanda E. Kowalski (2014), "The Early Impact of the Affordable Care Act, State By State," Brookings Paper on Economic Activity, Fall 2014, p. 301, available at: http://www.brookings.edu/~/media/Projects/BPEA/Fall%202014/Fall2014BPEA_Kowalski.pdf.

5. CBO, "Updated Estimates of the Effects of the Insurance Coverage Provisions of the Affordable Care Act," p. 7.

6. 6. As the April 2014 CBO report explains: "In November 2013, the Administration announced that states could accept renewals of noncompliant policies for a policy year starting between January 1, 2014, and October 1, 2014. In March 2014, that transitional relief was extended for two more years" (p. 9).

7. CBO, "Updated Estimates of the Effects of the Insurance Coverage Provisions of the Affordable Care Act," p. 12.

8. CBO, p. 8. In case the subsidy figures seem implausibly high, the report explains in a footnote: "The average exchange subsidy per subsidized enrollee includes premium subsidies and cost-sharing subsidies and thus may exceed the average benchmark premium in the exchanges."

9. We remind the reader to not confuse health coverage with health *care*. The people added to the rolls of Medicaid, for example, may discover that they still cannot access quality care.

10. The figures for US population and Medicare enrollment come from Tables 1 and 17 of CMS, "National Health Expenditure Projections 2012-2022," available at: http://www.cms.gov/Research-Statistics-Data-and-Systems/Statistics-Trends-and-Reports/NationalHealthExpendData/downloads/proj2012.pdf.

11. John Goodman, *Priceless*, pp. 221-222.

12. John Goodman, *Priceless*, p. 114.

13. Alain Enthoven and Leonard Schaeffer, quoted in John Goodman, *Priceless*, p. 113.

14. CBO, "Updated Estimates of the Effects of the Insurance Coverage Provisions of the Affordable Care Act," p. 16.

15. See http://www.hhs.gov/healthcare/facts/timeline/timeline-text.html#2010. Accessed September 28, 2014.

16. Julian Pecquet, "Health insurers drop coverage for children ahead of new rules," The Hill, September 20, 2010, available at: http://thehill.com/policy/health-care/119823-insurers-drop-childrens-insurance-plans-ahead-of-new-rules.

17. Patricia Borns, "Complainants say health insurers used high drug co-pays to discourage people with HIV/AIDS from enrolling," Miami Herald, May 29, 2014, available at: http://www.miamiherald.com/news/business/article1965143.html.

18. Paul Krugman, "Why Is Obamacare Complicated?" New York Times blog post, October 26, 2013, available at: http://krugman.blogs.nytimes.com/2013/10/26/why-is-obamacare-complicated/.

19. 19. Sarah Kliff, "Limited doctor choice plans don't mean worse care," Vox, September 8, 2014, available at: http://www.vox.com/2014/9/8/6119669/narrow-networks-quality-care-jon-gruber.

20. The NPR exchange was reported on by the time here, for example: Karoun Demirjian, "Reid says Obamacare just a step toward eventual single-payer system," Las Vegas Sun, August 10, 2013, available at: http://www.lasvegassun.com/news/2013/aug/10/reid-says-obamacare-just-step-toward-eventual-sing/. The transcript of the interview contained in the text above comes from this YouTube video: https://www.youtube.com/watch?v=SXgSKwYMnWo. Both accessed September 29, 2014.

21. The video of the question and Krugman's answer is available at: https://www.youtube.com/watch?v=kyeMnaAOQL8. Accessed September 29, 2014.

22. Albert Q. Maisel, "Bedlam 1946: Most US Mental Hospitals Are a Shame and a Disgrace," *Life* magazine, May 6, 1946. A transcript of the article (with some typos) is available at this PBS site, in relation to a story on lobotomies: http://www.pbs.org/wgbh/americanexperience/features/primary-resources/lobotomist-bedlam-1946/.

23. See the AP story, "VA Head: 18 more vets left off waiting list in Phoenix area died," June 6, 2014, available at: http://www.cbsnews.com/news/va-head-18-more-vets-left-off-waiting-list-in-phoenix-area-died/.

Chapter 9

1. Hanson, Robin. *Priceless*, Independent Institute, 2012.

2. Moore, H. "Why Is Thomas Piketty's 700-page book a bestseller?" *The Guardian*. September 21, 2014. http://www.theguardian.com/money/2014/sep/21/-sp-thomas-piketty-bestseller-why.

3. Konner, M and Eaton, "Paleolithic nutrition: twenty-five years later." Nutrition in Clinical Practice (2010) Dec; 25(6): 594-602.

4. National Health Council. *About Chronic Disease*. http://www.nationalhealthcouncil.org/sites/default/files/AboutChronicDisease.pdf

5. American Diabetes Association. *Economic Cost of Diabetes in the US in 2012*. http://care.diabetesjournals.org/content/early/2013/03/05/dc12-2625

6. American Diabetes Association. *The Cost of Diabetes.* http://www.diabetes.org/advocacy/news-events/cost-of-diabetes.html#sthash.Lzvs5n0v.dpuf

7. Yamanouchi, K et al., "Daily Walking Combined with Diet Therapy Is a Useful Means for Obese NIDDM Patients Not Only to Reduce Body Weight But Also to Improve Insulin Sensitivity." Diabetes Care (1995), 18:6:775-778.

8. O'Dea, K. "Marked improvement in carbohydrate and lipid metabolism in diabetic Australian aborigines after temporary reversion to traditional life-style." US National Library of Medicine National Institutes of Health (1984), 33(6):596-603. www.ncbi.nlm.nih.gov/pubmed/6373464/

9. Klonoff, David C. "The Beneficial Effects of a Paleolithic Diet on Type 2 Diabetes and Other Risk Factors for Cardiovascular Disease." Journal of Diabetes Science and Technology 3.6 (2009): 1229–1232. http://www.ncbi.nlm.nih.gov/pmc/articles/PMC2787021/

10. Centers for Disease Control and Prevention. Heart Disease Facts. http://www.cdc.gov/heartdisease/facts.htm

11. Centers for Disease Control and Prevention. *Cost of hospital discharges with common hospital operating room procedures in nonfederal community hospitals, by age and selected principal procedure: United States, selected years 2000–2011.* http://www.cdc.gov/nchs/data/hus/2012/115.pdf

12. Simopoulos, AP. "The omega-6/omega-3 fatty acid ratio, genetic variation, and cardiovascular disease." Asia Pac J Clin Nutr. 2008;17 Suppl 1:131-4. http://www.ncbi.nlm.nih.gov/pubmed/18296320

13. Frassetto, LA et al. "Metabolic and physiologic improvements from consuming a paleolithic, hunter-gatherer type diet." *European Journal of Clinical Nutrition* (2009) 63, 947–955. http://www.nature.com/ejcn/journal/v63/n8/full/ejcn20094a.html

14. American Cancer Society. *Cancer Facts & Figures 2015.* http://www.cancer.org/acs/groups/content/@editorial/documents/document/acspc-044552.pdf

15. Ibid.

16. Anand, P et al. "Cancer is a Preventable Disease that Requires Major Lifestyle Changes." Pharm Res. 2008 Sep; 25(9): 2097–2116. www.ncbi.nlm.nih.gov/pmc/articles/PMC2515569/

17. Anand, P et al. "Cancer is a Preventable Disease that Requires Major Lifestyle Changes." Pharm Res. 2008 Sep; 25(9): 2097–2116. www.ncbi.nlm.nih.gov/pmc/articles/PMC2515569/

18. Blask, David E. "Melatonin, sleep disturbance and cancer risk." Sleep Medicine Reviews Journal (2009), no. 4, vol. 3: 257-264. http://www.smrv-journal.com/article/S1087-0792(08)00078-6/abstract

19. Lappe, Joan M et al. "Vitamin D and calcium supplementation reduces cancer risk: results of a randomized trial." American Society for Clinical Nutrition (2007), no.6, vol. 85: 1586-1591. http://ajcn.nutrition.org/content/85/6/1586.short

20. Courneya, Kerry S and Friedenreich, Christine M. "Physical Activity and Cancer: An Introduction." Springer Link (2011) vol. 186:1-10. http://link.

springer.com/chapter/10.1007/978-3-642-04231-7_1

21. Rose, David P and Connolly, Jeanne M. "Omega-3 fatty acids as cancer chemopreventive agents." Science Direct (1999), no.3, vol. 83:217-244. http://www.sciencedirect.com/science/article/pii/S0163725899000261

22. Sasaki, YF et al. "The comet assay with 8 mouse organs: results with 39 currently used food additives." Mutat Res. 2002 Aug 26;519(1-2):103-19. http://www.ncbi.nlm.nih.gov/pubmed/12160896

23. John, EM et al. "Meat consumption, cooking practices, meat mutagens, and risk of prostate cancer." Nutr Cancer. 2011;63(4):525-37. http://www.ncbi.nlm.nih.gov/pubmed/21526454

24. Navarro, A et al. "Meat cooking habits and risk of colorectal cancer in Córdoba, Argentina." Nutrition. 2004 Oct;20(10):873-7. www.ncbi.nlm.nih.gov/pubmed/15474875

25. National Cancer Institute. *Chemicals in Meat Cooked at High Temperatures and Cancer Risk.* http://www.cancer.gov/cancertopics/causes-prevention/risk/diet/cooked-meats-fact-sheet

26. Sengupta, A et al. "Allium vegetables in cancer prevention: an overview." Asian Pac J Cancer Prev. 2004 Jul-Sep;5(3):237-45. http://www.ncbi.nlm.nih.gov/pubmed/15373701

27. Talalay, Paul and Fahey, Jed W. "Phytochemicals from Cruciferous Plants Protect against Cancer by Modulating Carcinogen Metabolism." The Journal of Nutrition (2001), no.11, vol. 131: 3027S-3033S. http://jn.nutrition.org/content/131/11/3027S.short

28. Burge, R et al. "Incidence and economic burden of osteoporosis-related fractures in the United States, 2005-2025." J Bone Miner Res. 2007 Mar;22(3):465-75. http://www.ncbi.nlm.nih.gov/pubmed/17144789

29. Iwamoto, J et al. "Effects of vitamin K2 on osteoporosis." Curr Pharm Des. 2004;10(21):2557-76. http://www.ncbi.nlm.nih.gov/pubmed/15320745

30. Rheaume-Bleue, Kate. *Vitamin K2 and the Calcium Paradox.* Harper, 2013.

31. International Osteoporosis Foundation. *Osteoporosis Prevention.* http://www.iofbonehealth.org/osteoporosis-musculoskeletal-disorders/osteoporosis/prevention/vitamin-d

32. Nelson, Miriam E et al. "Effects of High-Intensity Strength Training on Multiple Risk Factors for Osteoporotic Fractures." JAMA. 1994;272(24):1909-1914. http://jama.jamanetwork.com/article.aspx?articleid=384959

33. National Institute of Diabetes and Digestive and Kidney Diseases. *Overweight and Obesity Statistics.* http://win.niddk.nih.gov/statistics/

34. Finkelstein, Eric A et al. "Annual Medical Spending Attributable To Obesity: Payer-And Service-Specific Estimates." Health Affairs, 28, no.5 (2009):w822-w831. http://content.healthaffairs.org/content/28/5/w822.full.pdf+html

35. Partnership to Fight Chronic Disease. *New Data Shows Obesity Costs Will Grow to $344 Billion by 2018.* www.fightchronicdisease.org/media-center/releases/new-data-shows-obesity-costs-will-grow-344-billion-2018

36. Österdahl, M et al. "Effects of a short-term intervention with a paleolithic diet in healthy volunteers." European Journal of Clinical Nutrition (2008) 62, 682–685. http://www.nature.com/ejcn/journal/v62/n5/abs/1602790a.html

37. Jönsson, Tommy et al. "A paleolithic diet is more satiating per calorie than a mediterranean-like diet in individuals with ischemic heart disease." Nutrition & Metabolism 2010, 7:85. www.nutritionandmetabolism.com/content/7/1/85

38. Finkelstein, Eric A et al. "Annual Medical Spending Attributable To Obesity: Payer-And Service-Specific Estimates." Health Affairs, 28, no.5 (2009):w822-w831. http://content.healthaffairs.org/content/28/5/w822.full.pdf+html

39. Smith, Robyn N et al. "The effect of a high-protein, low glycemic–load diet versus a conventional, high glycemic–load diet on biochemical parameters associated with acne vulgaris: A randomized, investigator-masked, controlled trial." JAAD (2007), no.2, vol.57:247-256. http://www.jaad.org/article/S0190-9622%2807%2900414-8/abstract

40. National Institute of Mental Health. *Any Mental Illness (AMI) Among Adults.* http://www.nimh.nih.gov/health/statistics/prevalence/any-mental-illness-ami-among-adults.shtml

41. Insel, Thomas. "Director's Blog: Antidepressants: A complicated picture." *National Institute of Mental Health.* http://www.nimh.nih.gov/about/director/2011/antidepressants-a-complicated-picture.shtml

42. Addolorato, G. "Anxiety But Not Depression Decreases in Coeliac Patients After One-Year Gluten-free Diet: A Longitudinal Study." Scandinavian Journal of Gastroenterology (2001), no.5, vol.36:502-506. http://www.informahealthcare.com/doi/abs/10.1080/00365520119754

43. Stathopoulou, G et al. "Exercise Interventions for Mental Health: A Quantitative and Qualitative Review." Clinical Psychology: Science and Practice (2006), no.2, vol.13:179-193. http://onlinelibrary.wiley.com/doi/10.1111/j.1468-2850.2006.00021.x/abstract;jsessionid=8FE-C2209398A803A9522E1BB0D32063E.f03t01?deniedAccessCustomisedMessage=&userIsAuthenticated=false

44. Ledochowski, M et al. "Fructose- and Sorbitol-reduced Diet Improves Mood and Gastrointestinal Disturbances in Fructose Malabsorbers." Scandinavian Journal of Gastroenterology (2000), no.10, vol.35:1048-1052. informahealthcare.com/doi/abs/10.1080/003655200451162

45. C. Brand and B.K. Pederson, "The role of exercise-induced myokines in muscle homeostasis and the defense against chronic diseases." *J Biomed Biotechnol.* 2010; 2010:520258.

46. To reiterate, in the text I am only providing a starting point. Readers must consult marksdailyapple.com and/or bodybyscience.net for more resources.

Chapter 10

1. Note that in the text, we will often use male pronouns to refer to a generic doctor. Naturally, this is done to avoid the cumbersome "his or her" and "he or she"; we do not mean to suggest that the ideal doctor must be a man.

2. It is possible to combine a cash-practice and catastrophic insurance plan with the popular Health Savings Account (HSA), Health Reimbursement Account (HRA), and Flexible Spending Account (FSA). Our only caution here is that these programs have restrictions that partially defeat the purpose of gaining your medical freedom by "opting out" of the conventional system.

Chapter 11

1. Daniela Drake, "You Can't Yelp Your Doctor," The Daily Beast, May 21, 2014, available at: http://www.thedailybeast.com/articles/2014/05/21/the-mask-your-doctor-hides-behind.html.

Chapter 12

1. Sarah Glynn, "Alarm Fatigue Is Putting Patients' Lives At Risk," Medical News Today, April 10, 2013, available at: http://www.medicalnewstoday.com/articles/258855.php.

2. See "To Err Is Human," Institute of Medicine, November 1999, available at: https://www.iom.edu/Reports/1999/To-Err-is-Human-Building-A-Safer-Health-System.aspx.

Chapter 13

1. Cram, P. et al., "The impact of a celebrity promotional campaign on the use of colon cancer screening: the Katie Couric effect." *Archives of Internal Medicine* 2003 Jul 14;163(13):1601-5.

2. Gina Kolata, "Study Questions Colonoscopy Effectiveness," The New York Times, December 14, 2006, available at: http://www.nytimes.com/2006/12/14/health/14colon.html.

3. American Cancer Society, *Cancer Facts and Figures* (2007), p. 4.

4. Strictly speaking, there is a third logical possibility: actual cancer rates increased for some other reasons, coincidentally as the screening campaign came online.

5. The quote is taken from a January 31, 2007 Medscape summary given by David A. Johnson, referring to T.R. Levin et al., "Complications of colonoscopy in an integrated health care delivery system," *Annals of Internal Medicine* 2006;145:880-886.

6. Mi-Young Kim et al., "Tumor Self-Seeding by Circulating Cancer Cells," *Cell* 139 (2009) Issue 7: 1315–1326.

7. For a discussion of how even medical professionals often make mistakes in interpreting such probabilities, see Gerd Gigerenzer, *Calculated Risks: How to Know When Numbers Deceive You* (Simon and Schuster, 2002), pp. 5-6. We should clarify that the approximate figure of 9 percent in the text above is *not* implying that if a healthy woman undergoes a mammogram, that there is a 91

percent chance she will receive a false positive. To repeat, the situation is that *if* a woman receives a positive mammogram, then there is (approximately) a 91 percent chance that it was a false positive. However, it *is* also true that healthy women will likely (eventually) receive a false positive with extensive screening. For example, a recent study in the *Annals of Internal Medicine* studied nearly 170,000 US women and concluded that if they received annual mammograms over the course of a decade, a majority of women would see at least one false-positive result during this period. See Elizabeth Fernandez, "High Rate of False-Positives with Annual Mammogram," University of California San Francisco Post, October 17, 2011, available at: http://www.ucsf.edu/news/2011/10/10778/high-rate-false-positives-annual-mammogram.

8. John Brodersen and Volkert Dirk Siersma, "Long-Term Psychosocial Consequences of False-Positive Screening Mammography," *Annals of Family Medicine* 11 (2013): vol. 11, no. 2, pp. 106-115.

9. The 2008 summary is quoted in a 2012 edition of the Cochrane report, available at: http://www.cochrane.dk/screening/mammography-leaflet.pdf.

10. P.C. Gøtzsche and K.J. Jørgensen, "Screening for breast cancer with mammography (Review)," The Cochrane Collaboration, *The Cochrane Library* 2013 Issue 6, available at: http://www.cochrane.dk/research/Screening%20for%20breast%20cancer%202013%20CD001877.pdf.

11. Genetic tests (such as "23andMe") may offer help in this regard, but here too it is a matter of weighing benefits and costs; genetic tests have their version of false-positives as well. See the discussion later in this chapter.

12. For example see A. Bleyer and H.G. Welch, "Effect of three decades of screening mammography on breast-cancer incidence." *New England Journal of Medicine* 2012. Nov 22:367(21):1998-2005.

13. D. Ilic D, M. M. Neuberger, M. Djulbegovic, and P. Dahm. (2013) "Screening for prostate cancer (review)," The Cochrane Collaboration, available at: http://www.bibliotecacochrane.com/pdf/CD004720.pdf .

14. See: https://www.auanet.org/common/pdf/education/clinical-guidance/Prostate-Cancer-Detection.pdf .

Chapter 14

1. There are many state-based regulations that operate in tandem with federal rules regarding both raw milk and many types of occupational licensure. On raw milk, see: http://www.ncsl.org/documents/agri/NCSL_Raw_Milk_Memo.pdf.

2. Alex Tabarrok, "Life-Saving Incentives: Consequences, Costs and Solutions to the Organ Shortage," EconLib featured article, August 3, 2009, available at: http://econlib.org/library/Columns/y2009/Tabarroklifesaving.html.

INDEX

1906 Pure Food and Drugs Act, 47
1942 Stabilization Act, 24–25
1992 Prescription Drug User Fee Act (PDUFA), 56, 63
23andMe, 308
30-day readmission rule, 177–179

A

ACA. *See* Affordable Care Act (ACA)
adverse selection, 129
advertising, FDA regulation, 58–60
Affordable Care Act (ACA), 1–2, 7, 105–108
 CBO estimated cost of ACA, 118, 121–123, 143–144, 146
 CBO estimated individual mandate penalties, 134
 CBO estimated job reduction, 136
 child coverage, 169–170
 community rating, 111, 115–116, 127–129
 electronic medical records (EMRs), 39
 employer mandate, 114, 120, 145–148
 essential health benefits, 111–112, 116, 130–132
 flaws
  community rating, 127–129
  employer mandate, 145–148

 essential health benefits, 130–132
 government subsidies for the poor, 135–141
 guarantees to health insurance companies, 144–145
 individual mandate, 133–134
 tax hikes on the rich, 141–144
 universal coverage, 125–127
 government subsidies for the poor, 113, 117, 135–141
 guarantees to health insurance companies, 113, 118–120, 144–145
 health insurance costs before passage, 108–109
 health insurance premium increase, 152–158
 impact on long-term Medicare unfunded obligations, 164
 individual mandate, 112, 116–117, 133–134
 new taxes, 117–118
 "pay for performance" program, 254
 repeal of, 121–123, 327
 RomneyCare, 105
 single-payer system. *See* single-payer system
 tax hikes on the rich, 113, 117–118, 141–144
 universal coverage, 110–111, 115, 125–127

 failure leads to rationed care, 161–169
AIDS patients, 171
alcohol withdrawal, 265
alternative providers of health care, 251
 osteopathy, 12
AMA. *See* American Medical Association
Ambien, 254
American Cancer Society colorectal cancer statistics, 297
American Hospital Association support of Medicare, 26
American Medical Association (AMA), 10
 origins of, 10–11
 reduction of doctors, 12–13
anti-anxiety medicines
 life events, 253-254
 withdrawal symptoms, 265
The Archives of Internal Medicine colonoscopy study, 294
aspirin, 58–60
Ativan, 265
Avoid Poisonous Things (Primal Blueprint law #2), 220
Avoid Stupid Mistakes (Primal Blueprint law #9), 222

B

Baycol, 64
benzodiazepine withdrawal, 265
Bextra, 64
Big Pharma, 67, 101
 possible actions to improve situation, 329–331

blood pressure
Ken Korg, 190, 194, 200, 203, 205
primal lifestyle, 224–226
Blue Cross/Blue Shield (the Blues), 19
community rating, 19–21
origin of, 19
support of Medicare, 26
Body by Science, 234
Body by Science website, 234
Boehner, John, 122–123
breast cancer screening (mammography), 300–305
British Medical Journal, 8
Brookings Institution insurance premiums study, 155–156

C

CA-A Cancer Journal for Clinicians colonoscopy study, 297
Cadillac medical training, 11
Cadillac insurance plans, 117, 123
taxation, 117, 142, 157, 168
cancer
benefits of primal lifestyle, 227–229
screening for. *See* medical screening
cardiovascular diseases, 224–226
cash payments to doctors, 244–245
cattle-car care, 166–167
CBO. *See* Congressional Budget Office
celiac disease, 233

The Center for Health Transformation, 39
Centers for Medicare and Medicaid Services (CMS), 160–161
30-day readmission rule, 177–179
cervical cancer tests (Pap smears), 96–98
Charaka, 8
children
child coverage, 169–170
Children's Health Insurance Program (CHIP), 158–160
chiropractors, 251
cholesterol, 225–226
choosing doctors, 239
3 desired characteristics, 242
cash payments, 244–245
concierge doctors, 245–246
free-market orientation, 243–244
kind of doctor/specialty, 248–250
Medicaid patients, 248
Medicare patients, 247
mid-level providers, 250–251
sherpas as a model, 240–242
wellness, 242–243
willingness to seek non-pharmacologic solutions, 253
Christopher Sercye Emergency Hospital Care Zone Act of 1998, 34
Clinton, Bill, 34, 41
Clonidine, 265
CMS (Centers for Medicare and Medicaid Services). *See* Centers for Medicare and Medicaid Services

COBRA (Congressional Omnibus Reconciliation Act), 30
colonoscopy, 294–299
Committee on the Costs of Medical Care, 15
Commonwealth Fund 2011 study, 108–109
community rating, 19–21
ACA, 111–116, 127–129
origin of, 19–21
concierge doctors, 245–246
Congressional Budget Office (CBO)
2009 forecast of federal spending in 2050, 77–78
2009 long-term budget outlook, 76
analysis of The Repeal of ObamaCare Act, 121–123
estimate of ACA impact on 2016 premiums, 153
estimated cost of ACA, 118, 121–123, 143–144, 146
estimated individual mandate penalties, 134
estimated job reduction due to ACA, 136
estimated sources of health insurance in 2018, 160–161
estimated subsidies, 158–160
projections of universal coverage, 163–164
reduced projections of coverage over time, 163

Congressional Omnibus
Reconciliation Act
(COBRA), 30
corruption, 144
costs. *See also* pricing
American health care
spending, 45
cancer, 227
CBO estimated cost of
ACA, 118, 121–
123, 143–144, 146
CBO estimated job
reduction due to
ACA, 136
Committee on the
Costs of Medical
Care, 15
community rating,
19–21
concierge doctors, 245
coronary bypass, 224
DRGs and price con-
trols, 27–28
drug development, 55,
100–101
end-of-life care,
99–100
Friedman's categories
of spending, 21–23
health insurance be-
fore passage of the
ACA, 108–109
lower-than-projected
premiums for ex-
changes, 167–168
mental health prescrip-
tions, 232
obesity, 230
office visits, cash pay-
ments, 244–245
osteoporosis, 229
subsidies for the poor,
113, 117, 135–141
Couric, Katie, 294–295
COX-2 inhibitors, 61
cronyism, 144

D

deadly caution (FDA),
52, 60
death panels, 181–182
demographics's role in
social insurance pro-
grams, 71–73
Derman, Emanuel, 217
diabetes (type II),
223–224
medication needs
when adopting pri-
mal lifestyle, 268
diagnosis-related groups
(DRGs), 27–28, 178
diet, benefits of primal
eating, 230–232
discharge planning, hos-
pitalization, 290–291
doctors. *See* physicians
dose-dependent recep-
tors, 261–262
DRGs (diagnosis-related
groups), 27–28, 178
drugs
advertising, 58–60
costs to develop, 55
COX-2 inhibitors, 61
development costs,
100–101
FDA approval process,
63
FDA's delay of drug
development,
51–58
FDA's allowing
dangerous drugs to
market, 60–64
getting off meds. *See*
getting off medica-
tions
inventing diseases to
fit medications, 65
Keaton's Laws of Phar-
macology, 49–50
lock-and-key reac-
tions, 261–263

medication lists, for
hospitalization,
286–287
Minoxidil, 65
need to continue
some prescriptions,
268–269
new molecular entities
(NMEs), 57
NNT (number needed
to treat), 48–51
prescriptions for life
events, 253–254
reduced availability of
emergency medi-
cine, 91–92
resistance (tachyphy-
laxis), 262–264
side effects
Ken Korg, 205–210
getting off medica-
tions, 266–268
thalidomide, 52–53,
56
Vioxx, 56–57, 61–62
"Worst Pills, Best
Pills" newsletter, 64
Duract, 64

E

E&M (Evaluation and
Management) coding,
37–39
Eat Lots of Plants and
Animals (Primal Blue-
print law #1), 220
economics, 46
economics of US medi-
cine, 83
conflating health care
with health insur-
ance, 83–84
drug development
costs, 100–101
end-of-life care,
99–100

health insurance isn't
really insurance,
84–86
malpractice suits,
95–98
predominance of
third-party pay-
ment, 88
price controls
creation of two-
tiered health care
system, 93–95
prices don't do their
job, 89–92
reimbursement formu-
las, 95–98
reliance on existing
employer, 86–88
education
Flexner Report, 12
medical education in
history, 8–9
Medicare funding of
graduate medical
education (GME),
29
residency, 29
elective procedures,
310–312
checking NNT web-
site, 312–313
consulting with an
expert, 313–315
consulting with family
doctor, 315
discussing with loved
ones, 316
infection rates, 318
post-operative compli-
cations, 320–322
pricing, 318–320
selecting a specialist,
316–318
electronic medical records
(EMRs), 36–41
electronic personal
health information
(ePHI), 42

HIPAA (The Health
Insurance Portabili-
ty and Accountabil-
ity Act), 41–43
electronic personal health
information (ePHI),
42
Emergency Medical
Treatment and Active
Labor Act (EMTALA),
29–36, 106
repealing, 331
emergency medicine,
reduced availability,
91–92
emergency room
complications with
medical screening
procedures, 296
Ken Korg visits,
189–192, 207–209
provider perspective,
272
vs. direct admission,
283–284
employer mandate, 114,
120
flaws, 145–148
employers
Cadillac plans, 117,
123
taxation, 117, 142,
157, 168
Ken Korg's HR meet-
ing, 197–199
reliance on existing
employer for insur-
ance, 86–88
EMRs (electronic medical
records), 36–41
electronic personal
health information
(ePHI), 42
HIPAA (The Health
Insurance Portabili-
ty and Accountabil-
ity Act), 41–43

hospitalization,
280–281
EMTALA (Emergency
Medical Treatment
and Active Labor Act),
29–36, 106
repealing, 331
end-of-life care, 99–100
enrollment difficulties,
167
ephedra, 66
ePHI (electronic personal
health information),
42
essential health benefits,
111–112, 116
flaws, 130–132
Evaluation and Manage-
ment (E&M) coding,
37–39
evangelism, caution
against, 335
exchanges, low-
er-than-projected
premiums, 167–168
exercise, 233–236
existing health insurance
plans, 130–131

F

fact sheets, for hospitalization, 285–286
fats
omega-3 fatty acids,
66, 226
omega-6 fatty acids,
226
polyunsaturated fats
(PUFAs), 226
FDA Consumer magazine,
52, 54
FDA. *See* Food and Drug
Administration (FDA)
Ferriss, Timothy, 320
Fetter, Robert B., 27
fines
employer mandate,
146–147

individual mandate.
See individual
mandate
Flexner Report, 12–13
Flexner, Abraham, 12
Food and Drug Adminis-
tration (FDA), 45–48
abolishment of,
327–328
advertising regulation,
58–60
allowing dangerous
drugs to market,
60–64
approval process, 63
big government and
big business, 65–66
COX-2 inhibitors, 61
deadly caution, 52, 60
delay of drug develop-
ment, 51–58
drug development
costs, 100–101
history of, 47
Minoxidil, 65
mission of, 47
New Drug Applica-
tions (NDAs), 56
new molecular entities
(NMEs), 57
number needed to
treat (NNT),
48–51
Nutrition Labeling
and Education Act
(NLEA), 57
orange juice labeling,
57
supplements, 66
thalidomide, 52–53,
56
Vioxx, 56–57, 61–62
The Four Hour Body, 320
Free to Choose, 55
free-market orientation,
doctors, 243–244
Friedman, Milton, 11–55
Cadillac medical train-
ing analogy, 11

categories of spending,
21–23
Fulton, John F., 8

G

genetic testing, 308–310
Get Adequate Sleep
(Primal Blueprint law
#6), 221
Get Adequate Sunlight
(Primal Blueprint law
#8), 222
getting off medications,
253–254
need to continue
some prescriptions,
268–269
physical consequences,
261–265
prescriptions for life
events, 253–254
psychological implica-
tions, 260–261
reviewing your med-
ications with your
doctor, 255–260
side effects of getting
off meds, 266–268
Gingrich, Newt, 36, 39
gluten, 233
GME (graduate medical
education), funding by
Medicare, 29
Golden Rule, 243
Goodman, John, 24, 85,
89, 94, 96, 164, 167
government
AMA, 10–11
big government and
big business, 65–66
community rating,
19–21
dangers of govern-
ment health care,
182–183
dependence on gov-
ernment for health
insurance, 158–161

effects of intervention
in health care mar-
ket, 46
impact of increased
government inter-
vention, 2
insurance subsidies for
the poor, 113, 117,
135–141
medical licensure,
10–11
Medicaid. *See* Med-
icaid
Medicare. *See* Medi-
care
ObamaCare. *See*
Affordable Care Act
(ACA)
physicians' embrace-
ment of regulation,
14
possible actions to take
to improve situa-
tion, 327–331
graduate medical educa-
tion (GME), funding
by Medicare, 29
Graham, David, 61–62
Great Depression, rise
of health insurance,
18–19
Grok, 187
Gruber, Jon, 173–174
guarantees to health
insurance companies,
113, 118–120
flaws, 144–145

H

hand sanitizer, during
hospitalization, 289
Hanson, Robin, 217
Hayek, Friedrich, 90
health care, 14
conflating with health
insurance, 83–84
vs. health insurance,
14–16

Health Care for America
Now (HCAN), 170
health care system, 1–3
history. *See* history of
US health care
ObamaCare. *See*
Affordable Care Act
(ACA)
The Health Insurance
Portability and
Accountability Act
(HIPAA), 41–43
health insurance. *See*
insurance
heart disease, 224–226
Henderson, David R.,
138–139
Heritage Foundation,
105–106, 144
HHS.gov website, 42
hikes under ACA, 152
HIPAA (The Health In-
surance Portability and
Accountability Act),
41–43
Hippocrates, 8, 48
Hippocratic oath, 42
doctor-patient rela-
tionship, 13
history of US health care,
5–8
Committee on the
Costs of Medical
Care, 15
community rating,
19–21
dismantling of doc-
tor-patient relation-
ship, 13
DRGs and price con-
trols, 27–28
electronic medical
records (EMRs),
36–41
Emergency Medical
Treatment and
Active Labor Act
(EMTALA), 29–36
Flexner Report, 12

Food and Drug
Administration.
See Food and Drug
Administration
(FDA)
Friedman's categories
of spending, 21–24
Great Depression,
18–19
health care vs. health
insurance, 14–16
HIPAA (The Health
Insurance Portabili-
ty and Accountabil-
ity Act), 41–43
Medicare, 25–26, 29
pre-20th century,
8–11
AMA, 10–11
early physicians,
8–9
medical education,
8–9
medical licensure,
10–11
rise of insurance com-
panies, 18–19
rise of third-party
payment, 13
standardization of
insurance industry,
21–24
timeline of key dates,
16–17
World War II wage
and price controls,
24–25
HIV/AIDS patients, 171
homeopaths, 251
hospitalization, 271–272
dangers of hospital
system, 279–281
elective procedures,
310–312
checking NNT
website, 312–
313
consulting with an
expert, 313–315

consulting with
family doctor,
315
discussing with
loved ones, 316
infection rates, 318
pricing, 318–320
selecting a special-
ist, 316–318
infection rates, 318
medical errors/hospital
safety, 273–278
post-operative compli-
cations, 320–322
protecting yourself
avoiding hospital-
ization, 283
be prepared for
rounds, 289
coughing, 288–289
deep breaths,
288–289
discharge planning,
290–291
ER vs. direct admis-
sion, 283–284
fact sheets, 285–
286
food, 290
hand sanitizer, 289
having an advocate,
284
Internet access,
284–285
medication lists,
286–287
personal physicians,
282
standing out, 288
testing nurses and
doctors, 287–
288
walking, 288–289
provider perspective,
272–273
hospitals
30-day readmission
rule, 177–179

Emergency Medical Treatment and Active Labor Act (EMTALA), 29–36
residency/internships, 29
Veterans Health Administration (VHA) scandal, 182–183

I

individual mandate, 112, 116–117
flaws, 133–134
Supreme Court ruling, 133
infection rates, surgical procedures, 318
Institute of Medicine (IOM) hospital safety report, 275–278
insurance, 14
1942 Stabilization Act, 24–25
cancellation of existing health insurance plans, 130–131
conflating health insurance with health care, 83–84
costs before passage of the ACA, 108–109
dependence on government for health insurance, 158–161
Friedman's categories of spending, 21–24
health care vs. health insurance, 14–16
health insurance isn't really insurance, 84–86
HIPAA (The Health Insurance Portability and Accountability Act), 41–43

history. *See also* history of US health care
community rating, 19–21
Great Depression, 18–19
rise of insurance companies, 18–19
standardization of industry, 21–24
timeline of key dates, 16–17
malpractice suits, 95–98
Medicare. *See* Medicare
moral hazard, 20–21
ObamaCare. *See* Affordable Care Act (ACA)
percent of population lacking health insurance, 109–110
portability, 330
predominance of third-party payment, 88
premium increase under ACA, 152–158
price controls
creation of two-tiered health care system, 93–95
prices don't do their job, 89–92
reimbursement formulas, 95–98
reliance on existing employer, 86–88
rise of third-party payment system, 13
single payer. *See* single-payer system
insurance companies, guarantees under ACA, 113, 118–120
flaws, 144–145
internship/residency, 29

J

job reduction due to ACA, CBO estimate, 136
Joint Committee on Taxation (JCT)
estimated cost of ACA, 143
estimated subsidies, 158–159

K

Keaton, T. Kent, 49
Keaton's Laws of Pharmacology, 49
Kefauver, Estes, 54
Kefauver-Harris Amendments, 54
Kelsey, Frances Oldham, 53–55
Kennedy, Edward (Ted), 30
Kennedy, John F., 52, 54–55
Kessler, David A., 57–58
Kevadon, 53
Kliff, Sarah, 173
Kolata, Gina, 297
Konczal, Mike, 172
Korg, Ken, 187
blood pressure, 190, 194, 200, 203, 205
commute/day at office, 195
CT scan, 210–215
diagnosis, 191
ER visit, 189–192, 207–209
grocery shopping, 200
heartburn, 194
HR meeting, 197–199
illness, 188–189
kidney stone, 191, 195
lab work, 204–205
pancreas nodule, 210
prescriptions, 205
primary care doctor

visit, 203–204
search for primary
care doctor, 192,
198–204
side effects, 206–210
urologist's office, 196
Kowalski, Amanda E.,
155–156
Krugman, Paul, 70, 138,
141–142, 171–172,
181–182

L

labeling, 57
lawsuits (malpractice),
95–98
LDL cholesterol,
225–226
Leap, Edwin, 33
legislation, 2
1906 Pure Food and
Drugs Act, 47
1942 Stabilization Act,
24–25
1992 Prescription
Drug User Fee Act
(PDUFA), 56, 63
Christopher Sercye
Emergency Hospi-
tal Care Zone Act
of 1998, 34
Emergency Medical
Treatment and
Active Labor Act
(EMTALA), 29–36,
106
HIPAA (The Health
Insurance Portabili-
ty and Accountabil-
ity Act), 41–43
Medicare Moderniza-
tion Act (MMA),
91–92
Medicare. See Medi-
care
Nutrition Labeling
and Education Act
(NLEA), 57

ObamaCare. See
Affordable Care Act
(ACA)
timeline of key dates,
16–17
licensure of physicians
abolishing licensing
and certification,
328–329
AMA, 10–11
Flexner Report, 12
in history, 10–11
Lift Heavy Things (Pri-
mal Blueprint law #4),
221
lock-and-key reactions,
261–263

M

Madoff, Bernie, 69
Maisel, Albert, 182
malpractice suits, 95–98
mammograms, 300–305
mandates
employer, 114, 120
flaws, 145–148
individual, 112,
116–117
flaws, 133–134
Supreme Court
ruling, 133
Manhattan Institute pre-
miums study, 155
marketplaces, low-
er-than-projected
premiums, 167–168
Mark's Daily Apple
website, 219, 220,
233, 236
McGuff, Doug, 3, 40,
92, 177, 178, 179,
233, 234, 235, 236,
296, 301
McKinsey and Co.
estimate of narrow
networks, 173
McKnight, Robin,
173–174

Medicaid
choosing doctors, 248
dependence on gov-
ernment for health
insurance, 158–160
lack of care for Medic-
aid patients, 167
medical education
Flexner Report, 12
in history, 8–9
medical licensure
abolishing licensing
and certification,
328–329
AMA, 10–11
Flexner Report, 12
in history, 10–11
medical records, electronic (EMRs), 40–41
electronic personal
health information
(ePHI), 42
The Health Insurance
Portability and
Accountability Act
(HIPAA), 41–43
medical screening, 293,
294
cervical cancer tests
(Pap smears),
96–98
colonoscopy, 294–299
complications requir-
ing treatment, 296
genetic testing,
308–310
mammogram,
300–305
overtesting, 95–98
prior probability, 307
PSA (prostate specific
antigen), 305–307
medical tourism, 320
Medicare, 25–26
2009 (pre-ACA) finan-
cial position, 76–78
2009 Trustee Report,
79–81
choosing doctors, 247

DRGs and price controls, 27–28
end-of-life care, 99–100
funding of graduate medical education (GME), 29
impact of ACA on long-term unfunded obligations, 164
importance of demographics, 71–73
lack of saving/investment of funds, 73–76
National Center for Policy Analysis study of impact of ACA, 165–166
opting out, 330
origins of, 25–26
Ponzi scheme, 69–71
ratio of OASDI-covered workers to beneficiaries, 75
Medicare Modernization Act (MMA), 91–92
medications. See also drugs
getting off meds. See getting off medications
medication lists, for hospitalization, 286–287
Mediterranean diet, 231
mental health, 232
Merck, 56, 61–62
Meridia, 64
Merritt, David, 39
mid-level providers, 250
Minoxidil, 65
Monahan, Jay, 294
moral hazard, 20–21, 128
Morgan, John, 9
Move Frequently at a Slow Pace (Primal Blueprint law #3), 221, 224

Mulligan, Casey, 139–140
Murphy, Robert P., 3

N

narcotics, withdrawal symptoms, 264
narrow networks, 173
National Center for Policy Analysis, study of impact of ACA on Medicare recipients, 165–166
National Colorectal Cancer Research Alliance, 294
naturopaths, 251
Nesbitt, Jeff, 58
New Drug Applications (NDAs), 56
new molecular entities (NMEs), 57
Nobel, Dr. Joel J., 45
number needed to treat (NNT), 48–51
elective procedures, 312–313
FDA approval process, 63
medical screenings, 295
side effects of getting off medications, 266–268
thennt.com website, 312–313
nurse practitioners, 250
Nutrition Labeling and Education Act (NLEA), 57
nutritionists, 251

O

OB/GYN doctors, 250
Obama, Barack, 45, 105, 144

promise to keep existing health care plans, 130–131
ObamaCare. See Affordable Care Act (ACA)
obesity, benefits of primal lifestyle, 230–232
omega-3 fatty acids, 226
supplementation, 66
omega-6 fatty acids, 226
organ sales, 329–330
osteopathy, 12
osteoporosis, benefits of primal lifestyle, 229–230
overtesting, 95–98

P

Page, James O., 45
Paine, Thomas, 126
Palin, Sarah, 181
Pap smears, 96–98
Patient Protection and Affordable Care Act. See Affordable Care Act (ACA)
"pay for performance" program, 254
payment
cash payments to doctors, 244–245
Committee on the Costs of Medical Care, 15
rise of third-party payment, 13
single-payer system. See single-payer system
third-party payment, 88
PDUFA (Prescription Drug User Fee Act), 56, 63
Petzel, Robert, 183
physician assistants, 250

physicians
 advice on elective pro-
  cedures, 313–315
 choosing, 239
  3 desired character-
   istics, 242
  alternative provid-
   ers, 251
  cash payments,
   244–245
  concierge doctors,
   245–246
  free-market orienta-
   tion, 243–244
  kind of doctor/spe-
   cialty, 248–250
  Medicaid patients,
   248
  Medicare patients,
   247
  mid-level providers,
   250
  sherpas as a model,
   240–242
  wellness, 242–243
  willingness to seek
   non-pharmaco-
   logic solutions,
   253
 concierge doctors,
  245–246
 doctor-patient rela-
  tionship, disman-
  tling of, 13
 early physicians in
  history, 8–9
 embracement of govern-
  ment regulation, 14
 Ken Korg's search for
  a primary care phy-
  sician, 192–193,
  198–204
 medical education in
  history, 8–9
 medical licensure in
  history, 10–11
 personal physicians,
  benefits of for hos-
  pitalization, 282

provider perspective
 of hospitalization,
 272–273
reduction in doctors
 due to AMA/Flex-
 ner Report, 12–13
reviewing your medi-
 cations, 255–260
selecting specialists,
 316–318
plaque, 225–226
Play (Primal Blueprint
 law #7), 221–222
polyunsaturated fats
 (PUFAs), 226
Ponzi schemes, 69–71
post-operative complica-
 tions, 320–322
pre-existing conditions,
 169–171
premiums
 community rating,
  19–21
 lower-than-projected
  premiums for ex-
  changes, 167–168
 moral hazard, 20–21
 premium hikes under
  ACA, 153–158
 taxation and 1942
  Stabilization Act,
  24–25
Prescription Drug User
 Fee Act (PDUFA),
 56, 63
prescriptions
 getting off meds. See
  getting off medica-
  tions
 medication lists, for
  hospitalization,
  286–287
price ceilings, 28
price controls
 creation of two-tiered
  health care system,
  93–95
 DRGs (diagnosis-relat-
  ed groups), 27–28

prices don't do their
 job, 89–92
Priceless, 89, 96, 164, 167
pricing. See also costs
 adverse selection, 129
 Committee on the
  Costs of Medical
  Care, 15
 community rating,
  19–21
 DRGs and price con-
  trols, 27–28
 elective procedures,
  318–320
 Friedman's categories
  of spending, 21–23
 insurance premium in-
  crease under ACA,
  152–158
 reimbursement formu-
  las, 95–98
The Primal Blueprint,
 187, 219–221
The Primal Connection, 220
primal lifestyle, 2, 3,
 217–219
 10 Primal Blueprint
  laws, 220–221
 benefits of embracing
  independence,
  333–334
 cancer, 227–229
 cardiovascular diseases,
  224–226
 exercise, 233–236
 obesity, 230–232
 osteoporosis, 229–230
 other ailments,
  232–233
 side effects of getting
  off meds, 266–268
 type II diabetes,
  223–224
primary care physicians
 choosing. See choosing
  doctors
 Ken Korg's search for
  primary care doctor,
  192–193, 198–204

prior probability, medical
   tests, 307
   genetic testing, 308–310
Propulsid, 64
prostate cancer screening,
   PSA tests, 305–307
psychological implica-
   tions of getting off
   medications, 260–261
PUFAs (polyunsaturated
   fats), 226

R

rationed care, 161–169
Raxar, 64
Reagan, Ronald, 2, 30,
   36, 106
redistribution of "health",
   127–129
redistribution of wealth,
   130–132
   tax hikes on the rich,
      113, 117–118,
      141–144
Redux, 64
regulation. See also gov-
   ernment
   AMA, 10-13
   Evaluation and Man-
      agement (E&M)
      coding, 37–39
   medical licensure,
      10–11
   organ sales, 329–330
   physicians' embrace-
      ment of govern-
      ment regulation, 14
Reid, Harry, 179
   interview with Steve
      Sebelius, 180–181
Reinsurance Program,
   119–120
Renaissance, 9
residency, 29
Revenue Act of 1954, 17
reviewing your medica-
   tions with your doctor,
   255–260

Rezulin, 64
Richardson-Merrell phar-
   maceutical company,
   53
Risk Corridor Program,
   119–120
rofecoxib. See Vioxx
Rogaine
   advertising, 58–60
   Minoxidil, 65
Rome, Ethan, 170
Romney, Mitt, 105–106,
   110
RomneyCare, 105
Roy, Avik, 101
Rubin, Paul H., 58, 59
Ryan, Paul, 123

S

Salerno, Joseph, 119
SAM-e, 66
Samuelson, Paul, 70
Sebelius, Kathleen, 131
Sebelius, Steve, interview
   with Harry Reid,
   180–181
selective serotonin
   reuptake inhibitors
   (SSRIs), 66
Sercye, Christopher, 34
sherpas, as a model for
   doctors, 240–242
Shinseki, Eric, 183
Shippen, William, 9
side effects of medication
   getting off medica-
      tions, 266–268
   Ken Korg, 205–210
single-payer system, 2,
   151–152
   dangers of govern-
      ment health care,
      182–183
   dependence on gov-
      ernment for insur-
      ance, 158–161
   "failure" of free mar-
      ket, 169–172

failure of universal
   coverage leads
   to rationed care,
   161–169
Harry Reid interview
   with Steve Sebelius,
   179–181
health insurance pre-
   mium increase un-
   der ACA, 152–158
restrictions on patient
   choice, 172–177
Sisson, Mark, 3, 187,
   218, 219, 234
sleep, 221
Social Security
   2009 (pre-ACA) finan-
      cial position, 76–78
   2009 Trustee Report,
      79–81
   importance of demo-
      graphics, 71–73
   lack of saving/invest-
      ment of funds,
      73–76
   Ponzi scheme, 70–71
   ratio of OASDI-cov-
      ered workers to
      beneficiaries, 75
Sprint Once in Awhile
   (Primal Blueprint law
   #5), 221
states
   lower-than-projected
      premiums for ex-
      changes, 167–168
   Reinsurance Program,
      119–120
statins, 66
stress, 221–222
stroke, 224–226
subsidies for the poor,
   113, 117
   flaws, 135–141
sunlight, 222
supplements, 66
Supreme Court individu-
   al mandate ruling, 133

surgery. *See* elective procedures; hospitalization
Surgery Center of Oklahoma, 319

T

tachyphylaxis, 262–264
taxation
    1942 Stabilization Act, 24–25
    community rating, 19–21
    employer Cadillac plans, 117, 142, 157, 168
    individual mandate, 112, 116–117
        flaws, 133–134
        Supreme Court ruling, 133
    insurance premium exemption, 19
    new ACA taxes, 117–118
    tax code reforms needed, 331
    tax hikes on the rich, 113, 117–118
        flaws, 141–144
Tengs, Tammy O., 96
Tequin, 64
tests, 293–294
    cervical cancer tests (Pap smears), 96–98
    colonoscopies, 294–299
    complications from medical screenings, 296
    genetic testing, 308–310
    Ken Korg lab work, 204–205
    mammograms, 300–305
    overtesting, 95–98

prior probability, 307
PSA (prostate specific antigen), 305–307
thalidomide, 52–53, 56
third-party payment, 88
Thompson, John D., 27
Trustee Report for Social Security and Medicare, 79–81
two-tiered health care system, price controls, 93–95
type II diabetes, 223-224
    medication needs when adopting primal lifestyle, 268

U

Ultimate Exercise, 268
universal coverage, 110–111, 115
    failure leads to rationed care, 161–169
    flaws, 125–127
US health care system. *See* health care system
US Department of Agriculture (USDA) influence on American diet, 328
Use Your Brain (Primal Blueprint law #10), 222

V

Valium, 265
Veterans Health Administration (VHA) hospitals scandal, 182–183
Vioxx, 56–57, 61–62, 64
vitamin D
    bone health, 229
    sunlight, 222
vitamin K2, 229
Vox website, 173–174

W

wellness, 242–243
withdrawal when getting off medications, 261–265
World War II wage and price controls, 24–25
"Worst Pills, Best Pills" newsletter, 64

X

Xanax, 253-254, 265

Z

Zelnorm, 64

OTHER BOOKS BY
PRIMAL BLUEPRINT PUBLISHING

MARK SISSON

The Primal Connection: *Follow your genetic blueprint to health and happiness*

The Primal Blueprint: *Reprogram your genes for effortless weight loss, vibrant health, and boundless energy*

The Primal Blueprint 21-Day Total Body Transformation: *A step-by-step diet and lifestyle makeover to become a fat-burning machine!*

The Primal Blueprint 90-Day Journal: *A Personal Experiment (n=1)*

COOKBOOKS BY MARK SISSON AND JENNIFER MEIER

The Primal Blueprint Cookbook: *Primal, low carb, paleo, grain-free, dairy-free and gluten-free meals*

The Primal Blueprint Quick and Easy Meals: *Delicous, Primal-approved meals you can make in under 30 minutes*

The Primal Blueprint Healthy Sauces, Dressings, and Toppings: *Plus rubs, dips, marinades and other easy ways to transform basic natural foods into Primal masterpieces*

OTHER AUTHORS

Hidden Plague: *A field guide for surviving and overcoming hidradenitis suppurativa,* by Tara Grant

Rich Food, Poor Food: *The Ultimate Grocery Purchasing System (GPS),* by Mira Calton, CN, and Jayson Calton, Ph.D.

Death by Food Pyramid: *How shoddy science, sketchy politics and shady special interests ruined your health,* by Denise Minger

The South Asian Health Solution: *A culturally tailored guide to lose fat, increase energy, avoid disease,* by Ronesh Sinha, MD

Paleo Girl: *A straight talk guide to navigating the challenges of adolescence with a sensible, stress-balanced, Primal approach,* by Leslie Klenke

Lil' Grok Meets the Korgs: *A prehistoric boy shows a high tech modern family how to live Primally,* by Janée Meadows

COOKBOOKS

The Paleo Primer: *A jump-start guide to losing body fat and living Primally,* by Keris Marsden and Matt Whitmore

Primal Cravings: *Your favorite foods made paleo,* by Brandon and Megan Keatley